W0036414

Current Topics in Microbiology and Immunology

Volume 321

Series Editors

Richard W. Compans
Emory University School of Medicine, Department of Microbiology and
Immunology, 3001 Rollins Research Center, Atlanta, GA 30322, USA

Max D. Cooper
Department of Pathology and Laboratory Medicine, Georgia Research Alliance,
Emory University, 1462 Clifton Road, Atlanta, GA 30322, USA

Tasuku Honjo
Department of Medical Chemistry, Kyoto University, Faculty of Medicine,
Yoshida, Sakyo-ku, Kyoto 606-8501, Japan

Hilary Koprowski
Thomas Jefferson University, Department of Cancer Biology, Biotechnology
Foundation Laboratories, 1020 Locust Street, Suite M85 JAH, Philadelphia,
PA 19107-6799, USA

Fritz Melchers
Biozentrum, Department of Cell Biology, University of Basel, Klingelbergstr.
50–70, 4056 Basel Switzerland

Michael B.A. Oldstone
Department of Neuropharmacology, Division of Virology, The Scripps Research
Institute, 10550 N. Torrey Pines, La Jolla, CA 92037, USA

Sjur Olsnes
Department of Biochemistry, Institute for Cancer Research, The Norwegian
Radium Hospital, Montebello 0310 Oslo, Norway

Peter K. Vogt
The Scripps Research Institute, Dept. of Molecular & Exp. Medicine, Division of
Oncovirology, 10550 N. Torrey Pines. BCC-239, La Jolla, CA 92037, USA

Bruce Beutler

Editor

Immunology, Phenotype First: How Mutations Have Established New Principles and Pathways in Immunology

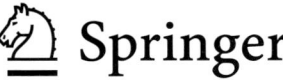 Springer

Editor
Bruce Beutler
Scripps Research Institute
Department of Immunology
10550 N. Torrey Pines Rd.
La Jolla CA 92037
USA
bruce@scripps.edu

ISBN 978-3-540-75202-8   e-ISBN 978-3-540-75203-5
DOI 10.1007/978-3-540-75203-5

Current Topics in Microbiology and Immunology ISSN 0070-217x

Library of Congress Catalog Number: 2008926501

© 2008 Springer-Verlag Berlin Heidelberg

This work is subject to copyright. All rights reserved, whether the whole or part of the material is concerned, specifically the rights of translation, reprinting, reuse of illustrations, recitation, broadcasting, reproduction on microfilm or in any other way, and storage in data banks. Duplication of this publication or parts thereof is permitted only under the provisions of the German Copyright Law of September, 9, 1965, in its current version, and permission for use must always be obtained from Springer-Verlag. Violations are liable for prosecution under the German Copyright Law.

The use of general descriptive names, registered names, trademarks, etc. in this publication does not imply, even in the absence of a specific statement, that such names are exempt from the relevant protective laws and regulations and therefore free for general use.

Product liability: The publisher cannot guarantee the accuracy of any information about dosage and application contained in this book. In every individual case the user must check such information by consulting the relevant literature.

Cover design: WMX Design GmbH, Heidelberg, Germany

Printed on acid-free paper

9 8 7 6 5 4 3 2 1

springer.com

Preface

This monograph deals with the impact of classical genetics in immunology, providing examples of how large immunological questions were solved, and new fields opened to analysis through the study of phenotypes, either spontaneous or induced. As broad as biology has become, there are those who do not fully understand what the genetic approach is, and how it differs fundamentally from most of the methods available to natural scientists. They may hold the opinion that genetics has run its course since Mendel read his paper on peas in 1865. "Why bother with classical genetics," they may ask. "Won't all genes be knocked out soon anyway?" Or they are intimidated by genetics, with its heavy reliance on model organisms that seem so alien. "What has *C. elegans* to do with me?" the questioning might go. "It doesn't even have lymphocytes." Such skeptics may be unaware that the mouse is fast becoming as tractable a model organism as the fly, and that humans may not be too far behind. So I would like to introduce the topic with a few words about the power of genetics, and why it has contributed so much to immunology, and to biology in general.

Genetics, as the word is used here, is not merely the science of heredity, but much more than that. It is the science of exceptions: the science that takes note of heritable variation and seeks to explain it at the most fundamental level. It is the science that splits phenomena into phenotypes; then assigns them to individual genes and even portions of genes. Through genetics, unambiguous conclusions can be drawn about the function of every protein we have. Although all science seeks to explain phenomena, "phenotype" is available only to biologists. Only in biology is an organism's life-plan written in its genes, and subject to alteration by changing a letter here or a word there.

Geneticists do not shrink from applying the scientific method, but it is not their primary tool. They have something special, something that solves problems that are ineluctable through hypothesis and experimentation. Why is genetics so powerful? Several reasons might be cited.

First, genetic analysis is unbiased, while hypothesis-driven research is not. In principle, hypotheses are merely tools and there is nothing personal about them, and no reason to attach a bias to them. But people like to be right about things, even when being wrong might better serve the advancement of human understanding. Time and again, scientists try to "prove the hypothesis" (and occasionally even write that they have done so) though they have been taught from their earliest days that the goal is to "test the hypothesis."

Genetic inquiry is different. Either the phenotype exists or it does not; either the phenotype is strong enough to map or it is not; either the mutation is found or it is not Finding a mutation may be disappointing insofar as it may reside in a gene with well-known functions, in which case little progress may have been made. But there is no question of bending the rules. The geneticist is an explorer. His or her prior conceptions about how a biological system works will help in forming a decision as to whether a particular phenomenon is worth investigating, and may also help in deciding how to construct a screen. But preconceptions will not mislead.

Second, genetics is calculated to produce surprise. In foreswearing hypotheses, there is a certain humility, an admission that biological complexity outstrips our ability to guess at how a given process works. Instead, we surrender to the possibility of surprise, and even trust in surprise. Of course, it may be argued that hypothesis-driven research also produces surprise. One devises experiments to test hypotheses, and the outcome may run contrary to expectation. All the same, the genetic approach does not even ask a question. It merely seeks exceptions to the status quo. And some of those exceptions may be bizarre, or even undreamed of.

Third, genetics asks why things go wrong. It is a deconstructive process, rather than one of invention. It must be granted that looking at the effects of damage is not unique to genetics, but all the same, it is fundamental to genetics, and is a powerful approach whenever it is applied in biology. By studying the effects of strokes, tumors, and traumatic injuries, clinical neurologists and pathologists were able to deduce the function of many parts of the human brain. For example, they inferred that a "homunculus" must exist in the posterior frontal cortex (and close by it, a second homunculus in the anterior parietal cortex), wherein each part of the body is spatially reflected, so that a lesion might affect adjacent areas of the body: the face, neck, arm, and trunk, for example, or the trunk and the legs and feet; but never the face and feet without involvement of intermediate structures. Geneticists follow much the same practice as neurologists, focusing intently on the effects of spontaneous mutations or those induced at random by mutagens, brought to their attention because something has gone wrong. They are able to decipher the function of each part of the genome, which contains its own "homunculus" just as the brain does, but one that is enormously more fractured and complex. The proteins that are required for limb development (or innate immune sensing, or any complex function) each have their physical representation in the genome, and though the corresponding genes may be widely scattered, they can all be found through mutagenesis and careful phenotypic screening.

Fourth, genetic conclusions are comparatively solid. The reliability of genetic conclusions is derived from the reliability of the technology upon which genetic research is based (the unbiased mapping of phenotypes to critical regions, and ultimately, DNA sequencing). This is not to say that geneticists are never wrong, or that there was never a case in which a phenotype was incorrectly attributed to a particular mutation. But such mistakes are rare. When genetic data conflict with biochemical data, or data developed from immunological assays, or data from cell transfection studies, or any combination thereof, the genetic data are usually correct.

The stories told in this book are some of the most important in immunology. Each begins with a phenotype and comes to a profound conclusion about cause. In some cases autoimmunity was at issue; in others cancer; in others a failure to detect or respond to infection. But in all instances, the biological function of a given protein or protein family was discovered. Finding the mechanism through which that protein functions presents the next challenge, and in all cases, the challenge has yet to be met in full. Ultimately, the geneticist must usually make hypotheses after all. Usually he or she is not alone: the field has been opened to many other workers once the key genetic advance has been made.

Reverse genetic methods are among the most powerful tools to be used in testing these hypotheses. Again, the situation might be compared to that of the neuroscientist, who creates brain lesions in experimental animals in order to test the function of distinct parts of the brain, alone or in conjunction with one another. Reverse geneticists, who deliberately target genes for destruction, attempt to test the function of particular parts of the genome. In both cases, nothing may be found, either because of functional redundancy, or because the investigator simply does not know what to look for. But at times, concrete and specific understanding is gained.

The interpretation of phenotypes is facilitated when there is a strong conceptual framework within which to operate. This is certainly the case in immunology, a relatively sophisticated science that has taught us quite a lot, though enormously less than it has left to teach. We know of innate immunity and adaptive immunity; we know of humoral immunity and cellular immunity. We know of antibody and complement. And we know of T cells, B cells, T-regulatory cells, antigen-presenting cells, natural killer cells, macrophages, and granulocytes. Each has a distinct role to play in protecting us from infection, or conversely, in causing inflammatory disease. Mutations can make things go very wrong where every cell and protein just mentioned is concerned. Yet we still lack a fully coherent understanding of exactly why we reject cells from unrelated individuals yet tolerate the placental allograft. We do not know why some among us develop autoimmunity while the majority does not. We do not understand why all microbes are recognized (for some, recognition receptors have yet to be found), and why some defy the immune response so effectively even when they are detected. This is the perfect playground for a geneticist: a desirable mixture of ignorance and understanding. And it is likely to remain this way for a very long time.

Yes, all genes will soon be knocked out. But many knockout mutations will be embryonic lethal, or will have other effects that mask the essential immunological function of the proteins concerned. Others will present no obvious phenotype, not because the gene in question has no function, but because we simply do not know what to look for. There is no escape from starting with phenotype. Biologists will always return to the phenotype-first approach.

We live at the dawn of a golden age of genetics, in which a phenovariant may be seen in the morning and the causal mutation known by noon. Stories formally similar to the ones presented here may soon be increasingly common, and we must all hope that they will be. But it should not be forgotten that these particular discoveries—whether in mice or in humans, most of them pursued before the respective genomes were sequenced and some of them at a time when sequencing was performed mostly manually—were heroic in their own time and have laid the foundation for some of the most important concepts in immunology.

La Jolla, USA   Bruce Beutler

Contents

Contributors

M.W. Appleby
ZymoGenetics Inc., 1201 Eastlake Ave East, Seattle, WA 98102, USA

B. Beutler
Department of Genetics, The Scripps Research Institute, 10550 N. Torrey
Pines Road, La Jolla, CA 92037, USA
bruce@scripps.edu

N.G. Copeland
Institute of Molecular and Cell Biology, 61 Biopolis Drive, Proteos,
Singapore 138673

R.H. DeKruyff
Harvard Medical School, Division of Immunology and Allergy, Children's
Hospital Boston, Karp Laboratories, Rm 10127, 1 Blackfan Circle, Boston,
MA 02115, USA

P. Gros
Department of Biochemistry, McGill University, McIntyre Medical Building,
3655 Promenade Sir William Osler, Room 910, Montréal, QC H3G 1Y6, Canada
philippe.gros@mcgill.ca

J.-L. Guénet
Département de Biologie du Développement, Institut Pasteur, 75724
Paris Cedex 15, France

N.A. Jenkins
Institute of Molecular and Cell Biology, 61 Biopolis Drive, Proteos,
Singapore 138673

D.L. Kastner
Genetics and Genomics Branch, National Institute of Arthritis and
Musculoskeletal and Skin Diseases, Bethesda, MD 20892, USA
kastnerd@mail.nih.gov

I. Kramnik
Department of Immunology and Infectious Diseases, Harvard School of Public
Health, 677 Huntington Avenue, Boston, MA 02115, USA
ikramnik@hsph.harvard.edu

J.-F. Marquis
Department of Biochemistry, McGill University, McIntyre Medical Building,
3655 Promenade Sir William Osler, Room 910, Montréal, QC H3G 1Y6, Canada

T. Mashimo
Institute of Laboratory Animals, Kyoto University Graduate School of Medicine,
Yoshidakonoe-cho, Sakyo-ku, Kyoto 606-8501, Japan

L.E. Matesic
Department of Biological Sciences, University of South Carolina, Columbia, SC
29208, USA
lmatesic@biol.sc.edu

E.M.Y. Moresco
Department of Genetics, The Scripps Research Institute, 10550 N. Torrey Pines
Road, La Jolla, CA 92037, USA

G. Orth
Department of Virology, Institut Pasteur, 25 Rue du Docteur Roux,
75015 Paris, France
gorth@pasteur.fr

F. Ramsdell
ZymoGenetics Inc., 1201 Eastlake Ave East, Seattle, WA 98102, USA
ramsdelf@zgi.com

J.G. Ryan
Genetics and Genomics Branch, National Institute of Arthritis and
Musculoskeletal and Skin Diseases, Bethesda, MD 20892, USA

A.A. Scalzo
Immunology and Virology Program, Centre for Ophthalmology and Visual
Science, University of Western Australia, Lions Eye Institute, 2 Verdun Street,
Nedlands, WA 6009, Australia

D. Simon-Chazottes
Département de Biologie du Développement, Institut Pasteur, 75724 Paris Cedex 15,
France

D.T. Umetsu
Harvard Medical School, Division of Immunology and Allergy, Children's
Hospital Boston, Karp Laboratories, Rm 10127, 1 Blackfan Circle, Boston,
MA 02115, USA
dale.umetsu@childrens.harvard.edu

S.E. Umetsu
Harvard Medical School, Division of Immunology and Allergy, Children's
Hospital, Boston, Karp Laboratories, Rm 10127, 1 Blackfan Circle, Boston,
MA 02115, USA

W.M. Yokoyama
Howard Hughes Medical Institute, Division of Rheumatology, Campus Box 8045,
Washington University School of Medicine, 660 South Euclid Avenue, St. Louis,
MO 63110, USA
yokoyama@im.wustl.edu

Part I
Immunodeficiency

The Forward Genetic Dissection of Afferent Innate Immunity

B. Beutler(✉), E.M.Y. Moresco

Contents

Abstract Recognition of the microbial world is mediated chiefly by a small group of immune receptors that activate a characteristic host inflammatory response, the innate immune response. Known as the Toll-like receptors (TLRs), these molecules are represented among most metazoans. In mammals, forward genetic analysis of the lipopolysaccharide (LPS) response led to the identification of TLR4 as the LPS receptor. Through a combination of forward and reverse genetic studies, a relatively detailed understanding of the functions of mammalian TLRs has now been achieved. As discussed here, mutagenesis has revealed proteins that participate in TLR signaling pathways, and informed our understanding of the subtleties of these molecules' structure and function.

B. Beutler
Department of Genetics, The Scripps Research Institute, 10550 N. Torrey Pines Road, La Jolla, CA 92037, USA
bruce@scripps.edu

B. Beutler (ed.), *Immunology, Phenotype First: How Mutations Have Established New Principles and Pathways in Immunology.* Current Topics in Microbiology and Immunology 321. © Springer-Verlag Berlin Heidelberg 2008

Introduction

The molecular basis of mammalian innate immune perception remained obscure for many years after microbes were first identified as the causal agents of infectious disease. From the earliest decades of the twentieth century it was widely assumed that specific receptors must detect microbes or molecules that they manufacture. Some of the microbial molecules that served as targets for recognition were established at that time, and their structures elucidated soon thereafter, because they elicited powerful inflammatory effects evocative of an authentic infection. But the host receptors for these molecules proved highly elusive.

In recent times the terms "pattern recognition receptors," "pathogen-associated molecular patterns," and "danger signals" have been introduced into the innate immunity field. But while these were convenient and all-embracing terms for conserved molecules of microbial origin, they brought the field no nearer to finding the receptors. Whatever one called them ("pattern recognition receptors" or "danger receptors"), the primary molecular sensors of infection remained beyond reach until genetic methodologies advanced to the point that they could be found.

The question as to precisely how we sense microbes was an important one for several reasons. First and foremost, it went to the heart of self/non-self discrimination: a topic that is fundamental in immunology. Second, whatever the receptors were, they transduce the very first molecular events that transpire after the inoculation of microbes. These initial events "light the fuse" for all that follows during infection, including the development of the inflammatory response, which limits infection when circumscribed but can prove fatal when generalized. Third, the inflammatory response seen during infection is biochemically similar to the inflammatory response seen during sterile inflammatory diseases. The same gateways to inflammation that are triggered by microbes might be activated to our detriment in rheumatoid arthritis, systemic lupus erythematosus, and other diseases in which the immune system plays a destructive role. Simply put, these receptors orchestrate the most powerful inflammatory events we know of.

A pure genetic approach ultimately led to the identification of the Toll-like receptors (TLRs) as innate immune sensors. This approach is recounted here. It was followed by extensive mutagenic analysis of the TLR signaling pathways, which further informed us of the key proteins used by TLRs to elicit changes in gene expression, leading to the activation of an antimicrobial state. The genetic approach, which depends on identifying mutations that cause phenotypes rather than the formation and testing of hypotheses, has many advantages. Importantly, it leads one to discover the unexpected. In addition, because it is unbiased, it is not subject to the type of manipulation that besets experimentalists who want to "prove the hypothesis correct."

The LPS Receptor, and How We Know It Exists

The most potent and best-studied molecule of microbial origin that triggers innate immune responses is lipopolysaccharide (LPS), a major constituent of the outer membrane of gram-negative bacteria. Famous for its ability to cause fever and shock, LPS in fact recreates many of the effects of an infection. It does so through an effect on cells of hematopoietic origin (Michalek et al. 1980), and specifically, does so by eliciting cytokine production by these cells. In 1985, tumor necrosis factor (TNF), elaborated in large amounts by LPS-activated macrophages (Beutler et al. 1985a, b) was shown to be a major contributor to the lethal effect of LPS in vivo (Beutler et al. 1985c).

In 1965 it was noticed that mice of the C3H/HeJ substrain were impervious to the lethal effect of LPS (Heppner and Weiss 1965), a finding confirmed and extended by Sultzer, who also observed that C3H/HeJ mice do not mount a normal exudative response to LPS when injected intraperitoneally with the substance (Sultzer 1968). By 1975 the existence of a single locus governing responses to LPS had been established (Watson and Riblet 1975), and by 1978 this locus had been mapped to mouse chromosome 4 using classical phenotypic markers (Watson et al. 1977, 1978). Coutinho and colleagues subsequently identified a second LPS-resistant strain (C57BL/10ScCr), showing that the mutation responsible for resistance in this strain was allelic with the resistance mutation in the C3H/HeJ strain (Coutinho et al. 1977; Coutinho and Meo 1978). Depending on the assay used, the phenotype of LPS resistance was either recessive or co-dominant, and it extended to all aspects of the LPS response, including, for example, the adjuvant effects of LPS (Skidmore et al. 1975), and the ability of mice to make antibodies against LPS itself (Coutinho and Gronowicz 1975). The universal dependence of LPS effects on the *Lps* genotype spoke strongly in favor of a single, nonredundant pathway for LPS perception in mammals, no matter how many protein components that pathway might incorporate. The cytokine response to LPS was ultimately used as an endpoint in detecting LPS responses and in cloning the *Lps* locus. Some investigators used other endpoints [B-cell mitogenesis (Peavy et al. 1970; Andersson et al. 1972; Coutinho and Gronowicz 1975); changes in pulmonary compliance (Peiffer-Schneider et al. 1997)] in the attempt to confine the mutation to a manageable critical region.

Identification of TLR4 as the LPS Receptor

Before positional cloning was feasible in the mouse, many attempts were made to identify the LPS receptor, and some of these efforts made use of LPS nonresponder mice. In two early studies (Forni and Coutinho 1978; Coutinho et al. 1978), antibodies raised in rabbits against C3H/Tif (normal LPS responder) strain B cells and exhaustively absorbed using cells from C3H/HeJ mice were found to be differentially reactive with LPS responder strains and the nonresponder strains C3H/HeJ and C57BL/10ScCr. However, the antiserum was never successfully used to isolate an LPS receptor.

Using an endogenously ^{14}C-labeled LPS preparation, Kabir and Rosenstreich tested C3H/HeJ and C3H/HeN splenocytes for differences in binding, and found no significant difference (Kabir and Rosenstreich 1977). Similarly, Watson and Riblet found that ^{3}H LPS bound equally well to C3H/HeJ and C3HeB/FeJ spleen cells

(Watson and Riblet 1975). They concluded that while a membrane-associated signaling molecule was likely defective in C3H/HeJ mice, the primary interaction between LPS and the lymphocyte was not dependent upon this molecule, and likely occurred through hydrophobic interaction with the membrane.

Affinity chromatography was used to search for LPS binding sites on human erythrocytes (Yokoyama et al. 1978) and mouse lymphocytes (Yokoyama et al. 1979), with the finding that band III protein and PAS (Periodic Acid-Schiff)-1 glycoprotein bound LPS in the former instance, and class I MHC bound LPS in the latter instance. These were two rather early examples of approaches taken by many investigators, who sought to find the LPS receptor through biochemical means (Wright and Jong 1986; Lei and Morrison 1988a, b, 1993; Lei et al. 1990, 1993; Bright et al. 1990; Wright 1991). Some putative binding molecules were never identified; others (like those just mentioned) are now considered to be irrelevant to LPS responses. Of particular note was the theme that CD18, complexed with one or more of the CD11 integrins, was essential to LPS responses (Golenbock et al. 1990 Lynn et al. 1991; Ingalls and Golenbock 1995; Ingalls et al. 1997, 1998a, b, 1999 Flaherty et al. 1997; Bhat et al. 1999).

Highly informative biochemical studies of LPS activity established that a plasma protein called LPS binding protein (LBP) engages LPS (Wright et al. 1989; Schumann et al. 1990) and that LPS signaling subsequently depends upon CD14 (Wright et al. 1990). This conclusion depended upon antibody depletion studies, and was validated later by the phenotype of mice that lack CD14 (Haziot et al. 1996 Jiang et al. 2005). CD14 therefore seemed to be at least a key part of the LPS receptor. Because the protein had no transmembrane domain, however, and was instead tethered to the surface by a glycosylphosphoinositide anchor, it was believed that it must participate in a complex with another protein(s) in order to signal. Moreover, the *Cd14* locus maps to chromosome 18 in the mouse; the *Lps* locus was by that time known to reside on chromosome 4 (Watson et al. 1978).

The early confinement of *Lps* to a position between the major urinary protein (*Mup1*) and polysyndactyly (*Ps*) loci (Watson et al. 1978) encompassed the type I interferon (IFN) genes, and as we now know, covered approximately 35 Mb of genomic DNA within which approximately 205 annotated genes reside. At the time, however, the total number of genes was unknown, and the type I IFN genes were regarded as early candidates. They were ultimately excluded by genetic mapping.

Prior to the year 2000 the mouse genome was largely *terra incognita*, and not only the total number of genes, but their relative locations within the genome, were open to discovery. After the landmark work of Watson and colleagues (1977, 1978), mapping efforts remained in abeyance for nearly 15 years. Although loose confinement of the *Lps* locus was made by recurrent crossing of C3H/HeJ to BALB/c, with the development of a congenic interval approximately 5.5 cM in size (Vogel et al. 1994), efficient mapping through parallel examination of thousands of meioses was not undertaken until the mid-1990s. A series of deletion constructs, spanning a large part of chromosome 4 including the *brown* (*b*) locus (Rinchik et al. 1994), were also used in an attempt to narrow the location of the gene, but without success, and ultimately ended with the erroneous conclusion that the genotype Lps^d/Lps^0 supports normal LPS signal transduction (Vogel et al. 1999). It is not entirely clear why this effort failed, as it is now quite clear that the Lps^d/Lps^0 genotype actually yields a nonresponder phenotype. For whatever cause, the location of the gene was not tightly confined by these approaches, however promising they might have seemed.

As the density of markers in the mouse genome grew, several laboratories attempted to narrow the position of *Lps*. During this later phase of investigation, the construction of contigs (from YAC or BAC clones) was undertaken independently in at least two laboratories. The de novo search for genes was then attempted (in the early days) through exon trapping; later, as expressed sequence tag (EST) libraries grew more complete, the search continued through basic local alignment search tool (BLAST) analysis of shotgun sequences of genomic DNA, while at all times it continued through computer-aided recognition of coding regions (programs such as Genscan and GRAIL).

Malo and colleagues mapped *Lps* on 1,604 meioses to a position between a proximal cluster of genes including *Cd30l*, *Hxb*, and *Ambp*, and the distal markers D4Mit178 and D4Mit7, which at the time had not been resolved from one another (Qureshi et al. 1996). Schwartz and colleagues mapped the locus on the basis of changes in pulmonary compliance occurring following intratracheal administration of LPS (Peiffer-Schneider et al. 1997).

The *Lps* locus was mapped to maximum resolution (2.6 Mb) on 2,093 meioses and positionally cloned by Poltorak and colleagues, who first succeeded in finding the relevant gene in the *Lps* critical region (Poltorak et al. 1998b) and, within it, the mutation responsible for LPS resistance (Poltorak et al. 1998a). In C3H/HeJ mice a single nucleotide substitution altered the cytoplasmic domain of Toll-like receptor 4 (TLR4), while in the C57BL/10ScCr mice and in the C57BL/10ScN strain (from which the former substrain was derived), a small deletion removed the *Tlr4* gene entirely (Poltorak et al. 1998a, b). Later, the exact limits of this deletion were determined (Poltorak et al. 2000), and it was further shown that C57BL/10ScCr (but not C57BL/10ScN) had a point mutation in the interleukin (IL)-12 receptor β2 chain, which caused a different form of immunocompromise superimposed on the LPS sensing defect (Poltorak et al. 2001).

The identity of the *Lps* locus was subsequently confirmed by Malo and her co-workers (Qureshi et al. 1999a, b). Later, the *Tlr4* gene was targeted for deletion by Akira and colleagues, who found an LPS-resistant phenotype (Hoshino et al. 1999). In still later work, the gene was inserted into the genome of C57BL/10ScCr animals by bacterial artificial chromosome (BAC) transgenesis, which restored LPS sensing (Kalis et al. 2003). This latter study also revealed that the *Tlr4* locus is haploinsufficient; moreover, the gene copy number determines LPS signaling intensity over a fairly wide range (Kalis et al. 2003).

Prior to the positional cloning of *Lps*, the function of the *Tlr4* locus was unknown. TLR4 was one of several homologs of the *Drosophila* protein Tcll, which had been known since the early 1990s to exist in mammals (Nomura et al. 1994; Taguchi et al. 1996). Toll had initially been known for its developmental role in the fly, but was shown in 1996 to have an immunological function as well (Lemaitre et al. 1996), as described in detail in the following section. Pursuant to this realization, it was shown that TLR4 could activate nuclear factor (NF)-κB in mammalian cells (Medzhitov et al. 1997), and it was speculated that it might have a role in mammalian immunity (both innate and adaptive), just as Toll was known to be important in *Drosophila* immunity. However, the genetic demonstration that TLR4 served as the membrane-spanning component of the mammalian LPS receptor, required for surviving gram-negative infections, gave the key insight into how mammals sense infection.

Innate Immunity in *Drosophila melanogaster*

Concurrent with the *Lps* locus positional cloning effort, Jules Hoffmann and colleagues worked to understand resistance to infection in insects. Among the key effectors of insect immunity are antimicrobial peptides, seven classes of which were identified by the Hoffmann lab. These included the Drosocin, Diptericin, Drosomycin, Metchnikowin, Cecropin, Attacin, and Defensin classes of peptide. It was observed that the genes encoding these proteins had motifs similar to those known to recognize NF-κB in their promoter regions; subsequently, it was found that the promoters would in fact respond to NF-κB activating stimuli (Reichhart et al. 1992, Georgel et al. 1993; Kappler et al. 1993; Meister et al. 1994). Drosomycin was particularly important for the containment of fungal infections, and was induced by fungal infection, while Diptericin was important for the containment of gram-negative infections, and was induced by gram-negative infection.

Only three NF-κB variants (Dorsal, Dif, and Relish) exist in *Drosophila*. The Toll signaling pathway, found by Nüsslein-Volhard and colleagues to be required for dorsoventral patterning in the fly embryo, was known as a possible source of NF-κB activation, triggering the nuclear translocation of Dorsal. Indeed, Toll was found to be essential for Drosomycin production in adult flies challenged with fungus (Vitaerna et al. 1994). So too was the Toll ligand Spaetzle, which was generated by proteolytic cleavage from a precursor in response to a then-unknown cascade triggered by infection. The NF-κB analog Dif, however, was used in preference to Dorsal (Rutschmann et al. 2000).

On the other hand, the gram-negative response pathway was clarified by positional cloning of a spontaneous mutation called Immune deficiency (Imd), which proved to affect a receptor-interacting protein (RIP)-like cytoplasmic protein linked to a transmembrane peptidoglycan recognition protein (PGRP). The Imd pathway also involved *Drosophila* FADD, an ortholog of the Fas-associated death domain linker protein in mammals, DREDD, a homolog of Caspase 8 in mammals, and Tab2. The pathway ultimately triggered the activation of Relish. It was strongly evocative of the TNF signaling pathway (Georgel et al. 2001).

The identification of Toll as a mediator of immunity in *Drosophila* was completed in 1996, while the identification of Imd as a mediator of immunity was achieved in 2001. The fact that Toll and the mammalian TLRs (as recognized in 1998) have conserved defensive functions was interesting in its own right. But the added fact that the Imd pathway is in many ways similar to the TNF pathway indicated something else. While Imd and Toll pathways operate with complete independence in *Drosophila*, any stimulus that activates a mammalian TLR will also activate TNF production and thence the TNF signaling pathway (Fig. 1). The two pathways are linked to one another in mammals. The special importance of the TNF pathway in defense in mammals, where it clearly does protect against infection by mycobacteria (Kindler et al. 1989), *Listeria monocytogenes* (Havell 1987), and other microbes, is reflected by its existence as a major response pathway with its own sensing mechanism in *Drosophila*. The efficacy of interdiction of TNF in the treatment of inflammatory diseases such as rheumatoid arthritis, Crohn's disease, psoriasis, and other ailments also speaks to its key importance as a linker of pathways that, in some organisms, have each assumed large duties in the inflammatory response.

The General Role of the TLRs in Innate Immune Recognition, and Their Conserved Structure

TLR4 is a large, single-spanning type I membrane protein marked by leucine-rich repeats (LRRs) throughout the length of its ectodomain, except in a centrally placed "hinge" region (Kim et al. 2007). The cytoplasmic domain of the protein is almost entirely devoted to a single TIR (Toll/IL-1R/Resistance) domain—a fold also observed in the IL-1 receptor and IL-18 receptor subunits—and in certain other receptors that have immunoglobulin-type repeats in their ectodomains (SIGIRR, TIGIRR, and ST2 proteins). The TIR domain has been identified in many proteins; both in plants and animals it is associated with defensive function (McHale et al. 2006; Roach et al. 2005). Microbes have also captured the TIR motif, and may use it to thwart immune signaling (Stack et al. 2005).

In humans there are 10 TLR paralogs; in mice, 12; in both species combined, 13. While humans lack TLRs 11, 12, and 13, they express TLR10 (which mice lack) and have an active TLR8 (no known activity is associated with TLR8 in mice). The TLRs are probably all dimeric (or heterodimeric) in structure. All TLR ectodomains probably assume a "curved solenoid" shape characteristic of LRR proteins (Jin et al. 2007; Kim et al. 2007).

When the function of TLR4 was determined, other members of the TLR family were already known in mammals. TLR1 had been the first mammalian homolog of Toll to be identified (Nomura et al. 1994; Taguchi et al. 1996), and by 1998 TLRs 2, 3, and 5 had been found by homology searches. TLRs 6–10 followed soon after as mouse and human genomic sequences approached completion; in the mouse, TLRs 11–13 (not represented in humans) are now known to complete the family (Tabeta et al. 2004). Because each of the TLRs was endowed with a similar cytoplasmic domain, conserved in Toll, IL-1 receptor chains, and IL-18 receptor chains, it appeared that they might each transduce similar signals, but perhaps in response

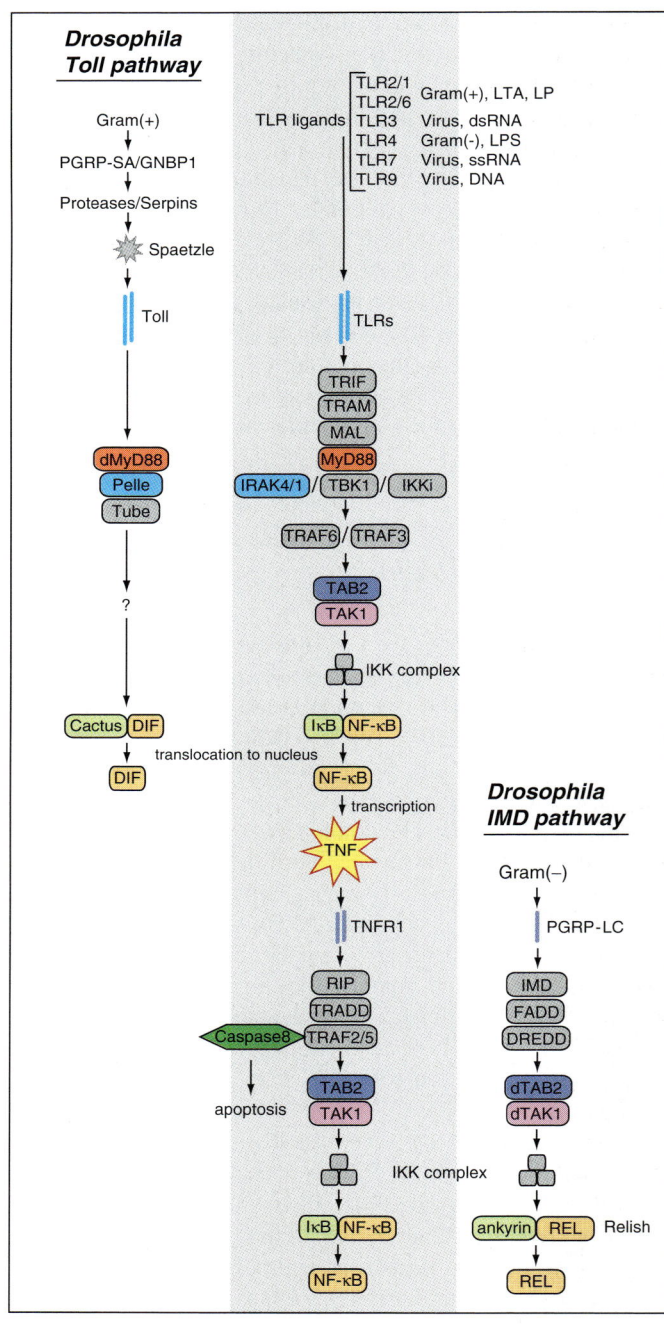

to different ligands. It made sense to hypothesize that the other TLRs each recognize various molecules of microbial origin as well.

When Akira and colleagues deleted TLR2 by gene targeting, they found that it was required for detection of lipopeptides (Takeuchi et al. 1999) and other components of gram-positive bacterial cell walls. TLR2 was found to operate in conjunction with TLRs 1 or 6 (Ozinsky et al. 2000), each heterodimeric complex showing a different ligand specificity (Takeuchi et al. 2001, 2002). TLR5 was eventually found to be a receptor for flagellin (Hayashi et al. 2001) while TLR3 was a receptor for poly I:C (Alexopoulou et al. 2001), TLR9 a receptor for unmethylated DNA (Hemmi et al. 2000), and TLR7 and TLR8 (the latter only active in humans) could detect ssRNA and the inflammatory nucleotide-based imidazoquinoline drugs resiquimod, imiquimod. and loxoribine (Hemmi et al. 2002; Heil et al. 2003).

In some cases (e.g., in the case of the TLR1/2 heterodimer), TLRs directly engage their microbial ligands; in other cases, the ligands probably interact first or exclusively with accessory proteins that then alter the shape of the TLRs and trigger a response. For example, TLR4 was shown to be tightly associated with MD-2 (Shimazu et al. 1999), a small protein later shown quite convincingly to bind LPS (Ohto et al. 2007) and presumably to transmit information about the LPS to the

---

Fig. 1 Mammalian TLR and *Drosophila* Toll and IMD pathways. The mammalian TLR and TNF pathways (schematized within the *gray bar*) are connected: any TLR-activating stimulus will lead to TNF production and subsequent TNF pathway activation. The Toll signaling pathway in flies (*left*) is homologous to the mammalian TLR pathway; the IMD pathway in flies (*right*) is homologous to the mammalian TNF pathway. TLR activation by various microbial ligands recruits between one and four of the adaptors TRIF, TRAM, MAL, and MyD88 in mammals and leads to the activation of IRAK family protein kinases or the TBK1 or Ikki family kinases, TRAF6 or TRAF3, and ultimately the IKK complex. The IKK complex phosphorylates IκB, which releases NF-κB for transcription of targets, including TNF. Activation of the TNF pathway then follows, stimulating TNF receptors to recruit RIP, TRADD, and TRAF2 and/or -5. These activate the TAB2/TAK1 complex, which leads to NF-κB activation in subsequent steps. Alternatively, TRAF2/5 may activate caspase 8, resulting in apoptosis. In the Toll pathway (*left*), the ligand for the Toll receptor is Spaetzle, which must first be cleaved by proteases or serpins initially activated through binding of gram-positive bacteria to PGRP-SA (peptidoglycan-recognition protein-SA) or GNBP1 (gram-negative binding protein 1). As in the TLR pathway, Toll requires the function of an adaptor, dMyD88, which forms part of the trimeric TISC (Toll-induced signaling complex) with Pelle (an IRAK homolog) and Tube. Through unknown mechanisms, TISC signals to Cactus (IκB homolog) to release DIF (dorsal-related immunity factor, an NF-κB homolog) for transcription activation. The IMD pathway (*right*) functions independently from the Toll pathway, is activated by gram-negative bacteria, and leads to activation of a distinct NF-κB homolog, Relish. PGRP-LC senses gram-negative peptidoglycan and recruits IMD (RIP homolog), FADD (FAS-associated death domain, a TRADD homolog) and DREDD (death-related ced-3/Nedd2-like protein), which in turn activate dTAB2 and dTAK1. As in the mammalian TNF pathway, dTAB2 and dTAK1 lead to Relish (NF-κB homolog) activation. In the case of Relish, the inhibitory C-terminal ankyrin repeats of Relish are cleaved, and remain in the cytoplasm. The active REL moiety translocates to the nucleus and stimulates transcription. *dsRNA*, double-stranded RNA; *LTA*, lipoteichoic acid; *LP*, lipopeptides; *ssRNA*, single-stranded RNA

TLR4 subunit (Kim et al. 2007). In the absence of any of three proteins: MD-2, CD14, or TLR4, responses to glycosylated LPS are abolished (Jiang et al. 2005). As described in "Requirements for TLR2 and TLR4 Complex Signaling", both CD36 and CD14 participate in signaling via TLR2 complexes (Hoebe et al. 2005; Jiang et al. 2005).

The Adaptors That Serve TLR Signaling

Muzio et al. (1997) observed that a cytoplasmic adaptor protein called MyD88 had homology to the IL-1 receptor cytoplasmic domains, and offered evidence that this protein participates in IL-1 signal transduction, an observation confirmed by the phenotype of the MyD88 knockout mouse (Adachi et al. 1998). MyD88 recruits members of the IL-1 receptor-associated kinase (IRAK) family to the activated complex via death domain interactions. MyD88 also supports signaling from most of the TLRs, with the exception of TLR3, which is fully MyD88 independent, and TLR4, which retains some signaling potential in the absence of MyD88. A total of four adaptors, however, are now known to be influential in mammalian TLR signaling: MyD88, MAL, TRIF, and TRAM (Fig. 2).

Two of these adaptors were sufficiently homologous to the TLRs to be identified by BLAST searches of EST databases. These were MyD88 and its closest homolog, MAL (also known as Tirap) (Fitzgerald et al. 2001; Horng et al. 2001). MyD88 is required for all signaling via the TLR2 complexes, TLR5, and TLRs 7, 8, and 9, as well as IL-1R and IL-18R. It is partly required for signaling via TLR4. It is not required for signaling via TLR3. MAL is partly required for signaling via the TLR2 complexes and TLR4, but no other TLRs (Fitzgerald et al. 2001).

Even when both MyD88 and MAL are targeted and a compound homozygous mutant is produced, residual signaling via TLR4 and unimpaired signaling via TLR3 are observed (Yamamoto et al. 2002). In particular, production of type I IFN (IFN-β) is unimpaired, suggesting that in the absence of MyD88 or MAL (or both), IRF-3 (interferon response factor-3), the transcription factor required for IFN-β production, undergoes phosphodimer formation and activates the IFN-β gene. This residual signaling occurs by way of the so-called "MyD88 independent pathway," which studies of the N-ethyl-N-nitrosourea (ENU)-induced phenotype Lps2 (See "TRIF is the MyD88-Independent Adaptor") and knockout mice demonstrated relies on the adaptor TRIF (Yamamoto et al. 2003a; Hoebe et al. 2003). IFNβ production is the hallmark of MyD88-independent signaling, and it is now known that TLR3 and TLR4 recruit TRIF and TBK1 (TRAF-family-member-associated NF-κB-activator-binding kinase 1), the critical kinase required for activation of IRF3 (McWhirter et al. 2004).

While the functions of MyD88 and MAL were first resolved by gene knockout work, the functions of the MyD88-independent adaptor proteins were deduced independently by both forward and reverse genetic methods, and in the former case, ENU mutagenesis was used to create the phenotypes of interest.

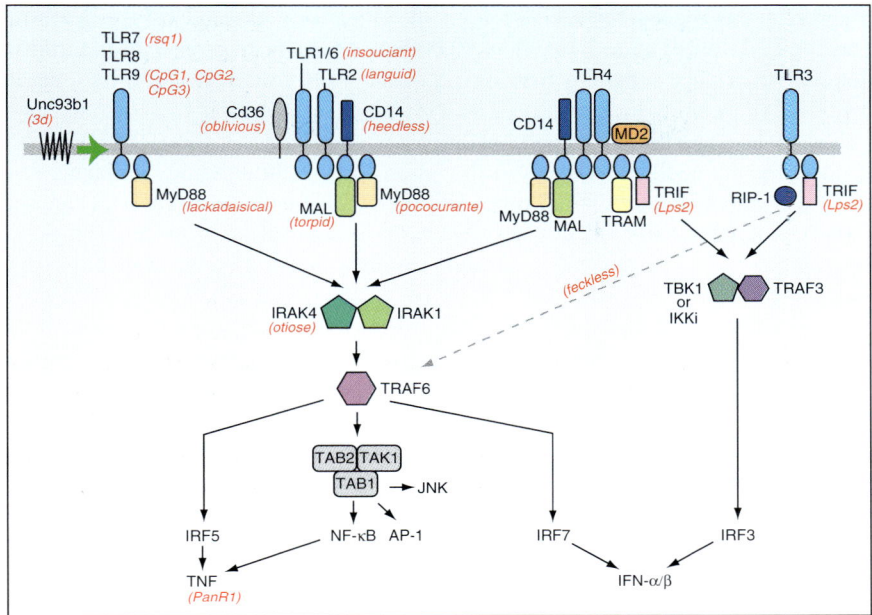

Fig. 2 Overview of TLR signaling pathways. The pathways represent data obtained from both forward and reverse genetic studies. *N*-Ethyl-*N*-nitrosourea (ENU)-induced phenotypes are shown in *red text*. Note that TLRs 3, 7, and 9 are endosomal proteins, while TLRs 1, 2, 6, and 4, as well as TLR5 (not shown), are expressed on the plasma membrane. Unc93b1 is an endoplasmic reticulum protein that influences endosome function. TLR activation recruits TRIF, TRAM, MAL, and/or MyD88 and leads to the activation of IRAK1 and IRAK4, or the TBK1 or Ikki family kinases. TRAF6 signaling to the TAB1/TAB2/TAK1 complex activates NF-κB, AP-1, and/or c-Jun N-terminal kinase (*JNK*). As mentioned in the text, IRF5 is another means by which signaling through MyD88 leads to TNF production. MyD88 and TRAF6 may interact directly with IRF5 in a complex, thereby activating IRF5 and promoting its translocation to the nucleus. Additionally, MyD88, together with TRAF6 and IRAK4, has also been shown to bind IRF7 directly in order to stimulate IFN-α production. This occurs downstream of TLR7, TLR8, and TLR9 in plasmacytoid dendritic cells and requires the phosphorylation of IRF7 by IRAK1 (Uematsu et al. 2005). In the MyD88-independent pathway, TLR3 or TLR4 recruit TRIF and TBK1, the critical kinase required for activation of IRF3. TRAF3 mediates the interaction between TRIF and TBK1. The kinase RIP-1 is required for NF-κB activation downstream of TRIF, and likely requires the direct interaction between TRIF and RIP-1. The point at which RIP-1 signaling impinges on the NF-κB pathway is unknown (*dashed gray arrow*)

ENU Mutagenesis in the Identification of TLR Signaling Proteins

The unbiased forward genetic approach to TLR signaling began in the year 2000 and has continued to the present time, with the production of more than 100,000 germline mutants over a 7-year time frame, most of them third generation (G3) offspring homozygous for a fraction of the mutations induced by the germline mutagen ENU in G0 mice. More than 30,000 mice have been screened for germline mutations that alter signaling from seven of the TLR complexes, causing impairment of TNF production as measured by a biological assay (L-929 cell cytotoxicity). A total of 19 transmissible mutations have been detected. Of these, 15 have been identified at the nucleotide level. Of the seven TLRs held under surveillance, four have been struck (one of them 3 times and the others once each). Three of the four adaptor proteins known to exist have been struck (one of them twice). Hence, an appreciable level of saturation—though certainly not complete saturation—has been achieved.

As described elsewhere in detail, ENU is the most widely used mutagen for the generation of phenotypical variance in mice, and is applied with the goal of positionally cloning the mutations responsible for phenotypes of interest (Beutler et al. 2007a). It causes mutations at a frequency sufficiently high to produce phenotype variance in abundance, low enough to permit unambiguous assignment of responsibility to a single mutation in the majority of cases, and to do so with only a modest amount of effort invested in mapping. A particular advantage of variant alleles produced by the ENU approach consists in the fact that they reside on a pure, defined genetic background (in our laboratory C57BL/6J). Knockouts, by contrast, generally exist on a rather poorly defined background, and this may sometimes create confusion in assessing phenotypes. ENU has the added virtue of producing viable alleles of genes for which null alleles are lethal in the homozygous state.

TRIF Is the MyD88-Independent Adaptor

An ENU-induced mutation called *Lps2* was the first germline mutation to affect MyD88-independent signaling (Fig. 2). Identified by Hoebe et al. after screening 4,000 mice, roughly half of them G3 and half G1 mutants, the *Lps2* phenotype was so named because it approximated the classical *Lps* phenotype (Hoebe et al. 2003). Mice showed a much diminished TNF response to LPS, and were entirely unable to produce type I IFN in response to LPS. Notably, however, TLR3 signaling was entirely abolished by the *Lps2* mutation (not a characteristic of the *Lps* mutation in Tlr4). It thus appeared that MyD88-independent signaling was selectively ablated. It also seemed clear that TLR4-driven TNF production was dependent partly on MyD88-independent signaling. Finally, it was clear that TLR3 and TLR4 must share a common transducer.

The *Lps2* mutation was mapped on more than 1,600 meioses to a 216-kb region of mouse chromosome 17, containing eight genes, one of which was annotated only as "novel," but on inspection proved to have a TIR domain and to be identical to a newly recognized TIR adaptor protein elsewhere called Ticam1 (Oshiumi et al. 2003a) or TRIF (Yamamoto et al. 2003a). This adaptor had been identified in one laboratory on the basis of two-hybrid system analyses using the TIR domain of TLR3 as bait to search for a novel binding protein (Oshiumi et al. 2003a), and in another laboratory by advanced homology searches (Yamamoto et al. 2003a). It was believed to support MyD88-independent signaling because, when overexpressed, it would drive type I IFN signaling. It was not at all clear, however, which TLRs depended upon it, with one group suspecting that it was utilized by all TLRs and another suggesting that it was utilized only by TLR3. In *Lps2* mutant mice, the TRIF coding region was disrupted by a single base pair deletion, leading to alteration and premature truncation of the protein. The product was, as a result, unstable and nonfunctional.

One interesting feature of the *Lps2* phenotype was observed on FACS analysis of macrophages from mice with the mutation. A fraction of cells were *Lps2*-independent, in the sense that when stimulated with LPS, they made TNF despite the mutation. No such population was evident when poly I:C was used as a stimulus. This implied that still another adaptor might substitute for TRIF in a fraction of macrophages, signaling downstream of TLR4 (but not TLR3) in the absence of TRIF.

Once TRIF was identified, its close homolog TRAM [initially called Adaptor X in our own laboratory (Hoebe et al. 2003) and also known as Ticam2 (Oshiumi et al. 2003b)] could easily be identified by BLAST searches. TRAM proved to be capable of substituting for TRIF in a fraction of macrophages (Hoebe et al. 2003), and to be primarily responsible for carrying the TLR4 signal initiated by certain ligands, notably glycoprotein G of vesicular stomatitis virus (Georgel et al. 2007).

The *Trif* (Yamamoto et al. 2003a), *Tram* (Yamamoto et al. 2003b), *MyD88* (Adachi et al. 1998), and *Tirap* (Yamamoto et al. 2002) genes have each been inactivated by targeting. Three of the four loci (*Trif*, *MyD88*, and *Tirap*) have been encountered through mutagenesis screening, and the ENU alleles have produced certain surprises, in that some are phenotypically distinguishable from the knockouts. While the *Trif* allele *Lps2* is essentially null, two hypomorphic and receptor-selective alleles of *Myd88* were produced by ENU mutagenesis (*pococurante* and *lackadaisical*; discussed in "The Nature of Receptor: Adaptor Interaction"). An allele of *Tirap* (*torpid*) was identified in screening and found to be rather different from the knockout in its effects: less drastic phenotypes than in the knockout are reported (see http://mutagenetix.scripps.edu for details).

More Distal Elements of the TLR Signaling Pathway

A mutation in *Irak4* (*otiose*) was identified through mutagenesis screening and, to all appearances so far, produces a phenotype identical to that caused by *Myd88* mutations (see http://mutagenetix.scripps.edu for details). A mutation in *Tnf* (used as the endpoint of screening) known as *PanR1* ("pan-resistance") was detected as a dominant phenovariant in G1 mice (Rutschmann et al. 2006). The *PanR1* allele does not affect the development of lymphoid organs as severely as knockout mutations of the *Tnf* locus do. On the one hand, minimal residual activity of the TNF protein may account for this. On the other hand, the knockout allele may affect neighboring genes such as the lymphotoxin-encoding locus, and may exert an effect on lymphoid development indirectly.

Requirements for TLR2 and TLR4 Complex Signaling

Further screening disclosed *oblivious*, a mutation that prevented signaling by some, but not all, TLR2/6 ligands (Hoebe et al. 2005). In particular, MALP-2 (a diacyl lipopeptide), lipoteichoic acid (a component of gram-positive bacteria that may well be contaminated with diacyl lipopeptides when obtained from commercial sources), and gram-positive peptidoglycan (another component of bacteria that generally is contaminated with lipopeptides) stimulated less than the normal amount of TNF production when added to *oblivious* macrophage cultures. Zymosan, the tri-acyl lipopeptide PAM_3CSK_4 (which signals entirely via TLR2/ TLR complexes) and the diacyl lipopeptide PAM_2CSK_4 (which signals partly via TLR2/1 complexes) stimulated normal TNF production. *Oblivious* mice were also hypersusceptible to infection with *Staphylococcus aureus*, and developed spontaneous infections of the surface of the eye, which became colonized with *Staphylococcus lentus* (Hoebe et al. 2005). The mutation proved to be a nonsense allele of *Cd36*, which encodes a class B scavenger receptor. CD36 thus acts as part of the TLR2/ TLR6 receptor complex, although its physical relationship to the other components of the complex remains unclear. *Oblivious* mice also show a defect of CD4 priming (Janssen et al. 2006), although the mechanism of this effect is unknown.

Heedless, a phenotype traced to a mutation of the CD14 protein (Jiang et al. 2005; Huber et al. 2006), had a dramatic effect on TLR4 signaling and a striking though partial influence on signaling from the TLR2/6 complex as well, although it did not affect TLR2/1 complex signaling. Remarkably, *heedless* influenced sensing of rough and smooth LPS variants differently. Rough LPS (minimally glycosylated) could activate MyD88-dependent signaling in *heedless* macrophages. Smooth LPS (luxuriantly glycosylated) could not. Neither LPS chemotype could activate MyD88-independent signaling in *heedless* macrophages.

The differential effects of both *Cd36* and *Cd14* mutations on the detection of specific ligands suggests that the encoded proteins may coordinate the tertiary structure of the TLR subunits, permitting them to respond to some ligands and not others, and influencing signaling in a qualitative manner as well. Possibly TLR2 and TLR4 can adopt multiple active conformations. Further to this hypothesis, the *pococurante* allele of MyD88 restricts signaling from some (but not all) TLR2 ligands (as discussed below in Sect. 6.5).

Insouciant (Jiang et al. 2006) and *languid* (http://mutagenetix.scripps.edu) were mutations of TLR6 and TLR2, respectively. Each produced a phenotype indistinguishable from that of the knockout mutations, produced in the Akira laboratory. To date, no functionally abnormal alleles of TLR1 or TLR4 have been identified in ENU mutagenesis screens.

The Nucleic Acid Sensing TLRs

TLRs 3, 7, 8, and 9, and very likely TLR13 (in the mouse), exist predominantly within the endosomes and endoplasmic reticulum rather than on the cell surface. TLRs 3, 7, 8, and 9 signal from acidified compartments (late endosomes or early lysosomes). A mutation termed *3d* ("triple defect") was found to suppress all signaling from these TLRs (Tabeta et al. 2006). *3d* mutant mice also failed to cross-present antigen, and had marked impairment (though not complete ablation) of class II restricted antigen presentation as well (Tabeta et al. 2006). Individual mutations affecting the TLR signaling apparatus (in TLR3, TLR9, TRIF, or MyD88) cause enhanced susceptibility to mouse cytomegalovirus (MCMV) (Tabeta et al. 2004). Almost certainly because of their inability to signal via TLRs 3 and 9, *3d* mutants were highly susceptible to MCMV infection. In addition, augmented susceptibility to *Listeria monocytogenes* and *Staphylococcus aureus* infection was observed (Tabeta et al. 2006).

The *3d* mutation was positionally cloned, and found to specify a missense error in *Unc93b1*, a gene encoding a 12-spanning protein restricted to the endoplasmic reticulum (ER) (Tabeta et al. 2006). Subsequent work revealed that UNC-93B is probably required to escort TLRs 3, 7, 9, and 13 to the endosomal compartment (Brinkmann et al. 2007). Hence, signaling does not occur in *3d* mutant mice because the TLRs do not encounter exogenously presented nucleic acids. In humans mutations of the orthologous gene were found to cause enhanced susceptibility to herpes simplex encephalitis, as well as the characteristic defect of nucleic acid sensing (Casrouge et al. 2006). The phenotype of humans with UNC-93B mutations is very similar to that of mice.

UNC-93B is one of three proteins of a small family that also includes UNC-93A and UNC-93C. The function of these remaining paralogs is unknown, but is being examined by gene targeting. In *Caenorhabditis elegans*, the UNC-93 protein fulfills a neurological function, as mutants are "uncoordinated." Based on suppression screens, it is possible (though uncertain) that the protein is a regulatory subunit of a two-pore potassium channel (de la Cruz et al. 2003). In mammals, the 12-spanning structure and the phenotype of the *3d* mutant, in which exogenous antigens are taken up by phagocytosis but not permitted access to the cell surface in conjunction with class I MHC proteins, suggests that a channel function may also exist. However, speculation holds that UNC-93B may comprise a channel for polypeptides rather than for ions.

The Nature of Receptor: Adaptor Interaction

There has been much speculation concerning the detailed interaction between TIR adaptor proteins and their receptors in vivo. Most commonly offered is a model of "bridging" in which the adaptors MAL and TRAM directly interact with TLR4 and permit MyD88 and TRIF to dock with them in turn. Some workers, however, have reported a direct interaction between MyD88 and TLR4, and it is not at all clear precisely how the four adaptors contact one another and the receptors themselves. This is despite the fact that the TIR domain structures of TLR1 and TLR2 have been solved (Xu et al. 2000; Jin et al. 2007), and other TIR domains may be modeled at low resolution based on these structures. All TIR domains consist of six α-helices (αA, αB, αC, αC′, αD, and αE) and five β-strands (βA, βB, βC, βD, and βE) that are connected by seven loops (named for the α-helix and β-strand they connect; e.g., AA connects βA with αA). The crystal structures of the TLR1 and TLR2 TIR domains reveal that they fold into a structure with a central five-stranded parallel β-sheet surrounded by five helices.

Molecular modeling studies, interpreted in the light of the *pococurante* ("*Poc*") phenotype caused by a point mutation within the TIR domain of MyD88, suggest that docking between MyD88 and TLR4 may indeed occur. The Poc site is located near to the site of the classical "Lps" mutation (corresponding to P712H in the TLR4 sequence), which resides within the BB loop. Poc and Lps mutations have identical effects, wherever they are engrafted. When introduced into MyD88 itself, the mutations prevent signaling from all of the MyD88-dependent TIR domain receptors except the TLR2/TLR6 complex. Similarly, when engrafted into TLR2, either mutation will permit residual signaling from the TLR2/TLR6 complex. But if both mutations are engrafted either into TLR2 or into MyD88, all signaling is abolished. It is clear that the Poc and Lps mutations prevent receptor:adaptor interaction because they prevent physical recruitment of MyD88 to those receptors for which signaling function is destroyed. On the other hand, mutations in the αE helices of receptors or adaptors (antipodal to the Poc and Lps sites) have different effects. In the case of the receptor, recruitment is abolished. In the case of MyD88, recruitment is observed, but signaling is abolished. This has been interpreted to mean that the αE helix is involved in receptor and adaptor oligomerization, while the Poc and Lps sites are involved in receptor:adaptor interaction (Jiang et al. 2006).

The *lackadaisical* phenotype is also caused by a receptor-selective MyD88 mutation, this time one that prevents signaling via TLRs 7 and 9 in part, but allows signaling via all other TLRs that require MyD88. The mutation, in this case, lies between the death domains of MyD88 and the TIR domain, a region for which there is no structural information. We can surmise that this part of the molecule is somehow important in choosing receptors, and may have direct contact with the receptors (Jiang et al. 2006).

How Far from Saturation, and How Far to Go?

A reasonably cohesive picture of the biochemical pathways required for TLR signaling has begun to emerge (Fig. 2). Not only ENU-induced mutations, but gene targeting as well, has helped us to assemble this picture. For example, gene targeting experiments have demonstrated that IRF5 (Takaoka et al. 2005) and IRF7 (Kawai et al. 2004; Honda et al. 2004) have specific roles to play in MyD88-dependent signaling; RIP-1 connects TLR3 signaling to the activation of NF-κB (Meylan et al. 2004); and TRAF3 signals in conjunction with TBK1 to allow MyD88-independent activation of IFN-β (Hacker et al. 2006). But surely the picture is incomplete, and some phenotypes induced with ENU have yet to be solved. *Feckless*, a mutation that prevents poly I:C-mediated activation of NF-κB but permits activation of IFN-β synthesis, has proved unusually stubborn (Z. Jiang, M. Berger, B. Beutler, unpublished data). Beyond this, there is the larger question of how far one should go with random germline mutagenesis. Ultimately, any screen is going to be exhausted, and there is less and less to be "mined" from the phenotype under analysis.

It is estimated, as a rule of thumb, that about 10% saturation results from the analysis of 10,000 G3 mice, produced in such a manner as to capture G1 mutations with 50% efficiency. Hence, about 30% of the targets that can cause phenotypical variations may now have been captured in the TLR signaling system. This assumes, however, that all aspects of the TLR signaling phenomenon have been maintained under surveillance, and this is almost certainly not true. Not all cytokine effectors have been monitored, nor all surface molecules induced. Only the core of the pathway has been studied with real attention. Therefore, there may be many molecules yet to find.

It is also true that some "secondary" phenotypes have much to tell and are not covered by the TLR signaling screen. For example, while we know that TLR signaling is important for the containment of MCMV, we do not know what role it may play in other physiologically important processes. It is here that the choice of screen (and the far-sightedness of the investigator) may determine the importance of what is ultimately discovered. Do TLRs play a role in inflammatory disease? Very likely so, and indeed, MyD88 mutations are known to suppress lupus-like disease in some mouse models (Christensen et al. 2006). But surely there is far more to be learned. It is also in combining mutations that much can be learned. In the absence of both MyD88 and TRIF, no TIR domain signaling can occur, and mice are severely immunocompromised. Yet to the surprise of many, they retain excellent adaptive immune competence (Gavin et al. 2006; Nemazee et al. 2006).

Concluding Thoughts on Immune Sensing and the Forward Genetic Approach

Forward genetics is a powerful approach in all aspects of biology, but it is particularly powerful in immunology, where a strong conceptual framework exists for the interpretation of new phenotypes. Yes, we knew that there was an LPS receptor, but it was seemingly impossible to isolate without genetics. Yes, we knew that there were endosomal and surface TLRs. But how did they reach their destinations? Many of the surprises that arise from forward genetics are easy to interpret, though this never diminishes their impact. Quite to the contrary, it enhances it.

Where the sensing pathways of the innate immune system are concerned, their beauty lies partly in their simplicity. Simple considerations suggested that there must be a limited number of germline-encoded receptors for innate immune recognition.

But there were other possibilities. Could alternative splicing be a means of generating diversity? Are there 100 receptors rather than only 10? Yet here is the situation as we see it: our most powerful inflammatory responses originate from an exceedingly small collection of molecules.

Not discussed in this chapter is that the retinoic-acid-inducible gene I (RIG-I)-like helicases and the NOD (nucleotide-binding oligomerization domain)/NALP family of proteins also serve sensing functions (Beutler et al. 2007b; Tschopp et al. 2003). The sequential dissection of all of these pathways is now a realistic prospect, as is the search for nonredundant pathways in adaptive immune activation.

References

Adachi O, Kawai T, Takeda K, Matsumoto M, Tsutsui H, Sakagami M, Nakanishi K, Akira S (1998) Targeted disruption of the MyD88 gene results in loss of IL-1- and IL-18-mediated function. Immunity 9:143–150

Alexopoulou L, Holt AC, Medzhitov R, Flavell RA (2001) Recognition of double-stranded RNA and activation of NF-kappaB by Toll-like receptor 3. Nature 413:732–738

Andersson J, Sjoberg O, Moller G (1972) Induction of immunoglobulin and antibody synthesis in vitro by lipopolysaccharides. Eur J Immunol 2:349–353

Beutler B, Greenwald D, Hulmes JD, Chang M, Pan YC, Mathison J, Ulevitch R, Cerami A (1985a) Identity of tumour necrosis factor and the macrophage-secreted factor cachectin. Nature 316:552–554

Beutler B, Mahoney J, Le Trang N, Pekala P, Cerami A (1985b) Purification of cachectin, a lipoprotein lipase-suppressing hormone secreted by endotoxin-induced RAW 264.7 cells. J Exp Med 161:984–995

Beutler B, Milsark IW, Cerami A (1985c) Passive immunization against cachectin/tumor necrosis factor (TNF) protects mice from the lethal effect of endotoxin. Science 229:869–871

Beutler B, Du X, Xia Y (2007a) Precis on forward genetics in mice. Nat Immunol 8:659–664

Beutler B, Eidenschenk C, Crozat K, Imler JL, Takeuchi O, Hoffmann JA, Akira S (2007b) Genetic analysis of resistance to viral infection. Nat Rev Immunol 7:753–766

Bhat N, Perera PY, Carboni JM, Blanco J, Golenbock DT, Mayadas TN, Vogel SN (1999) Use of a photoactivatable taxol analogue to identify unique cellular targets in murine macrophages: identification of murine CD18 as a major taxol-binding protein and a role for Mac-1 in taxol-induced gene expression. J Immunol 162:7335–7342

Bright SW, Chen TY, Flebbe LM, Lei MG, Morrison DC (1990) Generation and characterization of hamster-mouse hybridomas secreting monoclonal antibodies with specificity for lipopolysaccharide receptor. J Immunol 145:1–7

Brinkmann MM, Spooner E, Hoebe K, Beutler B, Ploegh HL, Kim YM (2007) The interaction between the ER membrane protein UNC93B and TLR3, 7, and 9 is crucial for TLR signaling. J Cell Biol 177:265–275

Casrouge A, Zhang SY, Eidenschenk C, Jouanguy E, Puel A, Yang K, Alcais A, Picard C, Mahfoufi N, Nicolas N, Lorenzo L, Plancoulaine S, Senechal B, Geissmann F, Tabeta K, Hoebe K, Du X, Miller RL, Heron B, Mignot C, de Villemeur TB, Lebon P, Dulac O, Rozenberg F, Beutler B, Tardieu M, Abel L, Casanova JL (2006) Herpes simplex virus encephalitis in human UNC-93B deficiency. Science 314:308–312

Christensen SR, Shupe J, Nickerson K, Kashgarian M, Flavell RA, Shlomchik MJ (2006) Toll-like receptor 7 and TLR9 dictate autoantibody specificity and have opposing inflammatory and regulatory roles in a murine model of lupus. Immunity 25:417–428

Coutinho A, Gronowicz E (1975) Genetical control of B-cell responses. III. Requirement for functional mitogenicity of the antigen in thymus-independent specific responses. J Exp Med 141:753–760

Coutinho A, Meo T (1978) Genetic basis for unresponsiveness to lipopolysaccharide in C57BL/10Cr mice. Immunogenetics 7:17–24

Coutinho A, Forni L, Melchers F, Watanabe T (1977) Genetic defect in responsiveness to the B cell mitogen lipopolysaccharide. Eur J Immunol 7:325–328

Coutinho A, Forni L, Watanabe T (1978) Genetic and functional characterization of an antiserum to the lipid A-specific triggering receptor on murine B lymphocytes. Eur J Immunol 8:63–67

de la Cruz I, Levin JZ, Cummins C, Anderson P, Horvitz HR (2003) sup-9, sup-10, and unc-93 may encode components of a two-pore K+ channel that coordinates muscle contraction in Caenorhabditis elegans. J Neurosci 23:9133–9145

Fitzgerald KA, Palsson-McDermott EM, Bowie AG, Jefferies CA, Mansell AS, Brady G, Brint E, Dunne A, Gray P, Harte MT, McMurray D, Smith DE, Sims JE, Bird TA, O'Neill LA (2001) Mal (MyD88-adapter-like) is required for Toll-like receptor-4 signal transduction. Nature 413:78–83

Flaherty SF, Golenbock DT, Milham FH, Ingalls RR (1997) CD11/CD18 leukocyte integrins: new signaling receptors for bacterial endotoxin. J Surg Res 73:85–89

Forni L, Coutinho A (1978) An antiserum which recognizes lipopolysaccharide-reactive B cells in the mouse. Eur J Immunol 8:56–62

Gavin AL, Hoebe K, Duong B, Ota T, Martin C, Beutler B, Nemazee D (2006) Adjuvant-enhanced antibody responses in the absence of toll-like receptor signaling. Science 314:1936–1938

Georgel P, Meister M, Kappler C, Lemaitre B, Reichhart JM, Hoffmann JA (1993) Insect immunity: the diptericin promoter contains multiple functional regulatory sequences homologous to mammalian acute-phase response elements. Biochem Biophys Res Commun 197:508–517

Georgel P, Naitza S, Kappler C, Ferrandon D, Zachary D, Swimmer C, Kopczynski C, Duyk G, Reichhart JM, Hoffmann JA (2001) Drosophila immune deficiency (IMD) is a death domain protein that activates antibacterial defense and can promote apoptosis. Dev Cell 1:503–514

Georgel P, Jiang Z, Kunz S, Janssen E, Mols J, Hoebe K, Bahram S, Oldstone MB, Beutler B (2007) Vesicular stomatitis virus glycoprotein G activates a specific antiviral Toll-like receptor 4-dependent pathway. Virology 362:304–313

Golenbock DT, Hampton RY, Raetz CR, Wright SD (1990) Human phagocytes have multiple lipid A-binding sites. Infect Immun 58:4069–4075

Hacker H, Redecke V, Blagoev B, Kratchmarova I, Hsu LC, Wang GG, Kamps MP, Raz E, Wagner H, Hacker G, Mann M, Karin M (2006) Specificity in Toll-like receptor signalling through distinct effector functions of TRAF3 and TRAF6. Nature 439:204–207

Havell EA (1987) Production of tumor necrosis factor during murine listeriosis. J Immunol 139:4225–4231

Hayashi F, Smith KD, Ozinsky A, Hawn TR, Yi EC, Goodlett DR, Eng JK, Akira S, Underhill DM, Aderem A (2001) The innate immune response to bacterial flagellin is mediated by Toll-like receptor 5. Nature 410:1099–1103

Haziot A, Ferrero E, Kontgen F, Hijiya N, Yamamoto S, Silver J, Stewart CL, Goyert SM (1996) Resistance to endotoxin shock and reduced dissemination of gram-negative bacteria in CD14-deficient mice. Immunity 4:407–414

Heil F, Ahmad-Nejad P, Hemmi H, Hochrein H, Ampenberger F, Gellert T, Dietrich H, Lipford G, Takeda K, Akira S, Wagner H, Bauer S (2003) The Toll-like receptor 7 (TLR7)-specific stimulus loxoribine uncovers a strong relationship within the TLR7, 8 and 9 subfamily. Eur J Immunol 33:2987–2997

Hemmi H, Takeuchi O, Kawai T, Kaisho T, Sato S, Sanjo H, Matsumoto M, Hoshino K, Wagner H, Takeda K, Akira S (2000) A Toll-like receptor recognizes bacterial DNA. Nature 408:740–745

Hemmi H, Kaisho T, Takeuchi O, Sato S, Sanjo H, Hoshino K, Horiuchi T, Tomizawa H, Takeda K, Akira S (2002) Small anti-viral compounds activate immune cells via the TLR7 MyD88-dependent signaling pathway. Nat Immunol 3:196–200

Heppner G, Weiss DW (1965) High susceptibility of strain A mice to endotoxin and endotoxin-red blood cell mixtures. J Bacteriol 90:696–703

Hoebe K, Du X, Georgel P, Janssen E, Tabeta K, Kim SO, Goode J, Lin P, Mann N, Mudd S, Crozat K, Sovath S, Han J, Beutler B (2003) Identification of Lps2 as a key transducer of MyD88-independent TIR signaling. Nature 424:743–748

Hoebe K, Georgel P, Rutschmann S, Du X, Mudd S, Crozat K, Sovath S, Shamel L, Hartung T, Zähringer U, Beutler B (2005) CD36 is a sensor of diacylglycerides. Nature 433:523–527

Honda K, Yanai H, Mizutani T, Negishi H, Shimada N, Suzuki N, Ohba Y, Takaoka A, Yeh WC, Taniguchi T (2004) Role of a transductional-transcriptional processor complex involving MyD88 and IRF-7 in Toll-like receptor signaling. Proc Natl Acad Sci U S A 101:15416–15421

Horng T, Barton GM, Medzhitov R (2001) TIRAP: an adapter molecule in the Toll signaling pathway. Nat Immunol 2:835–841

Hoshino K, Takeuchi O, Kawai T, Sanjo H, Ogawa T, Takeda Y, Takeda K, Akira S (1999) Cutting edge: Toll-like receptor 4 (TLR4)-deficient mice are hyporesponsive to lipopolysaccharide: evidence for TLR4 as the Lps gene product. J Immunol 162:3749–3752

Huber M, Kalis C, Keck S, Jiang Z, Georgel P, Du X, Shamel L, Sovath S, Mudd S, Beutler B, Galanos C, Freudenberg MA (2006) R-form LPS, the master key to the activation ofTLR4/MD-2-positive cells. Eur J Immunol 36:701–711

Ingalls RR, Golenbock DT (1995) CD11c/CD18, a transmembrane signaling receptor for lipopolysaccharide. J Exp Med 181:1473–1479

Ingalls RR, Arnaout MA, Golenbock DT (1997) Outside-in signaling by lipopolysaccharide through a tailless integrin. J Immunol 159:433–438

Ingalls RR, Arnaout MA, Delude RL, Flaherty S, Savedra R Jr, Golenbock DT (1998a) The CD11/CD18 integrins: characterization of three novel LPS signaling receptors. Prog Clin Biol Res 397:107–117

Ingalls RR, Monks BG, Savedra R Jr, Christ WJ, Delude RL, Medvedev AE, Espevik T, Golenbock DT (1998b) CD11/CD18 and CD14 share a common lipid A signaling pathway. J Immunol 161:5413–5420

Ingalls RR, Heine H, Lien E, Yoshimura A, Golenbock D (1999) Lipopolysaccharide recognition, CD14, and lipopolysaccharide receptors. Infect Dis Clin North Am 13:341–53, vii

Janssen E, Tabeta K, Barnes MJ, Rutschmann S, McBride S, Bahjat KS, Schoenberger SP, Theofilopoulos AN, Beutler B, Hoebe K (2006) Efficient T cell activation via a Toll-interleukin 1 receptor-independent pathway. Immunity 24:787–799

Jiang Z, Georgel P, Du X, Shamel L, Sovath S, Mudd S, Huber M, Kalis C, Keck S, Galanos C, Freudenberg M, Beutler B (2005) CD14 is required for MyD88-independent LPS signaling. Nat Immunol 6:565–570

Jiang Z, Georgel P, Li C, Choe J, Crozat K, Rutschmann S, Du X, Bigby T, Mudd S, Sovath S, Wilson IA, Olson A, Beutler B (2006) Details of Toll-like receptor:adapter interaction revealed by germ-line mutagenesis. Proc Natl Acad Sci U S A 103:10961–10966

Jin MS, Kim SE, Heo JY, Lee ME, Kim HM, Paik SG, Lee H, Lee JO (2007) Crystal structure of the TLR1-TLR2 heterodimer induced by binding of a tri-acylated lipopeptide. Cell 130:1071–1082

Kabir S, Rosenstreich DL (1977) Binding of bacterial endotoxin to murine spleen lymphocytes. Infect Immun 15:156–164

Kalis C, Kanzler B, Lembo A, Poltorak A, Galanos C, Freudenberg MA (2003) Toll-like receptor 4 expression levels determine the degree of LPS-susceptibility in mice. Eur J Immunol 33:798–805

Kappler C, Meister M, Lagueux M, Gateff E, Hoffmann JA, Reichhart JM (1993) Insect immunity. Two 17 bp repeats nesting a kappa B-related sequence confer inducibility to the diptericin gene and bind a polypeptide in bacteria-challenged Drosophila. EMBO J 12:1561–1568

Kawai T, Sato S, Ishii KJ, Coban C, Hemmi H, Yamamoto M, Terai K, Matsuda M, Inoue J, Uematsu S, Takeuchi O, Akira S (2004) Interferon-alpha induction through Toll-like receptors involves a direct interaction of IRF7 with MyD88 and TRAF6. Nat Immunol 5:1061–1068

Kim HM, Park BS, Kim JI, Kim SE, Lee J, Oh SC, Enkhbayar P, Matsushima N, Lee H, Yoo OJ, Lee JO (2007) Crystal structure of the TLR4-MD-2 complex with bound endotoxin antagonist Eritoran. Cell 130:906–917

Kindler V, Sappino AP, Grau GE, Piguet PF, Vassalli P (1989) The inducing role of tumor necrosis factor in the development of bactericidal granulomas during BCG infection. Cell 56:731–740

Lei MG, Morrison DC (1988a) Specific endotoxic lipopolysaccharide-binding proteins on murine splenocytes. I. Detection of lipopolysaccharide-binding sites on splenocytes and splenocyte subpopulations. J Immunol 141:996–1005

Lei MG, Morrison DC (1988b) Specific endotoxic lipopolysaccharide-binding proteins on murine splenocytes. II. Membrane localization and binding characteristics. J Immunol 141:1006–1011

Lei MG, Morrison DC (1993) Evidence that lipopolysaccharide and pertussis toxin bind to different domains on the same p73 receptor on murine splenocytes. Infect Immun 61:1359–1364

Lei MG, Flebbe L, Roeder D, Morrison DC (1990) Identification and characterization of lipopolysaccharide receptor molecules on mammalian lymphoid cells. Adv Exp Med Biol 256:445–466

Lei MG, Qureshi N, Morrison DC (1993) Lipopolysaccharide (LPS) binding to 73-kDa and 38-kDa surface proteins on lymphoreticular cells: preferential inhibition of LPS binding to the former by Rhodopseudomonas sphaeroides lipid A. Immunol Lett 36:245–250

Lemaitre B, Nicolas E, Michaut L, Reichhart JM, Hoffmann JA (1996) The dorsoventral regulatory gene cassette spatzle/Toll/cactus controls the potent antifungal response in Drosophila adults. Cell 86:973–983

Lynn WA, Raetz CR, Qureshi N, Golenbock DT (1991) Lipopolysaccharide-induced stimulation of CD11b/CD18 expression on neutrophils. Evidence of specific receptor-based response and inhibition by lipid A-based antagonists. J Immunol 147:3072–3079

McHale L, Tan X, Koehl P, Michelmore RW (2006) Plant NBS-LRR proteins: adaptable guards. Genome Biol 7:212

McWhirter SM, Fitzgerald KA, Rosains J, Rowe DC, Golenbock DT, Maniatis T (2004) IFN-regulatory factor 3-dependent gene expression is defective in Tbk1-deficient mouse embryonic fibroblasts. Proc Natl Acad Sci U S A 101:233–238

Medzhitov R, Preston-Hurlburt P, Janeway CA Jr (1997) A human homologue of the Drosophila Toll protein signals activation of adaptive immunity [see comments]. Nature 388:394–397

Meister M, Braun A, Kappler C, Reichhart JM, Hoffmann JA (1994) Insect immunity. A transgenic analysis in Drosophila defines several functional domains in the diptericin promoter. EMBO J 13:5958–5966

Meylan E, Burns K, Hofmann K, Blancheteau V, Martinon F, Kelliher M, Tschopp J (2004) RIP1 is an essential mediator of Toll-like receptor 3-induced NF-kappa B activation. Nat Immunol 5:503–507

Michalek SM, Moore RN, McGhee JR, Rosenstreich DL, Mergenhagen SE (1980) The primary role of lymphoreticular cells in the mediation of host responses to bacterial endotoxin. J Infect Dis 141:55–63

Muzio M, Ni J, Feng P, Dixit VM (1997) IRAK (Pelle) family member IRAK-2 and MyD88 as proximal mediators of IL-1 signaling. Science 278:1612–1615

Nemazee D, Gavin A, Hoebe K, Beutler B (2006) Immunology: Toll-like receptors and antibody responses. Nature 441:E4

Nomura N, Miyajima N, Sazuka T, Tanaka A, Kawarabayasi Y, Sato S, Nagase T, Seki N, Ishikawa K, Tabata S (1994) Prediction of the coding sequences of unidentified human genes. I. The coding sequences of 40 new genes (KIAA0001-KIAA0040) deduced by analysis of randomly sampled cDNA clones from human immature myeloid cell line KG-1. DNA Res 1:27–35

Ohto U, Fukase K, Miyake K, Satow Y (2007) Crystal structures of human MD-2 and its complex with antiendotoxic lipid IVa. Science 316:1632–1634

Oshiumi H, Matsumoto M, Funami K, Akazawa T, Seya T (2003a) TICAM-1, an adaptor molecule that participates in Toll-like receptor 3-mediated interferon-beta induction. Nat Immunol 4:161–171

Oshiumi H, Sasai M, Shida K, Fujita T, Matsumoto M, Seya T (2003b) TIR-containing adapter molecule (TICAM)-2, a bridging adapter recruiting to toll-like receptor 4 TICAM-1 that induces interferon-beta. J Biol Chem 278:49751–49762

Ozinsky A, Underhill DM, Fontenot JD, Hajjar AM, Smith KD, Wilson CB, Schroeder L, Aderem A (2000) The repertoire for pattern recognition of pathogens by the innate immune system is defined by cooperation between toll-like receptors. Proc Natl Acad Sci U S A 97 13766–13771

Peavy DL, Adler WH, Smith RT (1970) The mitogenic effect of endotoxin and staphylococcal enterotoxin B on mouse spleen cells and human peripheral lymphocytes. J Immunol 105:1453–1458

Peiffer-Schneider S, Schutte BC, Frees KL, Williamson K, Swartz SJ, Schwartz DA (1997) Genetic mapping of the Lps gene and construction of a physical map of the critical region at mid-chromosome 4. 11th International Mouse Genome Conference

Poltorak A, He X, Smirnova I, Liu M-, Van Huffel C, Du X, Birdwell D, Alejos E, Silva M, Galanos C, Freudenberg MA, Ricciardi-Castagnoli P, Layton B, Beutler B (1998a) Defective LPS signaling in C3H/HeJ and C57BL/10ScCr mice: mutations in Tlr4 gene. Science 282:2085–2088

Poltorak A, Smirnova I, He XL, Liu MY, Van Huffel C, McNally O, Birdwell D, Alejos E, Silva M Du X, Thompson P, Chan EKL, Ledesma J, Roe B, Clifton S, Vogel SN, Beutler B (1998b) Genetic and physical mapping of the Lps locus—identification of the toll-4 receptor as a candidate gene in the critical region. Blood Cells Mol Dis 24:340–355

Poltorak A, Smirnova I, Clisch R, Beutler B (2000) Limits of a deletion spanning Tlr4 in C57BL/10ScCr mice. J Endotoxin Res 6:51–56

Poltorak A, Merlin T, Nielsen PJ, Sandra O, Smirnova I, Schupp I, Boehm T, Galanos C, Freudenberg MA (2001) A point mutation in the il-12rbeta2 gene underlies the il-12 unresponsiveness of lps-defective c57bl/10sccr mice. J Immunol 167:2106–2111

Qureshi S, Zhang X, Clermont S, Lariviere L, Skamene E, Gros P, Eydoux P, Malo D (1996) Genetic and physical mapping of the Lps locus. 10th International Mouse Genome Conference

Qureshi ST, Larivière L, Leveque G, Clermont S, Moore KJ, Gros P, Malo D (1999a) Endotoxin-tolerant mice have mutations in toll-like receptor 4 (Tlr4) [correction]. J Exp Med 189:1519–1520

Qureshi ST, Lariviere L, Leveque G, Clermont S, Moore KJ, Gros P, Malo D (1999b) Endotoxin-tolerant mice have mutations in Toll-like receptor 4 (Tlr4). J Exp Med 189:615–625

Reichhart JM, Meister M, Dimarcq JL, Zachary D, Hoffmann D, Ruiz C, Richards G, Hoffmann JA (1992) Insect immunity: developmental and inducible activity of the Drosophila diptericin promoter. EMBO J 11:1469–1477

Rinchik EM, Bell JA, Hunsicker PR, Friedman JM, Jackson IJ, Russell LB (1994) Molecular genetics of the brown (b)-locus region of mouse chromosome 4. I. Origin and molecular mapping of radiation- and chemical-induced lethal brown deletions. Genetics 137:845–854

Roach JC, Glusman G, Rowen L, Kaur A, Purcell MK, Smith KD, Hood LE, Aderem A (2005) The evolution of vertebrate Toll-like receptors. Proc Natl Acad Sci U S A 102:9577–9582

Rutschmann S, Jung AC, Hetru C, Reichhart JM, Hoffmann JA, Ferrandon D (2000) The Rel protein DIF mediates the antifungal but not the antibacterial host defense in Drosophila. Immunity 12:569–580

Rutschmann S, Hoebe K, Zalevsky J, Du X, Mann N, Dahiyat BI, Steed P, Beutler B (2006) PanR1, a dominant negative missense allele of the gene encoding TNF-alpha (Tnf), does not impair lymphoid development. J Immunol 176:7525–7532

Schumann RR, Leong SR, Flaggs GW, Gray PW, Wright SD, Mathison JC, Tobias PS, Ulevitch RJ (1990) Structure and function of lipopolysaccharide binding protein. Science 249:1429–1431

Shimazu R, Akashi S, Ogata H, Nagai Y, Fukudome K, Miyake K, Kimoto M (1999) MD-2, a molecule that confers lipopolysaccharide responsiveness on Toll-like receptor 4. J Exp Med 189:1777–1782

Skidmore BJ, Chiller JM, Morrison DC, Weigle WO (1975) Immunologic properties of bacterial lipopolysaccharide (LPS): correlation between the mitogenic, adjuvant, and immunogenic activities. J Immunol 114:770–775

Stack J, Haga IR, Schroder M, Bartlett NW, Maloney G, Reading PC, Fitzgerald KA, Smith GL, Bowie AG (2005) Vaccinia virus protein A46R targets multiple Toll-like-interleukin-1 receptor adaptors and contributes to virulence. J Exp Med 201:1007–1018

Sultzer BM (1968) Genetic control of leucocyte responses to endotoxin. Nature 219:1253–1254

Tabeta K, Georgel P, Janssen E, Du X, Hoebe K, Crozat K, Mudd S, Shamel L, Sovath S, Goode J, Alexopoulou L, Flavell RA, Beutler B (2004) Toll-like receptors 9 and 3 as essential components of innate immune defense against mouse cytomegalovirus infection. Proc Natl Acad Sci U S A 101:3516–3521

Tabeta K, Hoebe K, Janssen EM, Du X, Georgel P, Crozat K, Mudd S, Mann N, Sovath S, Goode J, Shamel L, Herskovits AA, Portnoy DA, Cooke M, Tarantino LM, Wiltshire T, Steinberg BE, Grinstein S, Beutler B (2006) The Unc93b1 mutation 3d disrupts exogenous antigen presentation and signaling via Toll-like receptors 3, 7 and 9. Nat Immunol 7:156–164

Taguchi T, Mitcham JL, Dower SK, Sims JE, Testa JR (1996) Chromosomal localization of TIL, a gene encoding a protein related to the Drosophila transmembrane receptor Toll, to human chromosome 4p14. Genomics 32:486–488

Takaoka A, Yanai H, Kondo S, Duncan G, Negishi H, Mizutani T, Kano S, Honda K, Ohba Y, Mak TW, Taniguchi T (2005) Integral role of IRF-5 in the gene induction programme activated by Toll-like receptors. Nature 434:243–249

Takeuchi O, Hoshino K, Kawai T, Sanjo H, Takada H, Ogawa T, Takeda K, Akira S (1999) Differential roles of TLR2 and TLR4 in recognition of gram-negative and gram-positive bacterial cell wall components. Immunity 11:443–451

Takeuchi O, Kawai T, Muhlradt PF, Morr M, Radolf JD, Zychlinsky A, Takeda K, Akira S (2001) Discrimination of bacterial lipoproteins by Toll-like receptor 6. Int Immunol 13:933–940

Takeuchi O, Sato S, Horiuchi T, Hoshino K, Takeda K, Dong Z, Modlin RL, Akira S (2002) Cutting edge: role of Toll-like receptor 1 in mediating immune response to microbial lipoproteins. J Immunol 169:10–14

Tschopp J, Martinon F, Burns K (2003) NALPs: a novel protein family involved in inflammation. Nat Rev Mol Cell Biol 4:95–104

Uematsu S, Sato S, Yamamoto M, Hirotani T, Kato H, Takeshita F, Matsuda M, Coban C, Ishii KJ, Kawai T, Takeuchi O, Akira S (2005) Interleukin-1 receptor-associated kinase-1 plays an essential role for Toll-like receptor (TLR)7- and TLR9-mediated interferon-alpha induction. J Exp Med 201:915–923

Vitaterna MH, King DP, Chang AM, Kornhauser JM, Lowrey PL, McDonald JD, Dove WF, Pinto LH, Turek FW, Takahashi JS (1994) Mutagenesis and mapping of a mouse gene, Clock, essential for circadian behavior. Science 264:719–725

Vogel SN, Wax JS, Perera PY, Padlan C, Potter M, Mock BA (1994) Construction of a BALB/c congenic mouse, C. J Exp MedC3H-Lpsd, that expresses the Lpsd allele: analysis of chromosome 4 markers surrounding the Lps gene. Infect Immun 62:4454–4459

Vogel SN, Johnson D, Perera PY, Medvedev A, Larivière L, Qureshi ST, Malo D (1999) Functional characterization of the effect of the C3H/HeJ defect in mice that lack an Lpsn gene: in vivo evidence for a dominant negative mutation. J Immunol 162:5666–5670

Watson J, Riblet R (1975) Genetic control of responses to bacterial lipopolysaccharides in mice. II. A gene that influences a membrane component involved in the activation of bone marrow-derived lymphocytes by lipopolysaccharides. J Immunol 114:1462–1468

Watson J, Riblet R, Taylor BA (1977) The response of recombinant inbred strains of mice to bacterial lipopolysaccharides. J Immunol 118:2088–2093

Watson J, Kelly K, Largen M, Taylor BA (1978) The genetic mapping of a defective LFS response gene in C3H/HeJ mice. J Immunol 120:422–424

Wright SD (1991) Multiple receptors for endotoxin. Curr Opin Immunol 3:83–90

Wright SD, Jong MTC (1986) Adhesion-promoting receptors on human macrophages recognize Escherichia coli by binding to lipopolysaccharide. J Exp Med 164:1876–1888

Wright SD, Tobias PS, Ulevitch RJ, Ramos RA (1989) Lipopolysaccharide (LPS) binding protein opsonizes LPS-bearing particle for recognition by a novel receptor on macrophages. J Exp Med 170:1231–1241

Wright SD, Ramos RA, Tobias PS, Ulevitch RJ, Mathison JC (1990) CD14, a receptor for complexes of lipopolysaccharide (LPS) and LPS binding protein. Science 249:1431–1433

Xu Y, Tao X, Shen B, Horng T, Medzhitov R, Manley JL, Tong L (2000) Structural basis for signal transduction by the Toll/interleukin-1 receptor domains. Nature 408:111–115

Yamamoto M, Sato S, Hemmi H, Sanjo H, Uematsu S, Kaisho T, Hoshino K, Takeuchi O, Kobayashi M, Fujita T, Takeda K, Akira S (2002) Essential role for TIRAP in activation of the signalling cascade shared by TLR2 and TLR4. Nature 420:324–329

Yamamoto M, Sato S, Hemmi H, Hoshino K, Kaisho T, Sanjo H, Takeuchi O, Sugiyama M, Okabe M, Takeda K, Akira S (2003a) Role of adaptor TRIF in the MyD88-independent toll-like receptor signaling pathway. Science 301:640–643

Yamamoto M, Sato S, Hemmi H, Uematsu S, Hoshino K, Kaisho T, Takeuchi O, Takeda K, Akira S (2003b) TRAM is specifically involved in the Toll-like receptor 4-mediated MyD88-independent signaling pathway. Nat Immunol 4:1144–1150

Yokoyama K, Terao T, Osawa T (1978) Membrane receptors of human erythrocytes for bacterial lipopolysaccharide (LPS). Jpn J Exp Med 48:511–517

Yokoyama K, Mashimo J, Kasai N, Terao T, Osawa T (1979) Binding of bacterial lipopolysaccharide to histocompatibility-2-complex proteins of mouse lymphocytes. Hoppe Seylers Z Physiol Chem 360:587–595

Genetic Analysis of Resistance to Infections in Mice: A/J meets C57BL/6J

J.-F. Marquis, P. Gros(✉)

Contents

Abstract Susceptibility to infectious diseases has long been known to have a genetic component in human populations. This genetic effect is often complex and difficult to study as it is further modified by environmental factors including the disease-causing pathogen itself. The laboratory mouse has proved a useful alternative to implement a genetic approach to study host defenses against infections. Our laboratory has used genetic analysis and positional cloning to characterize single and multi-gene effects regulating inter-strain differences in the susceptibility of A/J and C57BL/6J mice to infection with several bacterial and parasitic pathogens. This has led to the identification of several proteins including Nramp1 (Slc11a1), Birc1e, Icsbp, C5a, and others that play critical roles in the antimicrobial defenses of macrophages against intracellular pathogens. The use of AcB/BcA recombinant congenic strains has further facilitated the characterization of single gene effects in complex traits such as susceptibility to malaria. The genetic identification of erythrocyte pyruvate kinase (Pklr) and myeloid pantetheinase enzymes (Vnn1/3) as

P. Gros
Department of Biochemistry, McGill University, McIntyre Medical Building,
3655 Promenade Sir William Osler, Room 910, Montréal, QC H3G 1Y6, Canada
philippe.gros@mcgill.ca

B. Beutler (ed.), *Immunology, Phenotype First: How Mutations Have Established*
New Principles and Pathways in Immunology. Current Topics in Microbiology
and Immunology 321. © Springer-Verlag Berlin Heidelberg 2008

key regulators of blood-stage parasitemia has suggested that cellular redox potential may be a key biochemical determinant of *Plasmodium* parasite replication. Expanding these types of studies to additional inbred strains and to emerging stocks of mutagenized mice will undoubtedly continue to unravel the molecular basis of host defense against infections.

Introduction

Infectious diseases continue to be a major cause of morbidity and mortality worldwide. In developing countries, infectious diseases are responsible for about half the burden of premature death and disability. Although antimicrobial drugs and vaccination programs have made headway in combating some pathogens, the absence of effective vaccines and the widespread emergence of microbial drug resistance continue to hamper the prevention and treatment of major foes such as malaria, tuberculosis, and human immunodeficiency virus (HIV). Additional socio-economic factors such as climate change, deforestation, floods, armed conflicts, population migration, and increased travel have contributed to the emergence and dissemination of novel viral and bacterial pathogens that constitute novel global health threats (reviewed in Khasnis and Nettleman 2005). The rapid microbial adaptation to antibiotics, together with the reduced interest of the pharmaceutical industry in the field of antimicrobial drug discovery (Norrby et al. 2005), are sure to compound the problem of infectious diseases in the years to come. On the other hand, most individuals coming in contact with an infectious agent do not develop disease, suggesting that the natural defenses of the body are generally well equipped to resist assault by microbial pathogens. A better understanding of such host defense mechanisms, therefore, may provide insight in understanding not only pathogenesis, but it may also suggest some novel host-based pathways and targets for pharmacological prevention and the treatment of the corresponding disease. Such defense mechanisms may manifest themselves as genetic variations in innate susceptibility to infections in humans and in animal models of disease.

In humans, an apparent heritability of infectious disease susceptibility has long been recognized. More recent population and epidemiological studies relating to geographic distributions, effect of race, first contact epidemics, and studies in twins have confirmed a genetic component to infection susceptibility in humans (Clementi and Di Gianantonio 2006; Cooke and Hill 2001; Frodsham and Hill 2004; Hill 2001, 2006). In the case of malaria, there is evidence of co-evolution of the pathogen and host genomes, with otherwise deleterious allelic variants in human erythrocyte proteins being retained in the population as they confer a protective advantage against the *Plasmodium* parasite (Min-Oo and Gros 2005). Except for some rare exceptions (Casanova and Abel 2007), the genetic component to susceptibility to infections is believed to be complex and multigenic, most probably because of the expected plurality in cell types and biochemical pathways ultimately involved in host response to a pathogen. In addition, the host:pathogen interaction is dynamic in nature with adaptive mechanisms at play on both sides of this interaction. Thus, the study of this genetic component in humans is complicated by many environmental factors, none of which is more important than pathogen-associated virulence determinants (strain, dose, co-infection, etc.). Such a complex gene–environment interaction results in apparent genetic heterogeneity, incomplete penetrance, and variable expressivity, all reducing the power of standard genetic association or linkage studies. Furthermore, ascertainment of disease status is sometimes difficult in field studies further complicating these types of studies. Nevertheless, numerous association studies with candidate genes identified in animal models have been published (Marquet and Schurr 2001). Obvious limitations of such studies are that many genes are left out of the analysis, and that only a single gene is analyzed at one time. More recently, genetic studies by whole genome scans have also been published for major diseases such as tuberculosis, leprosy, and malaria (Casanova and Abel 2007). Although major gene effects have been identified in a few studies (Baghdadi et al. 2006; Picard et al. 2006), the norm has been that the genetic control is complex and multigenic with an often modest contribution of individual loci.

The laboratory mouse has been extremely useful for genetic analysis in infectious diseases. First, there exist several excellent experimental mouse models of infection that mimic different aspects of the corresponding human infection. Second, pathogen-associated parameters such as strains, virulence, dose, and route of infection can be controlled. Third, there are many inbred, recombinant and naturally occurring or experimentally induced mutant mouse strains that are commercially available, which can be used to identify major gene effects influencing onset, progression, host response, and ultimate outcome of infection with a specific pathogen. Fourth, genetic analysis can be conducted in fairly easy-to-produce informative crosses that can be analyzed for the presence of major gene effects or quantitative trait loci (QTLs), using readily available single-nucleotide polymorphisms (SNP) or di-nucleotide markers. Additional mapping stocks such as recombinant inbred and recombinant congenic stocks can be used in large multi-strain intercrosses to break down multigenic effects into monogenic traits. Fifth, the mouse genome has been sequenced and annotated, and tissue expression data are available for most of the genes, facilitating the prioritization of positional candidates contained within a genetic interval of interest. Importantly, germ-line modification in transgenic mice can be used to generate gain- or loss-of-function mutants, and thereby validate the role of individual genes in host defenses against infection with a specific pathogen (Yap and Sher 2002). Finally, genes, proteins, and biochemical pathways identified in mouse studies provide candidate genes for validation in parallel genetic studies in human populations from areas of endemic disease (De Jong et al. 1998; Dupuis et al. 2003; Greenwood et al. 2000; Jouanguy et al. 1999).

Our laboratory has worked for the past 20 years on the mapping and characterization of host genes that affect susceptibility to various infectious diseases. Our approach has been to sample the genetic diversity of a small number inbred mouse strains to identify and clone major gene effects. In a few instances we have also succeeded in using AcB/BcA recombinant congenic mouse strains to identify single gene effects in complex traits. Our findings will be herein reviewed.

Simple Traits

Our definition of a simple trait corresponds to an infection-associated phenotype(s) that shows clear variation among inbred strains, with no overlap in quantitative evaluation of the phenotype or phenotypes between individuals of different such strains. Furthermore, when allowed to segregate in informative backcross or F_2 progeny, these traits show a classical Mendelian segregation pattern indicative of a single gene effect that can be identified by positional cloning. We have generally achieved further validation of positional candidates through direct sequence analysis, transfection studies in vitro, or through the creation of transgenic animals in vivo.

Mycobacterium *Species*

Nramp1

Susceptibility to infection by *Mycobacterium bovis* (bacillus Calmette-Guerin, BCG), as measured by early in vivo replication in the liver and spleen, is under simple genetic control in inbred strains, with resistance dominant over susceptibility. The locus responsible was detected some 30 years ago, and was mapped to the proximal part of chromosome 1 using recombinant inbred strains and classical crosses, and given the designation *Bcg*. It was immediately obvious that *Bcg* was either identical or tightly linked to two other previously mapped loci, *Ity* and *Lsh*, that independently control susceptibility to infection with *Salmonella typhimurium* and *Leishmania donovani* (Skamene et al. 1998). Experiments ex vivo demonstrated that macrophages are responsible for the phenotypic expression of infection resistance/susceptibility in mice (Gros et al. 1983). The *Bcg/Ity/Lsh* locus was identified by a laborious early positional cloning approach based on high-resolution linkage mapping, physical mapping by pulse-field gel electrophoresis, and the creation of a transcript map of the region using CpG clustering and exon trapping (Marquis et al. 2007; Poon and Schurr 2004). A positional candidate, designated as *Nramp1* (natural resistance associated macrophage protein, currently annotated as *Slc11a1*), was identified based on its exclusive expression in macrophages and macrophage-rich tissues. Sequence analysis showed that *Nramp1* encoded an integral membrane protein of 60 kDa composed of 12 transmembrane (TM) domains, and further revealed that susceptible inbred strains carried a single nonconservative Gly-to-Asp substitution at position 169 in (predicted) TM4 of the protein. This mutation was subsequently shown to impair protein folding, processing, and targeting, resulting in the absence of mature protein being expressed in the membrane compartment of susceptible macrophages (Vidal et al. 1993, 1996). Validation of the causal relationship between *Nramp1* and *Bcg/Ity/Lsh* came in the form of the construction and characterization of a null allele of *Nramp1* by gene targeting, which abrogated resistance to infection with all three infectious agents. Conversely, introduction of a wildtype, resistance-associated *Nramp1^{G169}* allele on the otherwise susceptible background of *Nramp1^{D169}* restored resistance to infection both in transfected RAW macrophages and in transgenic mice (reviewed in Lam-Yuk-Tseung and Gros 2003; Poon and Schurr 2004).

Nramp1 protein is not present at the plasma membrane but is exclusively expressed in the Lamp1-positive lysosomal compartment of macrophages and the gelatinase-positive granules of neutrophils (Canonne-Hergaux et al. 2002; Gruenheid et al. 1997). Upon phagocytosis of inert particles or live microorganisms including *Salmonella*, *Leishmania*, *Mycobacterium*, and *Yersinia* (Cuellar-Mata et al. 2002; Govoni et al. 1999; Searle et al. 1998), Nramp1 is quickly recruited to the membrane of the maturing phagosomes (Gruenheid et al. 1997). Subsequent studies by microfluorescence imaging using solid particles coupled to a metal sensitive fluorophore showed that Nramp1 in macrophages functions as a manganese transporter at the phagosomal membrane (Jabado et al. 2000). Nramp1 was shown to function as an efflux pump, moving Mn^{2+} ions down a concanamycin-sensitive proton gradient created by the vacuolar H^+/ATPase (Jabado et al. 2000). Subsequent studies in transfected cells expressing a mutant Nramp1 variant at the plasma membrane showed that Nramp1 can act both on Mn^{2+} and Fe^{2+}, although it appears to show a preference for the former (Forbes and Gros 2003). Finally, Nramp1 is part of a large family of metal transporters that has been highly conserved in evolution from bacteria to humans (Cellier et al. 1995). Of note is the Nramp2/Slc11a2 protein, which functions as the general Fe^{2+} acquisition system in humans for both nutritional iron at the duodenal brush border and more generally for transferrin iron at the membrane of recycling endosomes (Canonne-Hergaux et al. 1999). Mutations in human and mouse Nramp2/Slc11a2 cause a severe form of microcytic anemia (Lam-Yuk-Tseung et al. 2006).

Mycobacteria survive within macrophages by inhibiting the maturation of phagosomes into fully bactericidal phagolysosomes, as demonstrated by reduced recruitment of lysosomal enzymes and vacuolar H^+/ATPase and reduced acidification (Clemens and Horwitz 1995; Clemens et al. 2000a, b; Russell et al. 1996; Schaible et al. 1998; Sturgill-Koszycki et al. 1994, 1996). Early experiments by Hackam and colleagues (1998) using macrophages from *Nramp1^{-/-}* mice showed that recruitment of Nramp1 to the membrane of *M. bovis*-containing phagosomes caused a significant increase in acidification. Subsequent electron microscopy studies showed that recruitment of Nramp1 to the membrane of *M. avium*-containing phagosomes causes bacteriostasis, increased bacterial damage, increased acidification and increased fusion to lysosomes when compared to *Nramp1^{-/-}* phagosomes (Frehel et al. 2002; Hackam et al. 1998). A simple explanation of these results is that inhibition of phagosome maturation by mycobacteria requires a metal-dependent, active process that can be antagonized by Nramp1-mediated metal efflux from the phagosomal lumen. Globally, Nramp1-induced depletion of phagosomal iron could impair the ability of mycobacteria to modulate phagolysosomal fusion. Similar conclusions have been reached in the study of *Salmonella* and *Leishmania*-containing phagosomes (see the following section).

The human *NRAMP1* gene maps to chromosomal region 2q35, in close proximity to the interleukin 8 receptor gene (Cellier et al. 1994). The gene is composed of 15 exons including one that is alternatively spliced. Comparison of the human and mouse predicted NRAMP protein sequences revealed a remarkable degree of conservation between the two polypeptides, with 88% identical residues and 93% overall sequence similarity (Cellier et al. 1994). In humans, *NRAMP1* mRNA is expressed in spleen, lung, and at high levels in peripheral blood leukocytes, macrophages, and neutrophils (Canonne-Hergaux et al. 2002; Cellier et al. 1997). A possible role of *NRAMP1* in susceptibility to infectious diseases and to autoimmune disorders in humans has been intensely investigated (for complete reviews, please see Marquis et al. 2007; Poon and Schurr 2004). It suffices to note that *NRAMP1* has been consistently associated with pulmonary tuberculosis susceptibility in African and Asian populations but not in populations of European descent (Li et al. 2006), with direct genetic linkage data obtained during a tuberculosis outbreak in a Canadian aboriginal family (Greenwood et al. 2000) and in pediatric tuberculosis among children (Malik et al. 2005). Additional studies have shown that *NRAMP1* is involved in susceptibility to two other common mycobacterial diseases, leprosy (Abel et al. 1998; Alcais et al. 2000), and Buruli ulcer (Stienstra et al. 2006).

Together, these studies of Nramp1/Slc11a1 provide a clear example of how a gene discovered using genetic analysis in mice can subsequently be shown to contribute to a complex disease trait in humans.

Icsbp1

In inbred mouse strains, there is a strict correlation between allelic combination at *Nramp1* alleles and susceptibility to infection with *M. bovis* (BCG) (Malo et al. 1994) with the notable exception of the recombinant inbred strain BXH-2 (Skamene et al. 1982). BXH-2 is a recombinant inbred mouse strain derived from C3H/HeJ and C57BL/6J (Taylor 1978) that is known to develop a myelogenous leukemia by a two-step mutagenic process including an inherited mutation that causes a myeloproliferative syndrome, with a second retroviral-mediated insertion mutation resulting in clonal expansion of leukemic cells (Bedigian et al. 1981, 1984, 1993; Jenkins et al. 1982). Using splenomegaly as a phenotypic marker of myeloproliferation in F_2 crosses derived from BXH-2, we showed that this latter trait is determined by a single recessive locus in BXH-2 that we designated *Myls* (Turcotte et al. 2004). Positional cloning showed that the gene was located on the distal portion of chromosome 8 near marker *D8Mit13* [logarithm of differences (LOD)>44; map position 125 Mb (Turcotte et al. 2004)]. The *Myls* interval contains several positional candidates, including *Icsbp1* [interferon consensus sequence-binding protein 1, also known as interferon regulatory factor 8 (*IRF8*)]. Icsbp1 is a transcriptional regulator that plays an important role in transcriptional activation of interferon γ-responsive genes that bear an interferon-stimulated response element (ISRE) sequence element in their regulatory regions. BXH-2 mice carry an R294C mutation within the predicted interferon regulatory factor (IRF)-association domain of the protein. The R294C allele is associated with a complete failure of BXH-2 splenocytes to produce interleukin-12 and interferon-γ in response to activating stimuli.

Despite a C3H-derived resistance $Nramp1^{G169}$ allele, BXH-2 mice are susceptible to infection with *M. bovis* (BCG). Susceptibility appears somewhat variable, however, when tested at 3 weeks post-infection, with spleen colony-forming units (CFU) counts 5- and 100-fold (Skamene et al. 1982) superior to those seen in parental C3H controls, depending on the experiment. The effect of the R294C mutation in *Icsbp1* on susceptibility to *M. bovis* (BCG) was analyzed using a number of F_2 crosses between BXH-2 (*IRF-8*^{C294}, $Nramp1^{G169}$) and other inbred strains of known *Nramp1* genotype. These studies showed that the $Icsbp1^{R294C}$ mutation increased susceptibility to *M. bovis* (BCG), and this effect was most visible in segregating F_2 mice fixed for homozygosity or heterozygosity for resistance $Nramp1^{G169}$ alleles (Turcotte et al. 2005). Subsequent studies showed that BXH-2 mice cannot control *M. bovis* (BCG) replication during the late stages of infection, and display continuous growth in the spleen associated with complete absence of granuloma formation. Additional preliminary data also indicate that BXH-2 mice present a severe susceptibility phenotype to pulmonary tuberculosis following an intravenous challenge with highly virulent *M. tuberculosis* H37Rv (J.F. Marquis, R. LaCourse, L. Ryan, R.J. North, and P. Gros, unpublished data). In addition, the effect of the $Icsbp1^{R294C}$ mutation appears pleiotropic as BXH-2 mice also show susceptibility to infection with the unrelated pathogens *Salmonella typhimurium* and *Plasmodium chabaudi* (Turcotte et al. 2007). In the case of *P. chabaudi*, although BXH-2 can clear the initial burst of parasitemia, they fail to mount a long-term protective immune response since the animals develop multiple waves of recurring parasitemia late in the infection. These findings together suggest that *Icsbp1* plays a critical role in both innate and acquired immune responses to intracellular pathogens.

Genetic *Nramp1* Modifier Detected in *Mus spretus* Wild Mice

The presence of genetic modifiers of *Nramp1*-dependent susceptibility to *M. bovis* (BCG) infection was investigated in the wild-derived mouse strain *Mus spretus*. *Mus spretus* is a wild-derived inbred strain that is phylogenetically distant from *Mus musculus* from which common laboratory inbred strains are derived. The evolutionary distance and associated genetic diversity separating wild-derived mice, such as *M. spretus* and *M. musculus*, are advantageous for the identification of novel gene effects in crosses derived from the two strains. Despite the presence of a fixed $Nramp1^{G169}$ resistance allele, *M. spretus* (SPRET/EiJ) is quite susceptible to infection with a low dose of *M. bovis* (BCG). The presence of possible modifiers of the protective effect of $Nramp1^{G169}$ alleles in

SPRET/EiJ was investigated by whole-genome scans using 159 informative markers distributed along 19 autosomes and the X chromosome of 175 (SPRET/EiJ×B6) F_1 ×B6 backcross mice, using splenic *M. bovis* (BCG) bacterial load as a quantitative phenotype. As expected, *Nramp1* had a major effect (*D1Mcg4*) on splenic bacterial loads. Several additional weaker gene effects were noted, however, on chromosomes 4 (*D4Mit150*) and X (*DXMit249*) in male mice, and on chromosome 9 (*D9Mit77*) and 17 (*D17Mit81*) in female mice. The chromosome 17 QTL showed a strong interaction with *Nramp1* in female mice. It overlaps the major histocompatibility (MHC) locus, a region that contains many genes regulating early (innate) and late phase (acquired immunity) of host response to infection with mycobacteria including *M. bovis* (BCG) and *M. tuberculosis* (Lavebratt et al. 1999; Sanchez et al. 2003). The effect of chromosome 17 on host response to *M. tuberculosis* has recently been attributed to a functional polymorphism in the tumor necrosis factor (TNF)-α gene (Kahler et al. 2005), suggesting a possible modifying effect of this pleiotropic proinflammatory cytokine on *Nramp1*-mediated resistance.

QTLs detected as modifiers of Nramp1 action in mice may represent novel and valuable entry points for the parallel search for mycobacterial susceptibility loci in humans.

Salmonella typhimurium

Salmonella are facultative intracellular gram-negative bacteria of major global health importance. Almost all *Salmonella* serotypes belong to the same species designated *Salmonella enterica*. Over 2,500 serovars of *S. enterica* have been identified that are differentiated by their flagellar, carbohydrate, and lipopolysaccharide (LPS) structures (Fierer and Guiney 2001; Ochman and Groisman 1994). *S. enterica* species are typically orally acquired pathogens that cause one of four major syndromes: enteric fever (typhoid), enterocolitis/diarrhea, bacteremia, and chronic asymptomatic carriage (Fierer and Guiney 2001). In humans, serovars Typhi, Paratyphi, and Sendai cause enteric fever, while most serovars cause enterocolitis. While serovar Typhi is largely restricted to humans, serovar Typhimurium causes disease in both humans and other animals. *Salmonella typhimurium* infection in mice recapitulates the pathophysiology of the acute human infection with *Salmonella* Typhi or Paratyphi. Following infection by the oral or parenteral route, *S. typhimurium* localizes to the spleen and the liver where it replicates rapidly, causing death of the susceptible mice within a week of infection.

Tlr4 (Lps)

Bacterial LPS is a major constituent of the outer membrane of gram-negative bacteria and is essential for virulence of *Salmonella* in vivo (Rietschel et al. 1994).

In addition, bacterial LPS is a major mediator of pathogenesis in vivo, being a potent inducer of inflammatory responses in macrophages and mitogenic activity in B lymphocytes (Rosenberger et al. 2000; Royle et al. 2003). Inbred strains of mice vary dramatically in their degree of susceptibility and resistance to infection with *S. typhimurium* as determined by the extent of microbial replication in spleen and liver, and overall survival to the acute infection. In addition, a robust response to LPS is required in mice for survival to acute infection with *S. typhimurium*. Inbred mouse strains such as C3H/HeJ and C57BL/10ScCr do not respond to LPS in vitro and are susceptible to *S. typhimurium* infection (MacVittie et al. 1982; O'Brien et al. 1980, 1985; Vazquez-Torres et al. 2004; Weinstein et al. 1986). The acute susceptibility of C3H/HeJ mice was studied by linkage analysis and was found to be inherited in a recessive manner, which segregated as a monogenic trait (Watson and Riblet 1974; Watson et al. 1977). The locus was named *Lps*, and two alleles were defined: Lps^n and Lps^d for normal and defective response to LPS, respectively (Watson et al. 1978). High-resolution genetic, physical, and transcriptional maps of the area were used to identify the gene responsible for the *Lps* effect (Poltorak et al. 1998; Qureshi et al. 1996). These studies led to the identification of the gene encoding Toll-like receptor 4 (*Tlr4*) as the gene mutated at *Lps* (Poltorak et al. 1998; Qureshi et al. 1999). Tlr4 functions as a pattern recognition receptor that recognizes LPS of gram-negative bacteria such as *Salmonella*. Confirmation of the role of *Tlr4* in LPS hyporesponsiveness was obtained through examination of mice that had been rendered deficient for *Tlr4* (Hoshino et al. 1999). These studies were the first to show that the Tlr family plays a major role in innate defense mechanisms. In particular, they are critical for the recognition of microbial products based on a set of molecular determinants (leucine-rich repeats) unrelated to the immunoglobulin super-family.

Nramp1 (Ity)

Early studies in recombinant inbred strains together with direct progeny testing experiments strongly suggested that the *M. bovis* susceptibility locus *Bcg* was identical to two other host resistance loci, *Ity* and *Lsh*, independently described as affecting susceptibility to infection with *S. typhimurium* and *L. donovani*, respectively (Skamene et al. 1998). Subsequent gene targeting and transfection experiments formally demonstrated that *Nramp1*, *Bcg*, *Ity*, and *Lsh* were indeed the same locus controlling susceptibility to infection with unrelated intracellular pathogens (Govoni et al. 1996; Vidal et al. 1995).

The effect of Nramp1 on the biochemical composition and physiological properties of *Salmonella*-containing phagosomes formed in macrophages has been well studied and has proved useful in understanding the mechanistic basis of the protein's effect on intracellular pathogens. As with mycobacteria, *Salmonella* survive within macrophages by interfering with normal phagosome maturation (toward phagolysosome), and reside in specialized *Salmonella*-containing vacuoles (SCV), also known as "spacious" phagosomes (Knodler and Steele-Mortimer 2003). As opposed to phagosomes containing mycobacteria, SCVs formed in both *Nramp1⁺/⁺* and *Nramp1⁻/⁻* macrophages acidify fully and recruit the lysosomal marker Lamp-1. In *Salmonella*-permissive *Nramp1⁻/⁻* macrophages, however, SCV exhibit reduced incorporation of the late endosomal marker mannose-6-phosphate receptor (M6PR), remain negative for endosomal markers (EEA1), and are inaccessible to endosomal vesicles loaded with fluid-phase tracers after invasion. By contrast, SCVs formed in nonpermissive *Nramp1⁺/⁺* macrophages recruit M6PR and EEA1 (Cuellar-Mata et al. 2002) and show increased microbicidal activity (Govoni et al. 1999). Additional studies in vitro in explanted macrophages have shown that the addition of membrane-permeant iron chelators can recapitulate the Nramp1 effect, and stimulate recruitment of M6PR and EEA1 to SCVs formed in otherwise *Nramp1⁻/⁻* cells (Jabado et al. 2003). These studies show that Nramp1-mediated metal depletion at the phagosomal membrane antagonizes the ability of *Salmonella* to become secluded from the degradative pathways of macrophages (Cuellar-Mata et al. 2002). *Salmonella* included in SCVs have been found to respond to the presence of Nramp1 at the membrane by transcriptional induction of a number of virulence genes, including *ssrA* and *sseJ*, that map within *Salmonella* pathogenicity island 2 (*SPI2*) (Zaharik et al. 2002). Thus, Nramp1-mediated metal depletion at the membrane of SCV is associated with major changes in biochemical and fusogenic properties of these vesicles, resulting in increased bacteriostatic activity of macrophages. Indeed, adequate supplies of iron had been known to be essential for *Salmonella* virulence in vivo, and for intracellular replication in macrophages in vitro (Kehres and Maguire 2003; Ratledge 2004). *Salmonella* possess several high- or low-affinity, ATP-dependent or proton-coupled (*tonB*-dependent) iron transporters such as *fepBCDG, sitA-D, FeoABC, CorAD*, and the *Nramp* homolog *MntH* (Hantke 1997; Kammler et al. 1993; Kehres et al. 2002; Tsolis et al. 1996; Zhou et al. 1999). Many of these transporters have been shown to be essential for *Salmonella* virulence in vivo (Bearden and Perry 1999; Boyer et al. 2002; Janakiraman and Slauch 2000; Tsolis et al. 1996). Single mutations at *feoB* or *sitA-D* reduced virulence, while double mutations at *MntH, sitA-D*, or *feoB* completely abrogated *Salmonella* virulence in *Nramp1⁻/⁻* mutant 129 Sv mice in vivo. Together, these studies indicate that iron plays a critical role at the interface of host:pathogen interaction. Macrophage metal transporters such as Nramp1 and ferroportin (Nairz et al. 2007) thus represent major defenses acting to restrict intracellular access to this essential nutrient.

Finally, this hypothesis is in good agreement with results obtained with *L. donovani* (Huynh et al. 2006). Huynh and colleagues (2006) recently identified *LIT1* as a major Fe^{2+} transporter of *Leishmania*. LIT1 protein is expressed at the plasma membrane and is present only in the amastigote intracellular form of the parasite but is absent from the extracellular promastigote form. LIT1 was further shown to be a critical virulence determinant as its inactivation resulted in (1) reduced viability and impaired replication of the parasite in bone marrow macrophages in vitro and (2) reduced virulence in vivo in permissive BALB/c mice (*Nramp1^{D169}*). By comparing the timing and extent of expression of LIT1 protein following phagocytosis of *L. amazonesis* amastigotes by normal and Nramp1-defective macrophages, the authors observed accelerated LIT1 protein expression under iron-poor conditions of Nramp1-positive phagolysosomes

(Huynh et al. 2006). Therefore, LIT1 is an intracellular iron acquisition system essential for survival of *Leishmania* parasites in macrophages. LIT1 is subject to iron-specific regulation sensitive to the presence of Nramp1, confirming the critical role of this protein in regulating intra-phagosomal iron pools (Marquis and Gros 2007).

Modifiers of *Nramp1* Effect in *Salmonella* Infection

Genetic modifiers of *Nramp1*-mediated resistance to *Salmonella* were studied using the wild-derived mouse strains *M. musculus molossinus* (MOLF/Ei). MOLF/Ei mice are extremely susceptible to infection with *S. typhimurium* despite the presence of resistance alleles at *Nramp1* and *Tlr4*, with survival times comparable to that of C57BL/6J (*Nramp1^s*) controls. Linkage analysis using 252 (C57BL/6J × MCLF/Ei) F$_2$ animals identified two QTLs that significantly affect survival time following lethal infection with *S. typhimurium*, one on chromosome 11 (*Ity2*; LOD = 7.0; 10% of phenotypic the variance), and one on chromosome 1 (*Ity3*; LOD = 4.8; 7% of phenotypic variance) (Sebastiani et al. 1998, 2000). Several candidate genes were detected in the *Ity2* region, including granulocyte/macrophage colony-stimulating factor (*Csfgm*), interleukin 3 (*Il3*), myeloperoxidase (*Mpo*), and inducible nitric oxide synthase (*Nos2*). MOLF/Ei mice showed a decreased capacity to induce *Nos2* mRNA and to produce NO (Sebastiani et al. 2002) following *Salmonella* infection. The observations that *Nos2*-null mutant mice are unable to suppress bacterial growth in the late phase of the infection and eventually die from infection (Mastroeni et al. 2000) strengthen the candidacy of *Nos2* as the gene responsible for the *Ity2* effect. The *Ity3* region contains a number of positional candidates (*C4bp*, *Cfh*, *Ptgs2*, and *Daf1*), including the *Tlr5* gene (Sebastiani et al. 2000). mRNA expression studies during infection with *S. typhimurium* show that *Tlr5* mRNA levels in liver are consistently lower in MOLF/Ei (~50% reduction) compared to other inbred mouse strains including C57BL/6J, 129S6/SvEvTac, C3H/HeJ, and C57BL/10J. Finally, sequence analysis defined a unique *Tlr5* haplotype in MOLF/Ei mice (distinct from 47 other strains tested) associated with a lower level of *Tlr5* mRNA expression (Sebastiani et al. 2000). The subsequent demonstration that Tlr5 acts as a cellular receptor for *S. typhimurium* flagellin suggests a mechanism by which Tlr5 could underlie the effect of *Ity3* in response to infection in vivo (Gewirtz et al. 2001; Hayashi et al. 2001).

In an effort to identify additional modifiers of the *Nramp1* effect, 36 strains from the AcB/BcA set of recombinant congenics derived from A/J (*Salmonella*-resistant; *Nramp1^{G169}*) and C57BL/6J (*Salmonella*-susceptible; *Nramp1^{D169}*) were infected with 10^3 *S. typhimurium* intravenously, and bacterial replication in organs (spleen and liver) and overall survival to infection were used as measures of susceptibility (Roy et al. 2006). Several strains showed a phenotype that was deviant from that expected from their *Nramp1* genotype. Scoring for survival time, AcB61 were found to be susceptible despite an *Nramp1^{G169}* resistance allele, while AcB64 (*Nramp1^{G169}*) were significantly more resistant than the corresponding A/J parental control. Infected were 247 (AcB61×129S6) and 249 (AcB64×DBA/2J) informative F$_2$ mice (where *Nramp1^{G169}* alleles were fixed), and a whole genome scan was conducted using survival time as a measure of susceptibility. In the AcB64 cross, five novel *Salmonella* susceptibility QTLs mapping to chromosomes 3 (*Ity4*), 2 (*Ity5*), 14 (*Ity6*), 7 (*Ity7*), and 15 (*Ity8*) were detected. The genes underlying the effects of these QTLs remain unknown. In the AcB51 cross, a major QTL was detected (*Ity4*) on chromosome 3 that accounts for 42.1% of the phenotypic variance. The *Ity4* region contains an obvious candidate previously shown to affect susceptibility to malaria: the liver- and red blood cell-specific pyruvate kinase gene (*Pklr*), in which mutations cause a very severe anemia that protects mice against the lethal effects of *P. chabaudi* infection (Min-Oo et al. 2003).

Together, these studies demonstrate that susceptibility to acute infection with *S. typhimurium* is under complex genetic control in A/J and C57BL/6J strains, with a major role played by *Nramp1/Slc11a1*. They also provide an example of the usefulness of crosses with wild-derived mice and recombinant congenic lines in localizing some of these modifier loci.

Legionella pneumophila

Legionella pneumophila is a gram-negative bacterium that causes Legionnaire's disease, a severe form of pneumonia in humans. The intracellular survival of *L. pneumophila* in human macrophages depends on its ability to segregate into an endoplasmic reticulum (ER)-derived vacuole that does not mature, that does not acquire lysosomal markers, and that becomes studded with ribosomes. Macrophages from most inbred mouse strains are nonpermissive to intracellular replication of *L. pneumophila* ex vivo, with the exception of the A/J strain, which is uniquely permissive and which has been used as a model-system to better understand *L. pneumophila* pathogenesis in human cells. Genetic analyses in recombinant inbred mouse strains as well as in informative backcrosses derived from the A/J strain established that permissiveness to *L. pneumophila* replication in macrophages infected ex vivo was controlled by a single gene designated *Lgn1*, with nonpermissiveness completely dominant over permissiveness. High-resolution linkage mapping has located *Lgn1* to a 0.32-cM interval on mouse chromosome 13. This is a region of high genomic complexity that includes a large duplication that contains multiple intact and re-arranged copies of the *Birc1* (baculoviral inhibitor of apoptosis protein repeat-containing 1, formerly *Naip*) gene (reviewed by Fortier et al. 2005). The minimal physical 140-kb interval of *Lgn1* contains two such proteins, Birc1b (*Naip2*) and Birc1e (*Naip5*). Birc1 proteins were found expressed in macrophages and their levels of expression were shown to be upregulated following phagocytosis of infectious agents or inert particles. In addition, A/J macrophages (*Lgn1^s*) were found to express a lower level of Birc1 proteins compared to C57BL/6J macrophages (*Lgn1^r*). In vivo genetic complementation studies in A/J transgenic mice carrying genomic bacterial artificial chromosome (BAC) clones from the region were used to pin down the identity of *Lgn1*. Testing for complementation of the A/J-derived macrophage susceptibility phenotype indicated that the two BAC clones that rescued the phenotype both had the full-length *Birc1e* transcript in common (Diez et al. 2003). These results indicate that *Birc1e* is likely allelic with *Lgn1*. The possibility that transgenic rescue is caused by a gain-of-function on a haploid-insufficient background (overexpression of *Birc1e* by multiple BAC copies) remains to be determined. Parallel studies by W. Dietrich's group showed that morpholino-based antisense inhibition of *Birc1e* can partly reverse the nonpermissiveness of macrophages from mice containing a transgenic copy of *Birc1e* (Wright et al. 2003).

The term *Naip* (neuronal apoptosis inhibitory protein) was initially coined to reflect the candidacy of *Naip* for the human spinal atrophy locus. The Naip protein also has three BIR domains (baculovirus IAP repeats) that are present in other IAP family members, and that have been shown to interact with cellular caspases, thus implicating Naip in regulating cellular apoptosis (Maier et al. 2002; Martinon and Tschopp 2007). A role for Naip protein in survival of neurons following mechanical damage has been reported (Perrelet et al. 2000). On the other hand, Naip/Birc proteins have been recently re-classified as NBS-LRR proteins (now NLR) on the basis of their nucleotide-binding domain, and the presence of long leucine-rich repeats that are known to act as pattern recognition motifs in Toll-like receptor proteins. In fact, the NLR protein family includes nucleotide-binding oligomerization domains (NODs), Ipaf, and others, and has been shown to act as intracellular sensors for the presence of bacterial products (Fritz et al. 2006).

Recent studies have shed light on the ligand and signaling mechanism of Birc1e/Naip5 in macrophages (Molofsky et al. 2006; Ren et al. 2006; Zamboni et al. 2006). Zamboni and colleagues showed that infection with *L. pneumophila* induces caspase-1-dependent cell death in cells expressing the B6 (nonpermissive) but not the A/J (permissive) copy of *Birc1e/Naip5*. Studies of different *L. pneumophila* mutants indicated that activation of caspase-1 requires type IV secretion system-mediated transfer of products into the cytosol, but not intracellular replication or residency in the ER. Finally, macrophages from either caspase-1-deficient (*Casp1$^{-/-}$*) or Ipaf-deficient (*Card12$^{-/-}$*) mice were found to be more permissive to *L. pneumophila* replication than wildtype B6 mice, and co-immunoprecipitation studies demonstrated a direct interaction between Birc1e/Naip5 and Ipaf. A model was proposed in which recognition of *L. pneumophila* products by the LRR domain of Birc1e/Naip5 would cause caspase-1/Ipaf-mediated activation of the inflammasome, resulting in cell death and restriction of *L. pneumophila* replication in macrophages in nonpermissive strains. Recent genetic screens for *L. pneumophila* mutants capable of growing in nonpermissive B6 macrophages identified several mutations in the structural gene for flagellin (*flaA*) (Molofsky et al. 2006; Ren et al. 2006). The authors showed that flagellin is required to induce cell death in B6 macrophages, and A/J macrophages are resistant to flagellin-induced death. Therefore, the role of Birc1e/Naip5 in *Legionella* susceptibility may involve (1) regulation of Ipaf-dependent caspase-1 activation or (2) caspase-1 activation following a direct recognition of flagellin or another bacterial compound by Birc1e/Naip5, or (3) a caspase-1-independent mechanism. On the other hand, recent studies from our group using macrophages from A/J mice and from A/J transgenic mice harboring a functional *Birc1e* copy have suggested additional complexity and diversity in

Bircle protein function. Indeed, we found that *Legionella* phagosomes formed in the two types of macrophages differ markedly, and that presence of Bircle is associated with reduced acquisition of endoplasmic reticulum markers (calnexin) and enhanced acquisition of lysosomal markers (cathepsin D, Lamp1) (Fortier et al. 2007). The Bircle effect on phagosome maturation was very rapid, occurring within the first hour of infection, suggesting that Bircle-mediated activation of caspase-1 may affect early protein targets distinct from late targets associated with cell death or processing of IL-1. The nature of such targets is of great interest but still needs to be discovered.

Candida albicans

In humans, *Candida albicans* exists as a commensal in the gastrointestinal and genitourinary tracts but can also cause opportunistic infections in the immunocompromised host. It is a common cause of fungal infection in humans (Verduyn Lunel et al. 1999). Superficial candidiasis include thrush, chronic atrophic stomatitis, chronic mucocutaneous candidiasis, and vulvovaginitis (Eggimann et al. 2003). These infections tend to be self-limited in immunocompetent hosts (Eggimann et al. 2003). Invasive candidiasis refers to *Candida* infections that occur at sites other than the skin or mucous membranes, with most cases caused by bloodstream dissemination; this condition is almost exclusively limited to immunocompromised hosts (Kullberg and Filler 2002). The incidence of nosocomial infection with *Candida* has been on the rise, a problem compounded by the appearance of antifungal drug resistance (Verduyn Lunel et al. 1999). In disseminated severe forms of *Candida* infection, the major target organs are the digestive tract, lungs, kidney, heart, and brain (Odds 1988).

The pathogenesis of systemic and acute infection with *C. albicans* has been extensively studied in animal models (rats, rabbits, guinea pigs), with the mouse being the most widely used. Systemic infections in these animals resemble human candidiasis, with the kidney being the major target of infection (Ashman et al. 1995). Although *C. albicans* can cause systemic infection when introduced by the intra-peritoneal or gastrointestinal route, the intravenous route has been favored to induce acute infection (De Repentigny 2004) with major colonization of heart, kidney, liver, and brain. Additional models of cutaneous *C. albicans* infection (vaginitis) have also been used (Fidel and Sobel 1999). The median lethal dose (LD_{50}) for most *C. albicans* isolates introduced intravenously in immunocompetent mice is between 10^4 and 10^6 blastospores, depending on the strain of *C. albicans*, the growth conditions used to prepare the inoculum, and the genetic make-up of the murine host (Odds 1988; Odds et al. 2000). Besides time of survival, fungal burden and tissue damage in infected organs have been used as phenotypic markers of susceptibility in mouse (Ashman 1998). A correlation between kidney fungal load and mortality has been reported in some mouse strains, but not in others (Marquis et al. 1988; Mencacci et al. 1998; Salvin and Neta 1983). In other mouse strains, however, deleterious host response in the face of low to moderate fungal load has been associated with early death from acute *C. albicans* infection (Tuite et al. 2004).

A genetic approach in mice has been used to identify major determinants of susceptibility to acute infection with *C. albicans*. A reverse genetic approach, in which the effect of individual genes are assessed in gene knockout studies, and a forward genetic approach investigating natural differences in susceptibility to *C. albicans* infection in vivo have been undertaken (for a complete review, see Tuite et al. 2004). Early strain surveys showed that inbred strains such as C57BL/6J, BALB/cJ, CBA/J, and DBA/1 are resistant while A/J, DBA/2J, NZB/J, and AKR/J are susceptible. These studies further identified a partial correlation between the complement competence status (C5a) and susceptibility to infection (Wetsel et al. 1990). Recent studies using intravenous infection with *C. albicans* showed that A/J is highly susceptible while C57BL/6J is highly resistant to infection. Susceptibility was associated with increased fungal loads in kidney and heart, and very early death of A/J mice compared to B6. Histopathological analysis revealed that A/J did not mount a proper inflammatory response following infection and died within 48 h. By contrast, B6 mice developed much higher fungal loads over a 3-week period and ultimately died of renal failure (which was not seen in moribund A/J). Linkage analysis in 128 (A/J×B6) F_2 progeny using fungal load in kidney or heart and overall levels of TNF-α produced at 24 h as a readout showed that susceptibility behaved as an autosomal recessive monogenic trait which was mapped by whole genome scanning to the proximal part of chromosome 2, with the highest LOD score (LOD = 22.7) for a marker tightly linked to the structural gene for the C5 component of complement (Tuite et al. 2005). Up to 40% of the commonly used inbred mouse strains (Cinader et al. 1964) have a 2-bp deletion in an exon near the 5′-end of the mRNA, introducing a premature stop codon 4-bp downstream of the deletion (Wetsel et al. 1990). This leads to the production of a truncated 216-amino acid translation product compared to the wildtype 1,680-amino acid protein. This truncated protein is not secreted (Wetsel et al. 1990). Thus, C5 deficiency in mice is associated with severe susceptibility to acute *C. albicans* infection.

The functional consequences of a C5 deficiency on response to systemic candidiasis have been studied (Ashman et al. 2003; Lyon et al. 1986; Morelli and Rosenberg 1971). In our laboratory, we have used the recombinant congenic strain BcA70, which has the C5 mutant allele of A/J fixed on the genetic background of resistant C57BL/6J (B6) (Fortin et al. 2001b). BcA70 is as susceptible to infection as A/J. C5 is proteolytically processed to C5a, -b, and -c, which react with opsonized microbes to form a membrane attack complex (MAC) that creates pores in the membrane of invading microbes following binding of antibodies. In addition, C5a acts as a major chemoattractant to recruit neutrophils and macrophages at the site of infection, a response that is impaired in C5-deficient mice (Gerard and Gerard 1994; Mullick et al. 2006). Analysis of the profile of cytokines produced during infection of A/J and BcA70 shows a pattern of extreme inflammatory and allergic response, suggesting unregulated production of proinflammatory molecules including TNF-α, IL-6, monocyte chemoattractant protein-1 (MCP1), macrophage inflammatory protein (MIP2), tissue inhibitor of metalloproteinase (TIMP1), and keratinocyte-derived cytokine (KC) (Mullick et al. 2006). This results in cardiomyopathy (elevated creatine kinase and cardiac troponin I), hypoglycemia, and rapid death.

Finally, a systematic screening of AcB/BcA recombinant congenic lines for modifiers of the C5-deficiency effect on susceptibility to *C. albicans* infection identified two strains with discordant phenotypes (kidney fungal loads): BcA67 shows an intermediate level of susceptibility despite presence of wildtype C5-sufficient alleles, while BcA72 females are as resistant as B6 controls despite being genetically C5-deficient. These observations suggest additional complexity in the genetic control of susceptibility to *C. albicans* in A/J and B6 mice.

Complex Traits

Mycobacterium tuberculosis

Tuberculosis is caused by aerosol infection with the bacterial pathogen *Mycobacterium tuberculosis*. Although *M. tuberculosis* can infect and replicate in several organs, tuberculosis is almost exclusively a pulmonary disease. Tuberculosis still remains a global health problem of enormous proportions, with 32% of the world's population believed to be or certainly infected (WHO 2000), an estimated 8 million new cases of active disease per year (WHO 2002) and 1–1.5 million deaths annually. Globally, migration of populations from countries with endemic disease, HIV infection, poverty, unemployment, homelessness, overcrowding, and population aging have contributed to the persistence of tuberculosis in developed countries (Parry and Davies 1996). Moreover, the emergence of multidrug resistance also represents an increasing threat to tuberculosis control (Young and Duncan 1995).

Although the majority of people infected with *M. tuberculosis* remain asymptomatic, 5%–10% of them have a lifetime risk of developing active disease. Genetic factors have long been thought to play a role in onset, progression, and ultimate outcome of infection with *M. tuberculosis* (Levin and Newport 2000). This includes epidemiological data pointing to sex (Hinman et al. 1976; Rieder et al. 1991) and racial differences in susceptibility (Stead et al. 1990), as well as geographical distribution and familial aggregation of disease (Casanova and Abel 2002). In addition, population studies in endemic areas of disease and during first contact epidemics (Motulsky 1960; Sousa et al. 1997), together with studies in twins (Comstock 1978), have clearly established a genetic component of susceptibility to tuberculosis in humans. Moreover, case control studies in areas of endemic disease have pointed to several gene variants contributing to tuberculosis risk, including those encoding human leukocyte antigen (HLA) (Delgado et al. 2006; Goldfeld et al. 1998), the natural resistance-associated macrophage protein (*Nramp*) 1 (Bellamy et al. 1998; Cervino et al. 2000; Gao et al. 2000; Greenwood et al. 2000; Li et al. 2006; Malik et al. 2005; Ryu et al. 2000), the vitamin D receptor (Bellamy et al. 1999; Wilkinson et al. 2000), the mannose-binding protein (Selvaraj et al. 1999), the IL12/23-IFN pathway (Lio et al. 2002; Lopez-Maderuelo et al. 2003; Rossouw et al. 2003; Tso et al. 2005), and the genes encoding DC-SIGN (*CD209*) (Barreiro et al. 2006), chemokine monocyte chemoattractant protein-1 (MCP-1) (Flores-Villanueva et al. 2005), and *SP110* variants (Thye et al. 2006; Tosh et al. 2006). Whole-genome scanning experiments have also identified suggestive linkages on chromosomes 15 and X, identified in African families from The Gambia and South Africa (Bellamy et al. 2000), and on two regions of chromosomes 11 and 20 previously detected in Brazilian families (Miller et al. 2004). Of particular interest is the recent identification in a Moroccan population of a highly significant major locus on chromosome 8q12-q13 that confers predisposition to pulmonary tuberculosis in adults (Baghdadi et al. 2006).

The complex genetic component of susceptibility to tuberculosis is inherently difficult to study in humans. Mouse models of infection can provide a valuable alternative in which major gene effects and positional candidates can be detected, validated in vivo in gene transfer experiments, and ultimately tested for a parallel effect in human field studies. The mouse constitutes an excellent model to study human tuberculosis. Many key parameters of the host response to *M. tuberculosis* in the mouse closely parallel those observed in the human disease (see North and Jung 2004 for a recent review). The efficacy of the host response to pulmonary tuberculosis is under complex genetic control in the mouse, with a broad spectrum of disease severities observed among different strains. Genetic analyses have located a number of tuberculosis susceptibility loci (Kramnik et al. 2000; Lavebratt et al. 1999; Mitsos et al. 2000, 2003; Sanchez et al. 2003; Sapoval et al. 2002; Yan et al. 2006), but so far only a single such locus (*Ipr1*) has been identified (Pan et al. 2005). Please see Fortin et al. (2007) for a complete review of the genetic control of susceptibility to infection with mycobacteria in mice and humans.

Inbred strains have been classified as highly susceptible (CBA, C3H, DBA/2, 129SvJ) or highly resistant (C57BL/6J, BALB/c) to intravenous or aerosol infection with *M. tuberculosis* (Medina and North 1996, 1998). Replication of *M. tuberculosis* in the lungs of innately resistant (C57BL/6J) and susceptible (DBA/2) inbred strains follows a biphasic course. Following infection, *M. tuberculosis* initially (1–3 weeks) replicates rapidly in the lungs of both C57BL/6J and DBA/2 mice. The infection is subsequently (4 weeks to 5 months) held stationary in C57BL/6J while there is continuing microbial replication in the lungs of DBA/2 (Mitsos et al. 2003), which is accompanied by strong inflammatory response and premature death, with a mean survival time (MST) of 110 days. Resistant C57BL/6J mice can control the infection, although they ultimately succumb with a MST of 245 days (Medina and North 1998). Similar patterns of resistance and susceptibility were obtained following intravenous infection (1×10^5 CFU) (Mitsos et al. 2000).

The genetic basis for differential susceptibility of B6 and D2 strains was investigated in our laboratory by whole genome scanning in informative (C57BL/6J×DBA/2) F_2 mice infected by different routes and with different doses of *M. tuberculosis* H37Rv (Mitsos et al. 2000, 2003). An initial genome scan was conducted using survival time following intravenous infection with 10^5 CFU *M. tuberculosis* H37Rv as a phenotypic marker of susceptibility (Mitsos et al. 2000). Two significant linkages were identified: *Trl-1* on distal chromosome 1 (LOD = 4.80) and *Trl-3* (LOD=4.66) on proximal chromosome 7. A third suggestive linkage, *Trl-2* (LOD=3.93), was localized to proximal chromosome 3. For each of these loci, resistance was associated with homozygosity for the C57BL/6J alleles. The second genome scan used bacterial load in the lungs at 90 days post-infection following aerosol infection with 2×10^2 CFU as a measure of susceptibility (Mitsos et al. 2003). This scan confirmed the *Trl-3* locus (LOD=3.1) and also identified an additional locus, *Trl-4* (LOD = 5.6), that mapped to the distal portion of chromosome 19, with the C57BL/6J allele at this locus conferring resistance in a partially dominant manner. A strong genetic interaction was detected between *Trl-3* and *Trl-4*, with two-locus linkage analysis yielding a LOD=10.09 and explaining 38% of the variation in raw CFUs. Remarkably, F_2 mice homozygous for C57BL/6J alleles at both *Trl-3* and *Trl-4* were as resistant as C57BL/6J parents, whereas mice homozygous for DBA/2 alleles were as susceptible as DBA/2 parents (Mitsos et al. 2003). At present, the *Trl-3* and *Trl-4* QTLs affecting susceptibility to pulmonary tuberculosis have been retained and validated for the following reasons: (1) *Trl-3* appears to affect both the rate of pulmonary *Mtb* replication and survival to infection, (2) *Trl-4* is the strongest QTL detected to date in two genome scans, (3) the combined effect of both loci explains approx. 50% of the phenotypic variance in the (C57BL/6J×DBA/2) F_2 cross used, with (4) strong interaction between the loci.

Although QTL analysis has been successful in identifying loci involved in the control of susceptibility to *M. tuberculosis*, cloning the gene of interest remains an enormous challenge, not only because of the large size of the chromosomal regions and corresponding transcript maps but also because each locus often accounts only for a small fraction of the total phenotypic variance. To evaluate the individual contribution of *Trl-3* and *Trl-4* to the overall tuberculosis susceptibility phenotype, we generated individual mouse lines congenic for these loci by using a speed-congenic protocol (Bennett and Johnson 1998). In this protocol, successive F_1 backcross males are partially genotyped to identify those with the most biased parental genotype content for selection for further backcrossing. Once at the N4 generation, heterozygotes are intercrossed to generate the homozygote congenic lines and also to produce the double *Trl-3/Trl-4* congenic line, in order to test the separate and combined effects of C57BL/6J resistance alleles on the DBA/2 background. In these mice, the chromosome(s) carrying the QTL(s) of interest (chromosome 7 or 19) from C57BL/6J strain is transferred by breeding to the genetic background of the DBA/2 strain. For *Trl-3*, we are backcrossing a segment of the proximal half of chromosome 7 derived from C57BL/6J, and donated by the BXD19 strain, onto DBA/2 background. For *Trl-4*, we are backcrossing chromosome 19 from C57BL/6J, donated by the BXD9 strain, onto DBA/2 background. Recently, the breeding of both single congenic lines (BXD19 and BXD9) has been completed. Preliminary results have revealed that both congenic strains were about 50% less susceptible to aerosol infection than the DBA/2 parental strain (lung CFUs) (J.F. Marquis, R. LaCourse, L. Ryan, R.J. North, and P. Gros, unpublished data).

Plasmodium chabaudi

Malaria is caused by infection with members of the protozoan parasite family *Plasmodium*. *Plasmodium falciparum* and *Plasmodium vivax* are responsible for a large proportion of the human disease (Marsh and Snow 1997). Between 300 and 500 million cases of malaria are believed to occur each year, with a reported 1 million fatalities, mostly in young children from impoverished countries. Severe anemia and cerebral malaria are major disease manifestations of blood-stage malaria, especially in Africa, where transmission rates are high. There is no effective vaccine against malaria, and this global health problem has been exacerbated by the development of malarial drug resistance in the *Plasmodium* parasite and by insecticide resistance in the *Anopheles* insect vector (Marsh and Snow 1997). The malarial parasite has a complex life cycle in its mammalian host that involves sequential replication in the erythrocyte and sequestration in different tissues such as the liver and brain microvasculature, where it causes disease. Protective immunity against *Plasmodium* species is poorly understood but involves different cell types and physiological and biochemical pathways at each stage of the infection. An effective antimalarial vaccine, especially against the asexual, erythrocytic parasite that causes the symptoms associated with malaria, is still not available despite an enormous effort worldwide (Good 2005). Thus, a better understanding of the innate and adaptive immune mechanisms of host defense against the blood-stage *Plasmodium* parasite, which may manifest themselves as genetic determinants of susceptibility in endemic areas and during epidemics, may provide new targets for therapeutic intervention in this disease.

Malaria is one of the clearest manifestations of genetic control of disease. Population studies in areas of endemic disease indicate important three-way interactions among host genes, the environment, and the malaria parasite. It has also been recognized that normal or disease-associated alterations in certain erythrocyte proteins affect susceptibility to malaria in humans, with positive selection of these variants by the parasite in endemic areas (co-evolution). For a more comprehensive description of the genetic component of susceptibility to malaria in humans, the reader is referred to recent comprehensive reviews on this subject (Kwiatkowski 2000; Min-Oo and Gros 2005). The complex genetic control of susceptibility to malaria has been studied in mice where models for the blood-stage infection and for the cerebral disease have been developed using the murine parasites *Plasmodium chabaudi AS* and *Plasmodium berghei*, respectively. Mouse models of malaria, using *P. chabaudi*-parasitized erythrocytes, mimics several pathophysiological aspects of the blood-stage infection in humans, including host response, genetic control of parasitemia, and ultimate outcome of infection. This model has been effective in localizing several major QTLs, with the genes underlying two such QTLs recently identified by positional cloning. Infection in susceptible mouse strains such as A/J is characterized by heightened parasitemia at the peak of infection, muted inflammatory and erythropoietic responses, and a decreased survival time, compared to resistant strains such as C57BL/6J. Whole-genome scans have been conducted in backcross and F_2 mice bred from resistant and susceptible parents, and using peak parasitemia and mortality as quantitative phenotypes (Burt et al 1999; Foote et al. 1997; Fortin et al. 1997). These early studies led to the mapping of three major QTLs on distal chromosome 9 (*Char1*), central chromosome 8 (*Char2*), and chromosome 17 (*Char3*, H-2 locus). Large genetic intervals defired by these QTLs, coupled with the relatively small phenotypic variance explained by each locus have so far impeded cloning of the corresponding genes.

A parallel approach was used to help characterize the complex genetic factors determining the A/J (susceptible) vs B6 (resistant) inter-strain difference in susceptibility to infection with *P. chabaudi*. We phenotyped the AcB/BcA set of reciprocal recombinant congenic strains (derived from A/J and B6 by systematic inbreeding of a second backcross) (Fortin et al. 2001b) for susceptibility to malaria. The usefulness of recombinant congenic strains (RCS) for the study of complex traits has been discussed but can be summarized as follows. By virtue of the breeding scheme used in their derivation, individual AcB/BcA strains carry a small portion of one parental genome fixed as a set of congenic segments on the genetic background of the other strains. Individual genetic effects contributing to a complex trait may have segregated in individual RCS and can be studied in isolation, both for identifying the gene involved but also to elucidate unigenic contributions to the overall phenotype. The relatively small size of the congenic segments fixed in individual RCS facilitates the search and testing of candidate genes. In addition, secondary genetic effects can be detected in strains fixed for certain alleles at major mapped loci, but yet showing deviations from expected phenotypes. Furthermore, reassortment of parental haplotypes or appearance of novel mutations during the breeding of individual strains may generate "hyper-phenotypes" that segregate as simple traits and can be quickly cloned. With the advent of whole genome mRNA transcript profiling, AcB/BcA strains can be used to map *cis*-acting gene expression polymorphisms (eQTLs) and associated regulatory regions that genetically differ between A/J and B6.

A subset of 18 AcB/BcA strains was tested for susceptibility to malaria, using level of parasitemia at the peak of infection and overall survival as phenotypic traits. In general, there was a good correlation between resistance/susceptibility and haplotypes at *Char1* and *Char2* (Fortin et al. 2002). Strains AcB55 and AcB61, however, showed a discordant phenotype and were very resistant to *P. chabaudi* infection despite A/J-derived susceptibility alleles at *Char1* and *Char2* (Fortin et al. 2001a). Additional linkage studies to locate a possible B6-derived segment conferring resistance to AcB55 were carried out in 200 informative (AcB55×A/J) F_2 mice, leading to the identification of a locus (*Char4*) on chromosome 3 (LOD=6.57) that regulates peak parasitemia following infection. Phenotypic characterization of AcB55 and AcB61 strains identified splenomegaly in these mice, together with elevated reticulocyte numbers in peripheral blood and elevated numbers of Ter119[+] cells in the bone marrow. Additional transcript profiling using spleen RNA indicated that enhanced erythropoietic activity is a common phenotypic feature of both strains (Min-Oo et al. 2003). Reticulocytosis was found to be inherited as a monogenic trait in the aforementioned (AcB55×A/J) F_2 cross, co-segregating with *Char4* alleles and associated with resistance to malaria. Recombination between the

reticulocytosis trait and markers from the B6 congenic segment on chromosome 3 linked to *Char4*, however, suggested that the locus may map outside this B6 congenic segment. Further analysis in a fully informative (AcB55×DBA/2) F_2 cross showed that this was indeed the case. The transcript map of the chromosomal region contained a strong positional candidate liver- and red-cell specific pyruvate kinase (*Pklr*) based both on its essential role for ATP production in erythrocytes and the fact that mutations in *PKLR* cause hemolytic anemia in humans. Sequencing revealed the presence of an isoleucine-to-asparagine substitution at residue 90 of the Pklr protein in AcB55 and AcB61, a mutation that has also been described in a human case of pyruvate kinase deficiency (Min-Oo et al. 2004). Recently, a second mutant allele at the *Pklr* locus (G338D) was identified in a CBA/N mouse genetic background (CBA/N-*Pk^{slc}*). As for the I90N allele, this new allele was shown to cause severe hemolytic anemia, and also conferred dramatic protection against *P. chabaudi* infection (Min-Oo et al. 2007b). These findings indicate that loss of function at *Pklr* in mice protects against malaria.

Finally, we have obtained evidence indicating that the protective effect of pyruvate kinase deficiency may be further modulated by other host genetic factors. In addition to *Char4*, linkage analysis in (AcB55×A/J) F_2 mice identified a second suggestive QTL on chromosome 10 (*D10Mit189*) that maps to a 14-Mb C57BL/6J-derived congenic segment fixed in AcB55. C57BL/6J alleles at this locus are protective (reduced peak parasitemia), inherited in a co-dominant fashion, and show an additive effect with *Char4* (Fortin et al. 2001a). This locus was given the temporary designation *Char9* (Min-Oo et al. 2007a). The B6-derived 14-Mb congenic segment on chromosome 10 of AcB55 defining *Char9* is predicted to contain 77 genes that were characterized with respect to (1) tissue-specific expression, (2) the presence of strain-specific alterations in the level of gene expression, and (3) strain-specific polymorphic variants in coding and regulatory regions of positional candidates. *Vnn1/Vnn3* were identified as the likely candidates responsible for *Char9*. *Vnn1/Vnn3* map within a conserved haplotype block and show expression levels that are strictly *cis*-regulated by this haplotype. The absence of *Vnn* messenger RNA expression and lack of pantetheinase protein activity in tissues are associated with susceptibility to malaria and are linked to a complex rearrangement in the *Vnn3* promoter region. The A/J strain also carries a unique nonsense mutation that leads to a truncated protein. *Vanin* genes code for a pantetheinase involved in the production of cysteamine, a key regulator of host responses to inflammatory stimuli. Administration of cystamine in vivo partially corrects susceptibility to malaria in A/J mice, as measured by reduced blood parasitemia and decreased mortality. These studies suggest that pantetheinase is critical for the host response to malaria (Min-Oo et al. 2007a). They also raise the possibility that cysteamine may be a valid, host-based molecule for therapeutic intervention in malaria, alone or in combination with current "parasite-based" antimalarial drugs such as mefloquine. This example clearly illustrates the power of the AcB/BcA set to isolate a gene effect contributing to a complex phenotype in a single mouse strain. The small size of the syntenic fragment can in this case be a major advantage in restricting the size of the QTL. The positional cloning of the gene responsible can then be undertaken by a combination of haplotype mapping, transcript profiling, and nucleotide sequencing.

Conclusions and Future Perspectives

Genetic analyses in mice have proved extremely useful for identifying genes, proteins, and pathways playing a critical role in host defense against infections. In our laboratory we have focused our studies on two inbred mouse strains, A/J and C57BL/6J, and this has led to the identification of several monogenic traits and corresponding proteins, including *Nramp1*, *Birc1e*, *C5*, *Icsbp*, and others that are important determinants of innate immune responses to infection with several intracellular pathogens. We have also used recombinant congenic strains derived from these two parent strains to start studying more complex genetic traits. Although the genetic diversity represented by A/J and B6 is fairly modest, there exist a large number of commercially available and phylogenetically distant strains that may contain a large pool of hypomorphic or mutant alleles and that could similarly be used to identify additional genes and pathways participating in host response to infections. A limitation of this approach is that many of these gene effects may be partial and behave as QTLs for which the underlying gene or genes may be difficult to identify. The parallel production of large numbers of *N*-ethyl-*N*-nitrosourea (ENU)-mutagenized mice may alleviate this problem by providing mutants in which the effect on host response to infection can be readily studied and for which the corresponding mutant gene can be identified by direct sequencing. Genes discovered in the mouse can provide novel entry points to parallel studies in humans using populations at risk or focusing on areas of endemic disease. Finally, validated genes and metabolic pathways may also suggest novel strategies for therapeutic intervention in the corresponding infections.

Acknowledgements P.G. is a James McGill Professor of Biochemistry and a distinguished scientist of the Canadian Institutes of Health Research (CIHR). J.-F.M. is supported by a fellowship from the Fonds de Recherche en Santé du Québec.

References

Abel L, Sanchez FO, Oberti J, Thuc NV, Hoa LV, Lap VD, Skamene E, Lagrange PH, Schurr E (1998) Susceptibility to leprosy is linked to the human NRAMP1 gene. J Infect Dis 177:133–145
Alcais A, Sanchez FO, Thuc NV, Lap VD, Oberti J, Lagrange PH, Schurr E, Abel L (2000) Granulomatous reaction to intradermal injection of lepromin (Mitsuda reaction) is linked to the human NRAMP1 gene in Vietnamese leprosy sibships. J Infect Dis 181:302–308
Ashman RB (1998) Candida albicans: pathogenesis, immunity and host defence. Res Immunol 149:281–288; discussion 494–286
Ashman RB, Fulurija A, Papadimitriou JM (1996) Strain-dependent differences in host response to Candida albicans infection in mice are related to organ susceptibility and infectious load. Infect Immun 64:1866–1869
Ashman RB, Papadimitriou JM, Fulurija A, Drysdale KE, Farah CS, Naidoo O, Gotjamanos T (2003) Role of complement C5 and T lymphocytes in pathogenesis of disseminated and mucosal candidiasis in susceptible DBA/2 mice. Microb Pathog 34:103–113

Baghdadi JE, Orlova M, Alter A, Ranque B, Chentoufi M, Lazrak F, Archane MI, Casanova JL, Benslimane A, Schurr E, Abel L (2006) An autosomal dominant major gene confers predisposition to pulmonary tuberculosis in adults. J Exp Med 203:1679–1684

Barreiro LB, Neyrolles O, Babb CL, Tailleux L, Quach H, McElreavey K, Helden PD, Hoal EG, Gicquel B, Quintana-Murci L (2006) Promoter variation in the DC-SIGN-encoding gene CD209 is associated with tuberculosis. PLoS Med 3:e20

Bearden SW, Perry RD (1999) The Yfe system of Yersinia pestis transports iron and manganese and is required for full virulence of plague. Mol Microbiol 32:403–414

Bedigian HG, Taylor BA, Meier H (1981) Expression of murine leukemia viruses in the highly lymphomatous BXH-2 recombinant inbred mouse strain. J Virol 39:632–640

Bedigian HG, Johnson DA, Jenkins NA, Copeland NG, Evans R (1984) Spontaneous and induced leukemias of myeloid origin in recombinant inbred BXH mice. J Virol 51:586–594

Bedigian HG, Shepel LA, Hoppe PC (1993) Transplacental transmission of a leukemogenic murine leukemia virus. J Virol 67:6105–6109

Bellamy R, Ruwende C, Corrah T, McAdam KP, Whittle HC, Hill AV (1998) Variations in the NRAMP1 gene and susceptibility to tuberculosis in West Africans. N Engl J Med 338:640–644

Bellamy R, Ruwende C, Corrah T, McAdam KP, Thursz M, Whittle HC, Hill AV (1999) Tuberculosis and chronic hepatitis B virus infection in Africans and variation in the vitamin D receptor gene. J Infect Dis 179:721–724

Bellamy R, Beyers N, McAdam KP, Ruwende C, Gie R, Samaai P, Bester D, Meyer M, Corrah T, Collin M, Camidge DR, Wilkinson D, Hoal-Van Helden E, Whittle HC, Amos W, van Helden P, Hill AV (2000) Genetic susceptibility to tuberculosis in Africans: a genome-wide scan. Proc Natl Acad Sci USA 97:8005–8009

Bennett B, Johnson TE (1998) Development of congenics for hypnotic sensitivity to ethanol by QTL-marker-assisted counter selection. Mamm Genome 9:969–974

Boyer E, Bergevin I, Malo D, Gros P, Cellier MF (2002) Acquisition of Mn(II) in addition to Fe(II) is required for full virulence of Salmonella enterica serovar Typhimurium. Infect Immun 70:6032–6042

Burt RA, Baldwin TM, Marshall VM, Foote SJ (1999) Temporal expression of an H2-linked locus in host response to mouse malaria. Immunogenetics 50:278–285

Canonne-Hergaux F, Gruenheid S, Ponka P, Gros P (1999) Cellular and subcellular localization of the Nramp2 iron transporter in the intestinal brush border and regulation by dietary iron. Blood 93:4406–4417

Canonne-Hergaux F, Calafat J, Richer E, Cellier M, Grinstein S, Borregaard N, Gros P (2002) Expression and subcellular localization of NRAMP1 in human neutrophil granules. Blood 100:268–275

Casanova JL, Abel L (2002) Genetic dissection of immunity to mycobacteria: the human model. Annu Rev Immunol 20:581–620

Casanova JL, Abel L (2007) Human genetics of infectious diseases: a unified theory. EMBO J 26:915–922

Cellier M, Govoni G, Vidal S, Kwan T, Groulx N, Liu J, Sanchez F, Skamene E, Schurr E, Gros P (1994) Human natural resistance-associated macrophage protein: cDNA cloning, chromosomal mapping, genomic organization, and tissue-specific expression. J Exp Med 180:1741–1752

Cellier M, Prive G, Belouchi A, Kwan T, Rodrigues V, Chia W, Gros P (1995) Nramp defines a family of membrane proteins. Proc Natl Acad Sci USA 92:10089–10093

Cellier M, Shustik C, Dalton W, Rich E, Hu J, Malo D, Schurr E, Gros P (1997) Expression of the human NRAMP1 gene in professional primary phagocytes: studies in blood cells and in HL-60 promyelocytic leukemia. J Leukoc Biol 61:96–105

Cervino AC, Lakiss S, Sow O, Hill AV (2000) Allelic association between the NRAMP1 gene and susceptibility to tuberculosis in Guinea-Conakry. Ann Hum Genet 64:507–512

Cinader B, Dubiski S, Wardlaw AC (1964) Distribution, inheritance, and properties of an antigen, Mub1, and its relation to hemolytic complement. J Exp Med 120:897–924

Clemens DL, Horwitz MA (1995) Characterization of the Mycobacterium tuberculosis phago-some and evidence that phagosomal maturation is inhibited. J Exp Med 181:257–270

Clemens DL, Lee BY, Horwitz MA (2000a) Deviant expression of Rab5 on phagosomes contain-ing the intracellular pathogens Mycobacterium tuberculosis and Legionella pneumophila is associated with altered phagosomal fate. Infect Immun 68:2671–2684

Clemens DL, Lee BY, Horwitz MA (2000b) Mycobacterium tuberculosis and Legionella pneu-mophila phagosomes exhibit arrested maturation despite acquisition of Rab7. Infect Immun 68:5154–5166

Clementi M, Di Gianantonio E (2006) Genetic susceptibility to infectious diseases. Reprod Toxicol 21:345–349

Comstock GW (1978) Tuberculosis in twins: a re-analysis of the Prophit survey. Am Rev Respir D s 117:621–624

Cooke GS, Hill AV (2001) Genetics of susceptibility to human infectious disease. Nat Rev Genet 2:967–977

Cuellar-Mata P, Jabado N, Liu J, Furuya W, Finlay BB, Gros P, Grinstein S (2002) Nramp1 modi-fies the fusion of Salmonella typhimurium-containing vacuoles with cellular endomembranes in macrophages. J Biol Chem 277:2258–2265

de Jong R, Altare F, Haagen IA, Elferink DG, Boer T, van Breda Vriesman PJ, Kabel PJ, Draaisma JM, van Dissel JT, Kroon FP, Casanova JL, Ottenhoff TH (1998) Severe mycobacterial and Salmonella infections in interleukin-12 receptor-deficient patients. Science 280:1435–1438

de Repentigny L (2004) Animal models in the analysis of Candida host-pathogen interactions. Curr Opin Microbiol 7:324–329

Delgado JC, Baena A, Thim S, Goldfeld AE (2006) Aspartic acid homozygosity at codon 57 of HLA-DQ beta is associated with susceptibility to pulmonary tuberculosis in Cambodia. J Immunol 176:1090–1097

Diez E, Lee SH, Gauthier S, Yaraghi Z, Tremblay M, Vidal S, Gros P (2003) Birc1e is the gene within the Lgn1 locus associated with resistance to Legionella pneumophila. Nat Genet 33:55–60

Dupuis S, Jouanguy E, Al-Hajjar S, Fieschi C, Al-Mohsen IZ, Al-Jumaah S, Yang K, Chapgier A, Eidenschenk C, Eid P, Al Ghonaium A, Tufenkeji H, Frayha H, Al-Gazlan S, Al-Rayes H, Schreiber RD, Gresser I, Casanova JL (2003) Impaired response to interferon-alpha/beta and lethal viral disease in human STAT1 deficiency. Nat Genet 33:388–391

Eggimann P, Garbino J, Pittet D (2003) Epidemiology of Candida species infections in critically ill non-immunosuppressed patients. Lancet Infect Dis 3:685–702

Fidel PLJ, Sobel JD (1999) Murine models of Candida vaginal infections. In: Sande M, Zak O (eds) Handbook of animal models of infection. Academic Press, Guersney, pp 741–748

Fierer J, Guiney DG (2001) Diverse virulence traits underlying different clinical outcomes of Salmonella infection. J Clin Invest 107:775–780

Flores-Villanueva PO, Ruiz-Morales JA, Song CH, Flores LM, Jo EK, Montano M, Barnes PF, Selman M, Granados J (2005) A functional promoter polymorphism in monocyte chemoa-ttractant protein-1 is associated with increased susceptibility to pulmonary tuberculosis. J Exp Med 202:1649–1658

Foote SJ, Burt RA, Baldwin TM, Presente A, Roberts AW, Laural YL, Lew AM, Marshall VM (1997) Mouse loci for malaria-induced mortality and the control of parasitaemia. Nat Genet 17:380–381

Forbes JR, Gros P (2003) Iron, manganese, and cobalt transport by Nramp1 (Slc11a1) and Nramp2 (Slc11a2) expressed at the plasma membrane. Blood 102:1884–1892

Fortier A, Diez E, Gros P (2005) Naip5/Birc1e and susceptibility to Legionella pneumophila. Trends Microbiol 13:328–335

Fortier A, de Chastellier C, Balor S, Gros P (2007) Birc1e/Naip5 rapidly antagonizes modulation of phagosome maturation by Legionella pneumophila. Cell Microbiol 9:910–923

Fortin A, Belouchi A, Tam MF, Cardon L, Skamene E, Stevenson MM, Gros P (1997) Genetic con-trol of blood parasitaemia in mouse malaria maps to chromosome 8. Nat Genet 17:382–383

Fortin A, Cardon LR, Tam M, Skamene E, Stevenson MM, Gros P (2001a) Identification of a new malaria susceptibility locus (Char4) in recombinant congenic strains of mice. Proc Natl Acad Sci USA 98:10793–10798

Fortin A, Diez E, Rochefort D, Laroche L, Malo D, Rouleau GA, Gros P, Skamene E (2001b) Recombinant congenic strains derived from A/J and C57BL/6J: a tool for genetic dissection of complex traits. Genomics 74:21–35

Fortin A, Stevenson MM, Gros P (2002) Complex genetic control of susceptibility to malaria in mice. Genes Immun 3:177–186

Fortin A, Abel L, Casanova JL, Gros P (2007) Host genetics of mycobacterial diseases in mice and men: forward genetic studies of BCG-osis and tuberculosis. Annu Rev Genomics Hum Genet 8:163–192

Frehel C, Canonne-Hergaux F, Gros P, De Chastellier C (2002) Effect of Nramp1 on bacterial replication and on maturation of Mycobacterium avium-containing phagosomes in bone marrow-derived mouse macrophages. Cell Microbiol 4:541–556

Fritz JH, Ferrero RL, Philpott DJ, Girardin SE (2006) Nod-like proteins in immunity, inflammation and disease. Nat Immunol 7:1250–1257

Frodsham AJ, Hill AV (2004) Genetics of infectious diseases. Hum Mol Genet 13 Spec No 2: R187–194

Gao PS, Fujishima S, Mao XQ, Remus N, Kanda M, Enomoto T, Dake Y, Bottini N, Tabuchi M, Hasegawa N, Yamaguchi K, Tiemessen C, Hopkin JM, Shirakawa T, Kishi F (2000) Genetic variants of NRAMP1 and active tuberculosis in Japanese populations. International Tuberculosis Genetics Team. Clin Genet 58:74–76

Gerard C, Gerard NP (1994) C5A anaphylatoxin and its seven transmembrane-segment receptor. Annu Rev Immunol 12:775–808

Gewirtz AT, Navas TA, Lyons S, Godowski PJ, Madara JL (2001) Cutting edge: bacterial flagellin activates basolaterally expressed TLR5 to induce epithelial proinflammatory gene expression. J Immunol 167:1882–1885

Goldfeld AE, Delgado JC, Thim S, Bozon MV, Uglialoro AM, Turbay D, Cohen C, Yunis EJ (1998) Association of an HLA-DQ allele with clinical tuberculosis. JAMA 279:226–228

Good MF (2005) Vaccine-induced immunity to malaria parasites and the need for novel strategies. Trends Parasitol 21:29–34

Govoni G, Vidal S, Gauthier S, Skamene E, Malo D, Gros P (1996) The Bcg/Ity/Lsh locus: genetic transfer of resistance to infections in C57BL/6J mice transgenic for the Nramp1 Gly169 allele. Infect Immun 64:2923–2929

Govoni G, Canonne-Hergaux F, Pfeifer CG, Marcus SL, Mills SD, Hackam DJ, Grinstein S, Malo D, Finlay BB, Gros P (1999) Functional expression of Nramp1 in vitro in the murine macrophage line RAW264.7. Infect Immun 67:2225–2232

Greenwood CM, Fujiwara TM, Boothroyd LJ, Miller MA, Frappier D, Fanning EA, Schurr E, Morgan K (2000) Linkage of tuberculosis to chromosome 2q35 loci, including NRAMP1, in a large aboriginal Canadian family. Am J Hum Genet 67:405–416

Gros P, Skamene E, Forget A (1983) Cellular mechanisms of genetically controlled host resistance to Mycobacterium bovis (BCG). J Immunol 131:1966–1972

Gruenheid S, Pinner E, Desjardins M, Gros P (1997) Natural resistance to infection with intracellular pathogens: the Nramp1 protein is recruited to the membrane of the phagosome. J Exp Med 185:717–730

Hackam DJ, Rotstein OD, Zhang W, Gruenheid S, Gros P, Grinstein S (1998) Host resistance to intracellular infection: mutation of natural resistance-associated macrophage protein 1 (Nramp1) impairs phagosomal acidification. J Exp Med 188:351–364

Hantke K (1997) Ferrous iron uptake by a magnesium transport system is toxic for Escherichia coli and Salmonella typhimurium. J Bacteriol 179:6201–6204

Hayashi F, Smith KD, Ozinsky A, Hawn TR, Yi EC, Goodlett DR, Eng JK, Akira S, Underhill DM, Aderem A (2001) The innate immune response to bacterial flagellin is mediated by Toll-like receptor 5. Nature 410:1099–1103

Hill AV (2001) The genomics and genetics of human infectious disease susceptibility. Annu Rev Genomics Hum Genet 2:373–400

Hill AV (2006) Aspects of genetic susceptibility to human infectious diseases. Annu Rev Genet 40 469–486

Hinman AR, Judd JM, Kolnik JP, Daitch PB (1976) Changing risks in tuberculosis. Am J Epidemiol 103:486–497

Hoshino K, Takeuchi O, Kawai T, Sanjo H, Ogawa T, Takeda Y, Takeda K, Akira S (1999) Cutting edge: Toll-like receptor 4 (TLR4)-deficient mice are hyporesponsive to lipopolysaccharide: evidence for TLR4 as the Lps gene product. J Immunol 162:3749–3752

Huynh C, Sacks DL, Andrews NW (2006) A Leishmania amazonensis ZIP family iron transporter is essential for parasite replication within macrophage phagolysosomes. J Exp Med 203:2363–2375

Jabado N, Jankowski A, Dougaparsad S, Picard V, Grinstein S, Gros P (2000) Natural resistance to intracellular infections: natural resistance-associated macrophage protein 1 (Nramp1) functions as a pH-dependent manganese transporter at the phagosomal membrane. J Exp Med 192:1237–1248

Jabado N, Cuellar-Mata P, Grinstein S, Gros P (2003) Iron chelators modulate the fusogenic properties of Salmonella-containing phagosomes. Proc Natl Acad Sci USA 100: 6127–6132

Janakiraman A, Slauch JM (2000) The putative iron transport system SitABCD encoded on SPI1 is required for full virulence of Salmonella typhimurium. Mol Microbiol 35:1146–1155

Jenkins NA, Copeland NG, Taylor BA, Bedigian HG, Lee BK (1982) Ecotropic murine leukemia virus DNA content of normal and lymphomatous tissues of BXH-2 recombinant inbred mice. J Virol 42:379–388

Jouanguy E, Lamhamedi-Cherradi S, Lammas D, Dorman SE, Fondaneche MC, Dupuis S, Doffinger R, Altare F, Girdlestone J, Emile JF, Ducoulombier H, Edgar D, Clarke J, Oxelius VA, Brai M, Novelli V, Heyne K, Fischer A, Holland SM, Kumararatne DS, Schreiber RD, Casanova JL (1999) A human IFNGR1 small deletion hotspot associated with dominant susceptibility to mycobacterial infection. Nat Genet 21:370–378

Kahler AK, Persson AS, Sanchez F, Kallstrom H, Apt AS, Schurr E, Lavebratt C (2005) A new coding mutation in the Tnf-alpha leader sequence in tuberculosis-sensitive I/St mice causes higher secretion levels of soluble TNF-alpha. Genes Immun 6:620–627

Kammler M, Schon C, Hantke K (1993) Characterization of the ferrous iron uptake system of Escherichia coli. J Bacteriol 175:6212–6219

Kehres DG, Maguire ME (2003) Emerging themes in manganese transport, biochemistry and pathogenesis in bacteria. FEMS Microbiol Rev 27:263–290

Kehres DG, Janakiraman A, Slauch JM, Maguire ME (2002) SitABCD is the alkaline Mn(2+) transporter of Salmonella enterica serovar Typhimurium. J Bacteriol 184:3159–3166

Khasris AA, Nettleman MD (2005) Global warming and infectious disease. Arch Med Res 36:689–696

Knodler LA, Steele-Mortimer O (2003) Taking possession: biogenesis of the Salmonella-containing vacuole. Traffic 4:587–599

Kramnik I, Dietrich WF, Demant P, Bloom BR (2000) Genetic control of resistance to experimental infection with virulent Mycobacterium tuberculosis. Proc Natl Acad Sci USA 97:8560–8565

Kullberg BJ, Filler SG (2002) Candidemia. In: Calderone RA (ed) Candida and candidiasis. ASM Press, Washington DC, pp 327–340

Kwiatkowski D (2000) Genetic susceptibility to malaria getting complex. Curr Opin Genet Dev 10:320–324

Lam-Yuk-Tseung S, Gros P (2003) Genetic control of susceptibility to bacterial infections in mouse models. Cell Microbiol 5:299–313

Lam-Yuk-Tseung S, Camaschella C, Iolascon A, Gros P (2006) A novel R416C mutation in human DMT1 (SLC11A2) displays pleiotropic effects on function and causes microcytic anemia and hepatic iron overload. Blood Cells Mol Dis 36:347–354

Lavebratt C, Apt AS, Nikonenko BV, Schalling M, Schurr E (1999) Severity of tuberculosis in mice is linked to distal chromosome 3 and proximal chromosome 9. J Infect Dis 180:150–155

Levin M, Newport M (2000) Inherited predisposition to mycobacterial infection: histcrical considerations. Microbes Infect 2:1549–1552

Li HT, Zhang TT, Zhou YQ, Huang QH, Huang J (2006) SLC11A1 (formerly NRAMP1) gene polymorphisms and tuberculosis susceptibility: a meta-analysis. Int J Tuberc Lung Dis 10 3–12

Lio D, Marino V, Serauto A, Gioia V, Scola L, Crivello A, Forte GI, Colonna-Romano G, Candore G, Caruso C (2002) Genotype frequencies of the +874T→A single nucleotide polymorphism in the first intron of the interferon-gamma gene in a sample of Sicilian patients affected by tuberculosis. Eur J Immunogenet 29:371–374

Lopez-Maderuelo D, Arnalich F, Serantes R, Gonzalez A, Codoceo R, Madero R, Vazquez JJ, Montiel C (2003) Interferon-gamma and interleukin-10 gene polymorphisms in pulmonary tuberculosis. Am J Respir Crit Care Med 167:970–975

Lyon FL, Hector RF, Domer JE (1986) Innate and acquired immune responses against Candida albicans in congenic B10.D2 mice with deficiency of the C5 complement component. J Med Vet Mycol 24:359–367

MacVittie TJ, O'Brien AD, Walker RI, Weinberg SR (1982) Inflammatory response of LPS-hyporesponsive and LPS-responsive mice to challenge with gram-negative bacteria Salmonella typhimurium and Klebsiella pneumoniae. Adv Exp Med Biol 155:325–334

Maier JK, Lahoua Z, Gendron NH, Fetni R, Johnston A, Davoodi J, Rasper D, Roy S, Slack RS, Nicholson DW, MacKenzie AE (2002) The neuronal apoptosis inhibitory protein is a direct inhibitor of caspases 3 and 7. J Neurosci 22:2035–2043

Malik S, Abel L, Tooker H, Poon A, Simkin L, Girard M, Adams GJ, Starke JR, Smith KC, Graviss EA, Musser JM, Schurr E (2005) Alleles of the NRAMP1 gene are risk factors for pediatric tuberculosis disease. Proc Natl Acad Sci USA 102:12183–12188

Malo D, Vogan K, Vidal S, Hu J, Cellier M, Schurr E, Fuks A, Bumstead N, Morgan K, Gros P (1994) Haplotype mapping and sequence analysis of the mouse Nramp gene predict susceptibility to infection with intracellular parasites. Genomics 23:51–61

Marquet S, Schurr E (2001) Genetics of susceptibility to infectious diseases: tuberculosis and leprosy as examples. Drug Metab Dispos 29:479–483

Marquis G, Montplaisir S, Pelletier M, Auger P, Lapp WS (1988) Genetics of resistance to infection with Candida albicans in mice. Br J Exp Pathol 69:651–660

Marquis JF, Gros P (2007) Intracellular Leishmania: your iron or mine? Trends Microbiol 15:93–95

Marquis JF, Forbes JR, Canonne-Hergaux F, Horth C, Gros P (2008) Metal transport genes. In: Genetic susceptibility to infectious diseases. Kaslow R, McNicholl J, Hill A (eds) Oxford University Press, New York USA. pp175–189

Marsh K, Snow RW (1997) 30 years of science and technology: the example of malaria. Lancet 349:1–2

Martinon F, Tschopp J (2007) Inflammatory caspases and inflammasomes: master switches of inflammation. Cell Death Differ 14:10–22

Mastroeni P, Vazquez-Torres A, Fang FC, Xu Y, Khan S, Hormaeche CE, Dougan G (2000) Antimicrobial actions of the NADPH phagocyte oxidase and inducible nitric oxide synthase in experimental salmonellosis. II. Effects on microbial proliferation and host survival in vivo. J Exp Med 192:237–248

Medina E, North RJ (1996) Evidence inconsistent with a role for the Bcg gene (Nramp1) in resistance of mice to infection with virulent Mycobacterium tuberculosis. J Exp Med 183:1045–1051

Medina E, North RJ (1998) Resistance ranking of some common inbred mouse strains to Mycobacterium tuberculosis and relationship to major histocompatibility complex haplotype and Nramp1 genotype. Immunology 93:270–274

Mencacci A, Cenci E, Bistoni F, Bacci A, Del Sero G, Montagnoli C, Fe d'Ostiani C, Romani L (1998) Specific and non-specific immunity to Candida albicans: a lesson from genetically modified animals. Res Immunol 149:352–361; discussion 517–359

Miller EN, Jamieson SE, Joberty C, Fakiola M, Hudson D, Peacock CS, Cordell HJ, Shaw MA, Lins-Lainson Z, Shaw JJ, Ramos F, Silveira F, Blackwell JM (2004) Genome-wide scans for leprosy and tuberculosis susceptibility genes in Brazilians. Genes Immun 5:63–67

Min-Oo G, Gros P (2005) Erythrocyte variants and the nature of their malaria protective effect. Cell Microbiol 7:753–763

Min-Oo G, Fortin A, Tam MF, Nantel A, Stevenson MM, Gros P (2003) Pyruvate kinase deficiency in mice protects against malaria. Nat Genet 35:357–362

Min-Oo G, Fortin A, Tam MF, Gros P, Stevenson MM (2004) Phenotypic expression of pyruvate kinase deficiency and protection against malaria in a mouse model. Genes Immun 5:168–175

Min-Oo G, Fortin A, Pitari G, Tam M, Stevenson MM, Gros P (2007a) Complex genetic control of susceptibility to malaria: positional cloning of the Char9 locus. J Exp Med 204:511–524

Min-Oo G, Tam M, Stevenson MM, Gros P (2007b) Pyruvate kinase deficiency: correlation between enzyme activity, extent of hemolytic anemia and protection against malaria in independent mouse mutants. Blood Cells Mol Dis 39:63–69

Mitsos LM, Cardon LR, Fortin A, Ryan L, LaCourse R, North RJ, Gros P (2000) Genetic control of susceptibility to infection with Mycobacterium tuberculosis in mice. Genes Immun 1:467–477

Mitsos LM, Cardon LR, Ryan L, LaCourse R, North RJ, Gros P (2003) Susceptibility to tuberculosis: a locus on mouse chromosome 19 (Trl-4) regulates Mycobacterium tuberculosis replication in the lungs. Proc Natl Acad Sci USA 100:6610–6615

Molofsky AB, Byrne BG, Whitfield NN, Madigan CA, Fuse ET, Tateda K, Swanson MS (2006) Cytosolic recognition of flagellin by mouse macrophages restricts Legionella pneumophila infection. J Exp Med 203:1093–1104

More li R, Rosenberg LT (1971) Role of complement during experimental Candida infection in mice. Infect Immun 3:521–523

Motu sky AG (1960) Metabolic polymorphisms and the role of infectious diseases in human evolution. Hum Biol 32:28–62

Mullick A, Leon Z, Min-Oo G, Berghout J, Lo R, Daniels E, Gros P (2006) Cardiac failure in C5-deficient A/J mice after Candida albicans infection. Infect Immun 74:4439–4451

Nairz M, Theurl I, Ludwiczek S, Theurl M, Mair SM, Fritsche G, Weiss G (2007) The co-ordinated regulation of iron homeostasis in murine macrophages limits the availability of iron for intracellular Salmonella typhimurium. Cell Microbiol 9:2126–2140

Norrby SR, Nord CE, Finch R; European Society of Clinical Microbiology and Infectious Diseases (2005) Lack of development of new antimicrobial drugs: a potential serious threat to public health. Lancet Infect Dis 5:115–119

North RJ, Jung YJ (2004) Immunity to tuberculosis. Annu Rev Immunol 22:599–623

O'Brien AD, Rosenstreich DL, Scher I, Campbell GH, MacDermott RP, Formal SB (1980) Genetic control of susceptibility to Salmonella typhimurium in mice: role of the LPS gene. J Immunol 124:20–24

O'Brien AD, Weinstein DA, Soliman MY, Rosenstreich DL (1985) Additional evidence that the Lps gene locus regulates natural resistance to S. typhimurium in mice. J Immunol 134:2820–2823

Ochman H, Groisman EA (1994) The origin and evolution of species differences in Escherichia coli and Salmonella typhimurium. EXS 69:479–493

Odds FC (1988) Candida and candidosis, 2nd edn. Bailliaere Tindall, London

Odds FC, Van Nuffel L, Gow NA (2000) Survival in experimental Candida albicans infections depends on inoculum growth conditions as well as animal host. Microbiology 146:1881–1889

Pan H, Yan BS, Rojas M, Shebzukhov YV, Zhou H, Kobzik L, Higgins DE, Daly MJ, Bloom BR, Kramnik I (2005) Ipr1 gene mediates innate immunity to tuberculosis. Nature 434:767–772

Parry C, Davies PD (1996) The resurgence of tuberculosis. Soc Appl Bacteriol Symp Ser 25:23S–26S

Perrelet D, Ferri A, MacKenzie AE, Smith GM, Korneluk RG, Liston P, Sagot Y, Terrado J, Monnier D, Kato AC (2000) IAP family proteins delay motoneuron cell death in vivo. Eur J Neurosci 12:2059–2067

Picard C, Casanova JL, Abel L (2006) Mendelian traits that confer predisposition or resistance to specific infections in humans. Curr Opin Immunol 18:383–390

Poltorak A, Smirnova I, He X, Liu MY, Van Huffel C, McNally O, Birdwell D, Alejos E. Silva M, Du X, Thompson P, Chan EK, Ledesma J, Roe B, Clifton S, Vogel SN, Beutler B (1998) Genetic and physical mapping of the Lps locus: identification of the toll-4 receptor as a candidate gene in the critical region. Blood Cells Mol Dis 24:340–355

Poon A, Schurr E (2004) The NRAMP genes and human susceptibility to common diseases. In: Cellier M, Gros P (eds) The NRAMP family. Kluwer Academic/Plenum Publishers, New York, pp 29–43

Qureshi ST, Lariviere L, Sebastiani G, Clermont S, Skamene E, Gros P, Malo D (1996) A high-resolution map in the chromosomal region surrounding the Lps locus. Genomics 31:283–294

Qureshi ST, Lariviere L, Leveque G, Clermont S, Moore KJ, Gros P, Malo D (1999) Endotoxin-tolerant mice have mutations in Toll-like receptor 4 (Tlr4). J Exp Med 189:615–625

Ratledge C (2004) Iron, mycobacteria and tuberculosis. Tuberculosis (Edinb) 84:110–130

Ren T, Zamboni DS, Roy CR, Dietrich WF, Vance RE (2006) Flagellin-deficient Legionella mutants evade caspase-1- and Naip5-mediated macrophage immunity. PLoS Pathog 2:e18

Rieder HL, Kelly GD, Bloch AB, Cauthen GM, Snider DE Jr (1991) Tuberculosis diagnosed at death in the United States. Chest 100:678–681

Rietschel ET, Kirikae T, Schade FU, Mamat U, Schmidt G, Loppnow H, Ulmer AJ, Zahringer U, Seydel U, Di Padova F, et al (1994) Bacterial endotoxin: molecular relationships of structure to activity and function. FASEB J 8:217–225

Rosenberger CM, Scott MG, Gold MR, Hancock RE, Finlay BB (2000) Salmonella typhimurium infection and lipopolysaccharide stimulation induce similar changes in macrophage gene expression. J Immunol 164:5894–5904

Rossouw M, Nel HJ, Cooke GS, van Helden PD, Hoal EG (2003) Association between tuberculosis and a polymorphic NFkappaB binding site in the interferon gamma gene. Lancet 361:1871–1872

Roy MF, Riendeau N, Loredo-Osti JC, Malo D (2006) Complexity in the host response to Salmonella typhimurium infection in AcB and BcA recombinant congenic strains. Genes Immun 7:655–666

Royle MC, Totemeyer S, Alldridge LC, Maskell DJ, Bryant CE (2003) Stimulation of Toll-like receptor 4 by lipopolysaccharide during cellular invasion by live Salmonella typhimurium is a critical but not exclusive event leading to macrophage responses. J Immunol 170:5445–5454

Russell DG, Dant J, Sturgill-Koszycki S (1996) Mycobacterium avium- and Mycobacterium tuberculosis-containing vacuoles are dynamic, fusion-competent vesicles that are accessible to glycosphingolipids from the host cell plasmalemma. J Immunol 156:4764–4773

Ryu S, Park YK, Bai GH, Kim SJ, Park SN, Kang S (2000) 3'UTR polymorphisms in the NRAMP1 gene are associated with susceptibility to tuberculosis in Koreans. Int J Tuberc Lung Dis 4:577–580

Salvin SB, Neta R (1983) Resistance and susceptibility to infection in inbred murine strains. I. Variations in the response to thymic hormones in mice infected with Candida albicans. Cell Immunol 75:160–172

Sanchez F, Radaeva TV, Nikonenko BV, Persson AS, Sengul S, Schalling M, Schurr E, Apt AS, Lavebratt C (2003) Multigenic control of disease severity after virulent Mycobacterium tuberculosis infection in mice. Infect Immun 71:126–131

Sapoval B, Filoche M, Weibel ER (2002) Smaller is better—but not too small: a physical scale for the design of the mammalian pulmonary acinus. Proc Natl Acad Sci USA 99:10411–10416

Schaible UE, Sturgill-Koszycki S, Schlesinger PH, Russell DG (1998) Cytokine activation leads to acidification and increases maturation of Mycobacterium avium-containing phagosomes in murine macrophages. J Immunol 160:1290–1296

Searle S, Bright NA, Roach TI, Atkinson PG, Barton CH, Meloen RH, Blackwell JM (1998) Localisation of Nramp1 in macrophages: modulation with activation and infection. J Cell Sci 111:2855–2866

Sebastiani G, Olien L, Gauthier S, Skamene E, Morgan K, Gros P, Malo D (1998) Mapping of genetic modulators of natural resistance to infection with Salmonella typhimurium in wild-derived mice. Genomics 47:180–186

Sebastiani G, Leveque G, Lariviere L, Laroche L, Skamene E, Gros P, Malo D (2000) Cloning and characterization of the murine toll-like receptor 5 (Tlr5) gene: sequence and mRNA expression studies in Salmonella-susceptible MOLF/Ei mice. Genomics 64:230–240

Sebastiani G, Blais V, Sancho V, Vogel SN, Stevenson MM, Gros P, Lapointe JM, Rivest S, Malo D (2002) Host immune response to Salmonella enterica serovar Typhimurium infection in mice derived from wild strains. Infect Immun 70:1997–2009

Selvaraj P, Narayanan PR, Reetha AM (1999) Association of functional mutant homozygotes of the mannose binding protein gene with susceptibility to pulmonary tuberculosis in India. Tuber Lung Dis 79:221–227

Skamene E, Gros P, Forget A, Kongshavn PA, St Charles C, Taylor BA (1982) Genetic regulation of resistance to intracellular pathogens. Nature 297:506–509

Skamene E, Schurr E, Gros P (1998) Infection genomics: Nramp1 as a major determinant of natural resistance to intracellular infections. Annu Rev Med 49:275–287

Sousa AO, Salem JI, Lee FK, Vercosa MC, Cruaud P, Bloom BR, Lagrange PH, David HL (1997) An epidemic of tuberculosis with a high rate of tuberculin anergy among a population previously unexposed to tuberculosis, the Yanomami Indians of the Brazilian Amazon. Proc Natl Acad Sci USA 94:13227–13232

Stead WW, Senner JW, Reddick WT, Lofgren JP (1990) Racial differences in susceptibility to infection by Mycobacterium tuberculosis. N Engl J Med 322:422–427

Stienstra Y, van der Werf TS, Oosterom E, Nolte IM, van der Graaf WT, Etuaful S, Raghunathan PL, Whitney EA, Ampadu EO, Asamoa K, Klutse EY, te Meerman GJ, Tappero JW, Ashford DA, van der Steege G (2006) Susceptibility to Buruli ulcer is associated with the SLC11A1 (NRAMP1) D543 N polymorphism. Genes Immun 7:185–189

Sturgill-Koszycki S, Schlesinger PH, Chakraborty P, Haddix PL, Collins HL, Fok AK, Allen RD, Gluck SL, Heuser J, Russell DG (1994) Lack of acidification in Mycobacterium phagosomes produced by exclusion of the vesicular proton-ATPase. Science 263:678–681

Sturgill-Koszycki S, Schaible UE, Russell DG (1996) Mycobacterium-containing phagosomes are accessible to early endosomes and reflect a transitional state in normal phagosome biogenesis. EMBO J 15:6960–6968

Taylor BA (1978) Recombinant inbred strains: use in gene mapping. In: Morse H 3rd (ed) Origins of inbred mice. Academic Press, New York, pp 423–438

Thye T, Browne EN, Chinbuah MA, Gyapong J, Osei I, Owusu-Dabo E, Niemann S, Rusch-Gerdes S, Horstmann RD, Meyer CG (2006) No associations of human pulmonary tuberculosis with Sp110 variants. J Med Genet 43:e32

Tosh K, Campbell SJ, Fielding K, Sillah J, Bah B, Gustafson P, Manneh K, Lisse I, Sirugo G, Bennett S, Aaby P, McAdam KP, Bah-Sow O, Lienhardt C, Kramnik I, Hill AV (2006) Variants in the SP110 gene are associated with genetic susceptibility to tuberculosis in West Africa. Proc Natl Acad Sci USA 103:10364–10368

Tso HW, Ip WK, Chong WP, Tam CM, Chiang AK, Lau YL (2005) Association of interferon gamma and interleukin 10 genes with tuberculosis in Hong Kong Chinese. Genes Immun 6:358–363

Tsolis RM, Baumler AJ, Heffron F, Stojiljkovic I (1996) Contribution of TonB- and Feo-mediated iron uptake to growth of Salmonella typhimurium in the mouse. Infect Immun 64:4549–4556

Tuite A, Mullick A, Gros P (2004) Genetic analysis of innate immunity in resistance to Candida albicans. Genes Immun 5:576–587

Tuite A, Elias M, Picard S, Mullick A, Gros P (2005) Genetic control of susceptibility to Candida albicans in susceptible A/J and resistant C57BL/6J mice. Genes Immun 6:672–682

Turcotte K, Gauthier S, Mitsos LM, Shustik C, Copeland NG, Jenkins NA, Fournet JC, Jolicoeur P, Gros P (2004) Genetic control of myeloproliferation in BXH-2 mice. Blood 103:2343–2350

Turcotte K, Gauthier S, Tuite A, Mullick A, Malo D, Gros P (2005) A mutation in the Icsbp1 gene causes susceptibility to infection and a chronic myeloid leukemia-like syndrome in BXH-2 mice. J Exp Med 201:881–890

Turcotte K, Gauthier S, Malo D, Tam M, Stevenson MM, Gros P (2007) Icsbp1/IRF-8 is required for innate and adaptive immune responses against intracellular pathogens. J Immunol 179:2467–2467

Vazquez-Torres A, Vallance BA, Bergman MA, Finlay BB, Cookson BT, Jones-Carson J, Fang FC (2004) Toll-like receptor 4 dependence of innate and adaptive immunity to Salmonella: importance of the Kupffer cell network. J Immunol 172:6202–6208

Verduyn Lunel FM, Meis JF, Voss A (1999) Nosocomial fungal infections: candidemia. Diagn Microbiol Infect Dis 34:213–220

Vidal S, Tremblay ML, Govoni G, Gauthier S, Sebastiani G, Malo D, Skamene E, Olivier M, Jothy S, Gros P (1995) The Ity/Lsh/Bcg locus: natural resistance to infection with intracellular parasites is abrogated by disruption of the Nramp1 gene. J Exp Med 182:655–666

Vidal SM, Malo D, Vogan K, Skamene E, Gros P (1993) Natural resistance to infection with intracellular parasites: isolation of a candidate for Bcg. Cell 73:469–485

Vidal SM, Pinner E, Lepage P, Gauthier S, Gros P (1996) Natural resistance to intracellular infections: Nramp1 encodes a membrane phosphoglycoprotein absent in macrophages from susceptible (Nramp1 D169) mouse strains. J Immunol 157:3559–3568

Watson J, Riblet R (1974) Genetic control of responses to bacterial lipopolysaccharides in mice. I. Evidence for a single gene that influences mitogenic and immunogenic respones to lipopolysaccharides. J Exp Med 140:1147–1161

Watson J, Riblet R, Taylor BA (1977) The response of recombinant inbred strains of mice to bacterial lipopolysaccharides. J Immunol 118:2088–2093

Watson J, Kelly K, Largen M, Taylor BA (1978) The genetic mapping of a defective LPS response gene in C3H/HeJ mice. J Immunol 120:422–424

Weinstein DL, Lissner CR, Swanson RN, O'Brien AD (1986) Macrophage defect and inflammatory cell recruitment dysfunction in Salmonella susceptible C3H/HeJ mice. Cell Immunol 102:68–77

Wetsel RA, Fleischer DT, Haviland DL (1990) Deficiency of the murine fifth complement component (C5). A 2-base pair gene deletion in a 5Î-exon. J Biol Chem 265:2435–2440

Wilkinson RJ, Llewelyn M, Toossi Z, Patel P, Pasvol G, Lalvani A, Wright D, Latif M, Davidson RN (2000) Influence of vitamin D deficiency and vitamin D receptor polymorphisms on tuberculosis among Gujarati Asians in west London: a case-control study. Lancet 355:618–621

World Health Organization (2000) The world health report 2000. Health systems: improving performance. WHO, Geneva

World Health Organization (2002) Global tuberculosis control: surveillance, planning, financing. WHO report. WHO, Geneva

Wright EK, Goodart SA, Growney JD, Hadinoto V, Endrizzi MG, Long EM, Sadigh K, Abney AL, Bernstein-Hanley I, Dietrich WF (2003) Naip5 affects host susceptibility to the intracellular pathogen Legionella pneumophila. Curr Biol 13:27–36

Yan BS, Kirby A, Shebzukhov YV, Daly MJ, Kramnik I (2006) Genetic architecture of tuberculosis resistance in a mouse model of infection. Genes Immun 7:201–210

Yap GS, Sher A (2002) The use of germ line-mutated mice in understanding host-pathogen interactions. Cell Microbiol 4:627–634

Young DB, Duncan K (1995) Prospects for new interventions in the treatment and prevention of mycobacterial disease. Annu Rev Microbiol 49:641–673

Zaharik ML, Vallance BA, Puente JL, Gros P, Finlay BB (2002) Host-pathogen interactions: host resistance factor Nramp1 up-regulates the expression of Salmonella pathogenicity island-2 virulence genes. Proc Natl Acad Sci USA 99:15705–15710

Zamboni DS, Kobayashi KS, Kohlsdorf T, Ogura Y, Long EM, Vance RE, Kuida K, Mariathasan S, Dixit VM, Flavell RA, et al (2006) The Birc1e cytosolic pattern-recognition receptor contributes to the detection and control of Legionella pneumophila infection. Nat Immunol 7:318–325

Zhou D, Hardt WD, Galan JE (1999) Salmonella typhimurium encodes a putative iron transport system within the centisome 63 pathogenicity island. Infect Immun 67:1974–1981

Host Defenses Against Human Papillomaviruses: Lessons from Epidermodysplasia Verruciformis

G. Orth

Contents

Abstract Epidermodysplasia verruciformis (EV) is a rare, autosomal recessive genodermatosis associated with a high risk of skin carcinoma (MIM 226400). EV is characterized by the abnormal susceptibility of otherwise healthy patients to infection by specific, weakly virulent human papillomaviruses (HPVs), including the potentially oncogenic HPV-5. Inactivating mutations in either of the related *EVER1/TMC6* and *EVER2/TMC8* genes cause most EV cases. New insights in EV pathogenesis have been gained from the following recent observations:

G. Orth

Department of Virology, Institut Pasteur, 25 Rue du Docteur Roux, 75015 Paris, France
gorth@pasteur.fr

B. Beutler (ed.), *Immunology, Phenotype First: How Mutations Have Established New Principles and Pathways in Immunology.* Current Topics in Microbiology and Immunology 321. © Springer-Verlag Berlin Heidelberg 2008

(1) EV-specific HPVs (betapapillomaviruses) are defective for an important growth-promoting function encoded by an E5/E8 gene present in other HPVs, and inactivation of EVER proteins may compensate for the missing viral function; (2) the transmembrane viral E5/E8 and cellular EVER proteins interact both with the zinc transporter ZnT1, and are likely to modulate zinc homeostasis. EV may thus represent a primary deficiency in intrinsic, constitutive immunity to betapapillomaviruses, or constitute a primary deficiency in innate immunity (or both). Keratinocytes, the home cells of HPVs, are likely to play a central role in both cases. An important issue is to establish which cellular genes involved in intrinsic and innate antiviral responses play a part in the outcome of infections with other HPV types, such as genital oncogenic HPVs.

Abbreviations EV: Epidermodysplasia verruciformis; HPV: Human papillomavirus; PID: Primary immunodeficiency disease; NMSC: Nonmelanoma skin cancer; ORF: Open reading frame; TGF-β: Tumor growth factor beta; CMI: Cell-mediated immunity; NK cell: Natural killer cell; TNF-α: Tumor necrosis factor alpha; SCID: Severe combined immune deficiency; γc: Common γc cytokine receptor subunit; JAK-3: Janus kinase-3; WHIM syndrome: Warts, hypogammaglobulinemia, infections, and myelokathexis syndrome; SCC: Squamous cell carcinoma; EGFR: Epidermal growth factor receptor; CRPV: Cottontail rabbit papillomavirus; ERK1/2: Extracellular signal-regulated kinase 1/2; AP-1: Activating protein-1; PCDH1: Protocadherin 1; MTF1: Metal-responsive element-binding transcription factor 1; cM: Centimorgan; TMC: Transmembrane channel-like; TLR: Toll-like receptor; PAMP: Pathogen-associated molecular pattern

Introduction

Epidermodysplasia verruciformis (EV) was clinically described in 1922 by Lewandowsky and Lutz, and first considered a congenital epidermal anomaly. The first patient, a 29-year-old woman born from a consanguineous marriage, presented with reddish scaly papules covering her whole skin (Fig. 1), which were allegedly present at birth. The patient developed an invasive carcinoma on her forehead at the age of 25 (Lewandowsky and Lutz 1922). The parental consanguinity and familial aggregation observed for a proportion of reported cases later led to the postulate, in 1933, that EV was probably transmitted by a recessive gene (Cockayne 1933). For a long time, EV was considered either as an inborn anomaly of epidermal differentiation, involving a predisposition to the development of skin cancers, or as a particular form of generalized verrucosis (reviewed in Orth 2006).

The viral etiology of the disease was established by autoinoculation and heteroinoculation experiments (Lutz 1946; Jablonska and Formas 1959) and the regular observation of wart virus particles in benign lesions (reviewed in Jablonska et al. 1972; Lutzner 1978; Majewski and Jablonska 1995; Orth 1987, 2006). This was further substantiated by the demonstration that EV was associated with specific, related human papillomavirus (HPV) types (Pass et al. 1977; Orth et al. 1978, 1979), and by the detection of the

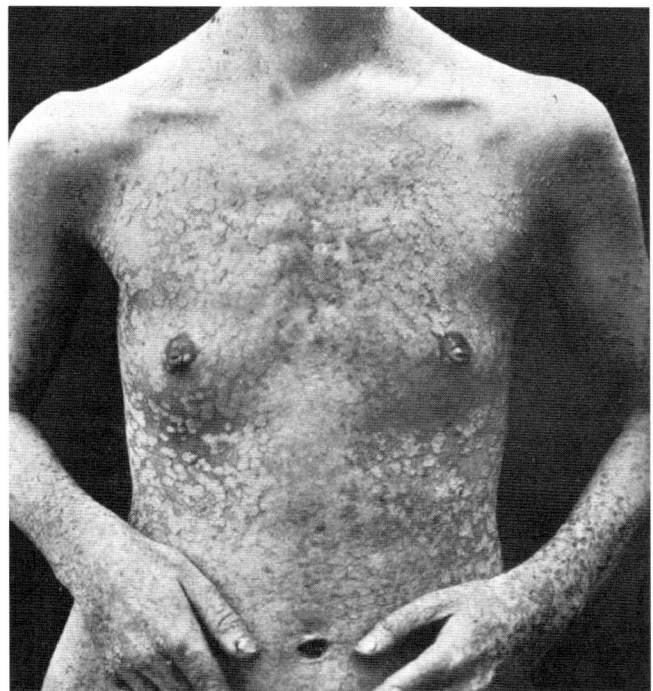

Fig. 1 First EV case described (Lewandowsky and Lutz 1922)

genome of HPV type 5 (HPV-5) in EV carcinomas (Orth et al. 1980; Ostrow et al. 1982; Pfister et al. 1983). Two susceptibility loci for EV were mapped to chromosomal regions 17q25 (*EV1*) and 2p21-p24 (*EV2*) (Ramoz et al. 1999, 2000), and this led to the identification of inactivating mutations that cause EV in either of two novel genes, *EVER1* and *EVER2*, located in the *EV1* locus (Ramoz et al. 2002).

EV can now be defined as a rare, lifelong, skin disease associated with a high risk of nonmelanoma skin cancer (NMSC), which results from a genetically deter- mined, recessively transmitted, abnormal susceptibility to a specific group of HPV genotypes and their carcinogenic potential, mainly that of HPV-5 (Orth et al. 2001). More than 100 HPV genotypes have been fully characterized to date. According to a recently adopted phylogenetic nomenclature, HPV types are grouped into five genera comprising a variable number (1 to 15) of species (de Villiers et al. 2004). The HPV types associated with EV (EV HPVs) are usually considered innocuous for the general population, and belong to the genus *Betapapillomavirus*. The genus *Alphapapillomavirus* comprises types differing by their genital, oral, or cutaneous tropism and by their pathogenicity. It includes the causative agents of genital warts (HPV types 6 and 11) and viruses etiologically related to the development of carcinomas of the uterine cervix and other anogenital cancers (mostly the potentially carcinogenic HPV types 16 and 18) (Bosch et al. 2002; Schiffman and Kjaer 2003).

The genera *Gammapapillomavirus*, *Mupapillomavirus*, and *Nupapillomavirus* comprise types associated with cutaneous warts (de Villiers et al. 2004). Infections caused by cutaneous and mucosal HPV types are widespread and often asymptomatic. HPV-associated diseases and asymptomatic infections usually clear spontaneously. Only persistent lesions associated with potentially carcinogenic types may evolve into invasive carcinomas. The host, viral, and environmental factors that determine the outcome of HPV infections remain poorly understood (Orth 2008).

EV is likely to represent the first identified primary immunodeficiency disease (PID), since this Mendelian condition was clinically described 30 years before the recognition of X-linked agammaglobulinemia (Bruton 1952; Casanova and Abel 2007). Recent advances in our understanding of the pathogenesis of EV provide some insights into mechanisms conditioning the outcome of HPV infections.

The EV Phenotype

EV HPVs can only express the full spectrum of their biological properties at the expense of individuals endowed with a genetically determined vulnerability (Orth et al. 2001). The corresponding phenotype is defined by a number of clinical, viral, and immunological features that characterize EV patients (EV phenotype).

Clinical Features

EV usually begins during infancy or early childhood. About 10% of the patients are born of consanguineous marriages. The disease is characterized by the presence of skin lesions presenting as flat warts or as scaly, reddish, brownish, or achromic plaques. Typical common warts are only occasionally observed, and anogenital warts only exceptionally. EV lesions are refractory to conventional wart treatments. In their second, third, or fourth decade, over half of EV patients start developing precancerous lesions of the skin (actinic keratoses, Bowen's carcinoma in situ) and invasive NMSCs (mostly squamous cell carcinomas), most frequently localized in sun-exposed areas of the skin. Cancers develop slowly, and are mainly locally destructive (reviewed in Lutzner et al. 1984; Jablonska and Orth 1985; Majewski and Jablonska 1995). In general, EV patients are otherwise healthy. It should be mentioned, however, that EV was found associated with mental retardation or other congenital abnormalities in a minority of cases (Lutzner 1978).

Virology

The genus *Betapapillomavirus* comprises 25 fully characterized HPV types, which are distributed into five species (de Villiers et al. 2004). Most of these viruses have been detected in benign EV lesions by molecular hybridization techniques:

HPV types 5, 8, 12, 14, 19, 20, 21, 24, 25, 36, 47 (species 1), 9, 15, 17, 22, 23, 37, 38 (species 2), and 49 (species 3). EV HPVs have a worldwide distribution, and HPV-5 is the most frequently found genotype. Patients are usually infected with multiple EV HPV types and, often, with HPV-3, an alphapapillomavirus that causes flat warts in the general population. A very high virus content characterizes the polymorphic benign EV lesions, and the viral genomes extracted from these lesions can even be identified by direct visualization of their restriction patterns in ethidium bromide-stained gels. This high level of intranuclear viral replication is associated with a specific cytopathic effect, namely the presence of large "dysplastic" keratinocytes with a pale-stained cytoplasm within the spinous and granular layers of the epidermis. This histological feature is pathognomonic of EV (Orth et al. 1980; Orth 1987, 2006).

Only a subset of betapapillomaviruses is associated with the malignant conversion of EV lesions, usually HPV-5 and occasionally, HPV types 8, 14, 17, 20, or 47. Viral genomes are maintained as high copy number episomes, and high levels of transcripts of the viral E6 and E7 open reading frames (ORFs) are detected in pre-malignant lesions and invasive carcinomas. This further indicates that this subset of betapapillomaviruses is endowed with an oncogenic potential. Recent in vitro studies have shown that the HPV-5 E6 protein, but not the E6 protein encoded by HPV-9, a nononcogenic EV HPV, represses the tumor growth factor beta (TGF-β) signaling pathway by binding to SMAD3, suggesting that a downregulation of this pathway could be involved in HPV-5-associated skin carcinogenesis (Mendoza et al. 2006). Most (but not all) EV carcinomas arise on sun-exposed areas of the skin. Sunlight represents the major risk factor for NMSC in the general population (Brash 1997; Ullrich 2005). The early development of EV carcinomas is likely to involve a synergistic carcinogenic role of HPV-5 and sunlight (reviewed in Orth 1987, 2006).

Immunology

The patients suffering from EV are not abnormally prone to bacterial, fungal, or viral infections. This includes infections caused by HPV types that induce genital diseases and skin warts in the general population, except HPV-3 and HPV-3-related types (Jablonska and Orth, 1985; Majewski et al. 1997). The risk for cancers other than NMSCs does not seem to be abnormally high in EV patients (Lutzner 1978). Humoral immunity appears to be preserved (Jablonska et al. 1979). Antibodies to the major L1 capsid protein of HPV-5 have been detected in all patients studied so far (Favre et al. 1998). Antibodies to the HPV-5 E6 or E7 (or both) oncoproteins were found in about 70% of EV patients with carcinomas (M. Favre, E. Mahé, S. Majewski, S. Jablonska, and G. Orth, unpublished results).

The first evidence for an impaired cell-mediated immunity (CMI) in EV patients was obtained 30 years ago (Glinski et al. 1976; Prawer et al. 1977). Most, but not all, EV patients studied since then were reported to have an impaired CMI on the basis of in vitro and in vivo tests. Decreased T lymphocyte counts and CD4+/CD8+ T cell ratios, as well as a reduced T cell responsiveness to mitogens, were reported for some patients. An anergy to common skin antigens was observed in most patients. The most common feature has been an anergy to sensitization to dinitro-chlorobenzene (Glinski et al. 1981; Majewski et al. 1986, 1997; Majewski and Jablonska 1992; Oliveira et al. 2003). Patients with EV were found to display normal or increased natural killer (NK) cell activity, using the standard K-562 cells as targets (Majewski et al. 1986). It should be mentioned that the normal number of Langerhans cells, the epidermal antigen presenting cells, appears to be preserved in EV patients (Majewski and Jablonska 1992).

HPV-associated lesions usually regress spontaneously, as a consequence of specific cell-mediated immune responses. Cytotoxic T lymphocyte responses or delayed-type hypersensitivity reactions (or the two together) directed against viral early proteins are thought to play a major role in this outcome (Tagami et al. 1985; Coleman et al. 1994; Stanley 2006). Potentially oncogenic genital HPV types, especially HPV-16, have evolved mechanisms to evade innate and adaptive immunity. This may allow the persistence of intraepithelial lesions, which is a prerequisite to the development of anogenital cancers (Frazer et al. 1999; Woodworth 2002; Stanley 2006). The complete regression of EV lesions has never been observed and innate or acquired cell-mediated immune responses toward keratinocytes infected with EV HPVs are still poorly understood. An increased expression of the tumor necrosis factor alpha (TNF-α) and TGF-β1 genes has been detected in keratinocytes of typical EV lesions, and this has been postulated to play a part in the impaired local immunosurveillance resulting in the persistence of the lesions (Majewski et al. 1991). Available data point to an unresponsiveness of T lymphocytes to autologous HPV-infected keratinocytes (Cooper et al. 1990), and to a reduced NK cell-mediated cytotoxicity against HPV-5-infected keratinocytes in patients with EV (Majewski et al. 1990). Further studies are needed to confirm these early data.

Little information is available on the immunological status of EV patients before the onset of their disease. A still unsolved issue is whether the immunological abnormalities observed to varying extents in most (but not all) patients are secondary to the chronic, massive HPV infection, or result from a primary immune deficiency involved in the pathogenesis of EV.

EV-Specific HPVs in Non-EV Individuals

Betapapillomaviruses Among Other HPVs

Betapapillomaviruses share many properties with the other HPV genotypes, including the general organization of their genome (a circular double-stranded DNA molecule of 7,500–8,000 base pairs), their strict tropism for keratinocytes, and the close link between their life cycle and the biology of their host cells (Howley and Lowy 2007). Generally speaking, cutaneous HPVs most likely target the slow-cycling, self-renewing epithelial stem cells located in the basal layer of the epidermis and in the bulge of hair follicles (Alonso and Fuchs 2003). HPV infections are often asymptomatic (latent) or may result in the development of a wart. The challenge shared by all papillomaviruses is to infect slow-cycling cells and to replicate in nondividing terminally differentiating keratinocytes. Their strategy relies on the interaction between the viral early proteins E5, E6, and E7 to activate the host cellular DNA machinery and to prevent apoptosis in response to unscheduled DNA synthesis. This leads to the development of a productively infected lesion. The maintenance of the viral DNA as autonomous episomes in latently infected cells would only require the expression of the viral early proteins E1 and E2, which are involved in the replication and segregation of the viral genome (Longworth and Laimins 2004; Münger et al. 2004; Howley and Lowy 2007; Orth 2008).

EV HPVs cause widespread asymptomatic infections in the general population. Our hypothesis is that betapapillomaviruses are defective for an essential growth-promoting function (Nonnenmacher et al. 2006; Orth 2006).

Betapapillomaviruses as Commensals of the Skin

The use of sensitive PCR approaches, designed to detect a broad range of known EV HPVs or putative novel EV HPV-related genotypes, has brought a wealth of information about the epidemiology and biology of betapapillomaviruses. An impressive diversity of putative novel betapapillomaviruses has been disclosed, in addition to the 25 genotypes already characterized (Antonsson et al. 2000). Infections of the skin with EV HPVs or related putative genotypes are highly prevalent in healthy adults (Boxman et al. 1997; Astori et al. 1998; Antonsson et al. 2000), and these infections are acquired very early in infancy (Antonsson et al. 2003). However, the prevalence of antibodies to the L1 major capsid protein of HPV-5 and other EV HPV genotypes is low (lesser than 10%) in the general population (Favre et al. 1998; Stark et al. 1998; Feltkamp et al. 2003; Karagas et al. 2006). Considering that betapapillomaviruses are ubiquitous and cause widespread asymptomatic cutaneous infections, it has been proposed that these viruses are commensals of the human skin (Antonsson et al. 2000).

Rare Phenocopies of EV upon Immunosuppression

Immunosuppression per se is not sufficient to allow EV HPVs to express their pathogenic and oncogenic potentials. This is illustrated by the scarcity of an EV-like syndrome (persistent cutaneous lesions with specific histologic features and a high level of EV HPV DNA replication) among patients with genetic, acquired, or induced depression or suppression of CMI. An increased incidence of warts and skin cancers is observed among organ allograft recipients, who have been intentionally immunosuppressed to prevent rejection of the transplants (Koranda et al. 1974; Euvrard et al. 2003). Only rare cases of HPV-5- or HPV-8-associated EV-like syndrome have been reported among renal transplant recipients (Lutzner et al. 1980, 1983; Barr et al. 1989). There are few reports of the development of lesions typical of EV in patients infected with human immunodeficiency virus (reviewed in Carré et al. 2003).

That the vulnerability to betapapillomaviruses may require a specific immune dysfunction has been supported by a long-term follow-up study of 41 patients with severe combined immune deficiency (SCID) who had undergone hematopoietic stem cell transplantation early in life. Late-onset, severe cutaneous disease was observed only in patients with SCID associated with either common γc cytokine receptor subunit (γc) or Janus kinase-3 (JAK-3) deficiency. Four of nine such patients had lesions typical of EV associated with HPV types 5 and 14, indicating that γc/JAK-3 signaling in keratinocytes may play a role in immunity against EV HPVs (Laffort et al. 2004). Patients suffering from WHIM syndrome (warts, hypogammaglobulinemia, infections, and myelokathexis), which is associated with mutations in the gene encoding the CXCR4 chemokine receptor, are prone to chronic cutaneous and genital HPV disease, usually associated with alphapapillomaviruses (Gorlin et al. 2000; Hernandez et al. 2003). EV-like lesions have not been described in such patients.

Innocuousness of Betapapillomaviruses?

Whether EV HPVs and related genotypes are harmless in the general population is still a matter of debate (Kawashima et al. 1990; Harwood and Proby 2002; Pfister 2003; Orth 2004, 2005). HPV DNA sequences (most frequently betapapillomaviruses) were detected in low amounts (usually much less than one copy of viral genome per cell) in 25%–65% of basal cell carcinomas and squamous cell carcinomas (SCCs) in immunocompetent individuals and in up to 90% of SCCs in organ transplant recipients. Similar detection rates were found for premalignant skin lesions (reviewed in Harwood and Proby 2002; Pfister 2003). These data, as well as seroepidemiological studies (Feltkamp et al. 2003; Karagas et al. 2006) and functional studies involving ectopic expression of E6 and E7 proteins of cutaneous HPV genotypes (reviewed in Storey 2002), brought some support to the possible role of betapapillomaviruses in the development of NMSCs in non-EV patients. However, mutagenic and immunosuppressive ultraviolet radiations of the sun are considered the major risk factors for skin cancer (Brash 1997; Ullrich 2005), and such a role for HPV remains elusive (Harwood and Proby 2002; Pfister 2002; Orth 2005).

High detection rates of DNA sequences of betapapillomaviruses (especially HPV-5) in the lesional skin have been reported in patients suffering from psoriasis (Favre et al. 1998; Weissenborn et al. 1999). The prevalence of antibodies to HPV-5 L1 protein in these patients (25%) and in patients with extensive, second degree burns or in patients with cutaneous autoimmune bullous diseases (15%–25%) was found to be significantly higher than that in individuals with no known history of

HPV disease (5%) (Favre et al. 1998, 2000). This suggests that the extensive proliferation of keratinocytes involved in epidermal repair processes could favor the expression of betapapillomaviruses (Favre et al. 2000). Whether this could have beneficial (wound healing) or detrimental (psoriasis) consequences remains to be determined (Favre et al. 1998, 2000; Majewski et al. 1999).

Betapapillomaviruses as Defective HPVs

The genome of betapapillomaviruses is characterized by a shorter size, a specific organization of its noncoding regulatory region, and, most importantly, by the lack of an E5 or E8 ORF (Fig. 2) (Fuchs and Pfister 1996; Garcia-Vallvé et al. 2005; Nonnenmacher et al. 2006). The E5 ORF is located between the early (E) and late (L) regions of the genome of alphapapillomaviruses, such as the genital HPV types 6, 16, and 18 and the cutaneous HPV types 2 and 3. It encodes short hydrophobic proteins associated with intracellular membranes (DiMaio and Mattoon 2001; Garcia-Vallvé et al. 2005). The well-characterized HPV-16 E5 protein exhibits a weak transforming activity in vitro, mainly through its ability to upregulate the epidermal growth factor receptor (EGFR) signaling pathway in a ligand-dependent manner. Expression of HPV-16 E5 in the epidermal basal layer of transgenic mice induces epidermal hyperplasia (requiring EGFR signaling) and spontaneous skin papillomas (Genther Williams et al. 2005). The E5 protein is thus assumed to contribute

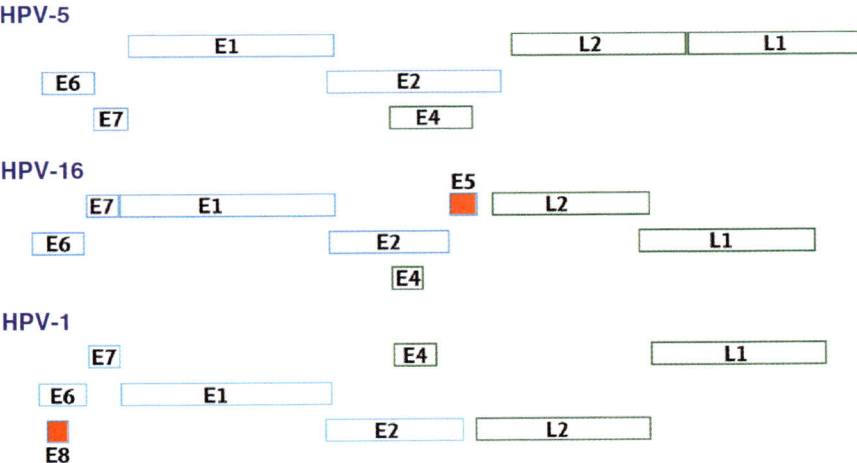

Fig. 2 Linear maps of the open reading frames of HPV-5 (*Betapapillomavirus* genus), HPV-16 (*Alphapapillomavirus* genus), and HPV-1 (*Mupapillomavirus* genus). ORFs are distributed downstream from a long regulatory noncoding region, within the early (*E*) and late (*L*) regions (Howley and Lowy 2007). Note the presence of an E5 ORF in the HPV-16 genome and an E8 ORF in the HPV-1 genome (*red boxes*), and the lack of either ORF in the HPV-5 genome

to the development of a lesion by stimulating cell division, together with the E6 and E7 proteins (DiMaio and Mattoon 2001; Maufort et al. 2007). Cutaneous HPV genotypes belonging to the genera *Gammapapillomavirus* (such as HPV-4) and *Mupapillomavirus* (HPV-1) induce skin warts, but lack an E5 ORF (de Villiers et al 2004; Garcia-Vallvé et al. 2005; Nonnenmacher et al. 2006). The E6 region of these viruses, however, harbors an E8 ORF with a coding potential for a small hydrophobic protein, structurally related to the E5 proteins (Garcia-Vallvé et al. 2005; Nonnenmacher et al. 2006). The HPV E8 proteins have not been studied yet, but recent in vivo and in vitro studies on the cottontail rabbit papillomavirus (CRPV) indicate that E8 plays a crucial role in viral pathogenesis (Nonnenmacher et al 2006)

CRPV E8 is a 50-amino acid, membrane-associated protein that shows little transforming activity in vitro (Harry and Wettstein 1996). However, E8-knockout CRPV genomes were found to display a dramatically reduced ability to induce warts upon biolistic inoculation into the skin of immunocompetent and immuno-suppressed rabbits. The scarce induced warts showed very slow growth despite sustained expression of E6 and E7 oncogenes. Intriguingly, E8 was found dispensable for wart induction (but not for growth) when the skin was first pretreated with turpentine, which promotes an acute inflammatory response, and then scarified prior to inoculation of E8-knockout genomes (Hu et al. 2002). This experimental procedure induces epidermal hyperplasia and wound healing and increases the susceptibility to CRPV infection (Friedewald 1944). Both epidermal hyperplasia and wound healing involve the release of the epidermal stem cells from their micro-environmental control (Fuchs et al. 2004; Blanpain et al. 2007), and this may allow wart induction by E8 mutants by substituting for E8 function. When expressed in cultured cells, CRPV E8, like HPV-16 E5, was found to increase the EGF-dependent extracellular signal-regulated kinase 1/2 (ERK1/2) phosphorylation, and both the EGF-dependent and the EGF-independent activity of activating protein-1 (AP-1) (Nonnenmacher et al. 2006).

E8 proteins are thus likely to be major players in the development of HPV-associated lesions, by disturbing epidermal homeostasis and promoting the proliferation of quiescent epidermal stem cells (Nonnenmacher et al. 2006). EV HPVs are usually harmless in the general population, and it can be proposed that they behave as defective viruses for an essential (E5/E8-like) growth-promoting function (Orth 2006).

The Missing Viral Function and Zinc Homeostasis

The CRPV E8 protein was found to bind to two cellular transmembrane proteins, the zinc transporter ZnT1 and protocadherin 1 (PCDH1) (Nonnenmacher et al. 2006). ZnT1 is a transporter involved in zinc efflux (Palmiter and Findley 1995) and PCDH1 is a poorly characterized protein potentially involved in cell–cell adhesion and signal transduction (Frank and Kemler 2002). This was an unexpected finding since neither protein had been linked previously to viral pathogenesis and cell transformation. Most interestingly, the HPV-16 E5 protein was also found to interact with ZnT1 and PCDH1, which supports the hypothesis that E5 and E8 proteins exert similar biological functions (Nonnenmacher et al. 2006). Both E8 and ZnT1 were found to colocalize with EGFR signaling complexes in endosomes, and CRPV E8–ZnT1 interaction was shown to be required for E8-induced AP-1 activation. Moreover, CRPV E8 was found to disrupt a complex formed by ZnT1 and PCDH1 (Nonnenmacher et al. 2006). These findings support the notion that the interaction between E8 and endogenous ZnT1 is required for the upregulation of EGFR signaling. Since zinc is a structural component of a great number of proteins, including signaling proteins and transcription factors, and is essential for their biological activities (Cousins et al. 2006), it may be expected that E8-ZnT1 interaction affects several unrelated cellular functions.

Zinc homeostasis relies on the balanced expression of the ZnT proteins, mediating zinc efflux from the cell or into intracellular organelles, and the Zip proteins, mediating zinc uptake, and on the activity of the cysteine-rich, zinc-storing metallothioneins. The regulation of the expression of ZnT1 and a number of zinc transporters and that of metallothioneins depends on a zinc-sensing protein, the metal-responsive element-binding transcription factor 1 (MTF1) (Cousins et al. 2006). Zinc homeostasis is modulated by various environmental signals, including microbial products, cytokines, antigens, oxidants, nitric oxide, and heavy metals (Spahl et al. 2003; Zhou et al. 2004; Liuzzi et al. 2005; Cousins et al. 2006; Kitamura et al. 2006; Kröncke 2007; Yamasaki et al. 2007). It has recently been proposed that zinc ions (Zn^{++}) act as an intracellular second messenger, with the potential to influence various aspects of cellular signaling (Cousins et al. 2006; Yamasaki et al. 2007).

The specific properties of EV HPVs may be explained, at least in part, by their inability to interact with mechanisms that modulate zinc homeostasis, which are likely to play a crucial role in the life cycle of these viruses. The EV phenotype would thus result from the inactivation of a cellular protein(s) or signaling pathway(s) that would compensate for the missing viral E5/E8 function(s).

The Genetic Etiology of EV: *EVER* Genes

EVER *Genes and EV*

About 10% of EV patients reported in the literature were born from consanguineous parents. About 10% of EV families have more than one affected sibling. The proportion of EV siblings approaches 25%, and the sex ratio for EV is close to one. These observations support the theory that EV is an autosomal recessive disease (MIM 226400) (Lutzner 1978). X-linked recessive inheritance was proposed for a well-documented EV family in which only males were affected (MIM 305350), pointing to a possible genetic heterogeneity of the disease (Androphy et al. 1985).

A genome-wide linkage study performed on consanguineous EV families (first-cousin marriages), using the homozygosity mapping approach, led to the mapping of a first susceptibility locus for EV (*EV1*) on chromosome 17q25, in a 1-cM region (Ramoz et al. 1999, 2000), which was narrowed to a region of about 180 kb (Ramoz et al. 2002). A second locus (*EV2*) was mapped on chromosomal region 2p21-p24, in an 8-cM interval, providing further evidence for nonallelic heterogeneity in the disease (Ramoz et al. 2000).

Mutation analysis of the genes and putative novel genes contained in the *EV1* region allowed identification of truncating mutations segregating with the disease in either of two novel related genes, which were named *EVER1* and *EVER2* (Ramoz et al. 2002). *EVER1* and *EVER2* are separated by 4.7 kb in an opposite orientation. Forty-one EV patients (either familial or sporadic cases) have now been analyzed in the course of a collaborative study between our group (N. Ramoz, C.J. Kim, P. Cassonnet, M. Favre) and B. Bouadjar (Algiers, Algeria), L.A. Rueda and L.S. Montoya (Bogota, Colombia), K. Fukai (Osaka, Japan), and S. Jablonska and S. Majewski (Warsaw, Poland). Homozygous truncating mutations in either gene were found in 31 (75.6%) cases, and four *EVER1* and six *EVER2* mutant alleles were identified in patients from Algeria, Colombia, Poland, and Japan (Ramoz et al. 2002; Orth 2006; B. Bouadjar, P. Cassonnet, M. Favre, K. Fukai, S. Jablonska, C.J. Kim, S. Majewski, L.S. Montoya, G. Orth, N Ramoz, L.A. Rueda, data to be published). The segregation of mutations in the families revealed a complete penetrance. No correlation between the genotype and the phenotype has been observed so far. Variable nucleotide positions leading to four amino acid substitutions in both EVER proteins were identified, but none of them was found to be associated with the disease. Inactivating mutations in either *EVER1* or *EVER2* have also been identified recently in one compound heterozygous Japanese patient (Tate et al. 2004) and four homozygous patients of Chinese (Sun et al. 2005; Zuo et al. 2006), Pakistani (Gober et al. 2007), and Hispanic (Berthelot et al. 2007) origin. This further stresses the worldwide association of *EVER* mutations with EV. No *EVER* mutations were detected in 25% of the EV patients of our series (including familial cases) and in a Turkish patient (Akgül et al. 2007). This brings further evidence for the genetic heterogeneity of the disease.

EVER *Genes and* TMC *Gene Family*

The *EVER* genes were found to belong to a novel gene family, the transmembrane channel-like (*TMC*) gene family, which comprises eight genes (*TMC1* to -*8*) (Kurima et al. 2003; Keresztes et al. 2003). *EVER1* and *EVER2* are identical to the *TMC6* and *TMC8* genes, respectively. All *TMC* genes are predicted to encode transmembrane proteins with six to ten membrane-spanning domains. The human *TMC* genes and their murine orthologs are highly conserved (75%–95% amino acid sequence identity, pairwise). Homologs of *TMC* genes have been identified in nonmammalian vertebrates and invertebrates (Kurima et al. 2003; Keresztes et al.

2003). All these genes encode a conserved 120-amino acid sequence. the TMC domain (Kurima et al. 2003). Dominant and recessive mutations of *TMCi* and its murine ortholog *tmc1* cause hearing loss (Kurima et al. 2002; Vreugde et al. 2002). *TMC1* and *tmc1* are expressed in cochlear hair cells of the inner ear, and *tmc1* was found to be required for the normal maturation and function of these cells (Kurima et al. 2002; Vreugde et al. 2002; Marcotti et al. 2006). The highly evolutionarily conserved *TMC* genes most likely encode proteins with important cellular roles. It has been speculated that TMC proteins could constitute a novel group of ion transporters or channels, or modifiers of such activities, and could be involved in signal transduction (Kurima et al. 2003; Keresztes et al. 2003).

EVER Proteins and Zinc Homeostasis

Transcripts spanning the full length of the ORFs of *EVER1/TMC6* (20 exons) and *EVER2/TMC8* (16 exons) encode putative proteins of 805 amino acids and 726 amino acids, respectively. Alternative splice events generate smaller *EVER1/TMC6* and *EVER2/TMC8* transcripts, which would encode protein isoforms of 454 amino acids and 503 amino acids, respectively (Ramoz et al. 2002). The EVER1 and EVER2 proteins share 28.4% of their amino acids, the less conserved regions being their amino- and carboxyl-termini. Both proteins are predicted to be integral membrane proteins with ten (EVER1) or eight (EVER2) putative transmembrane domains, two (EVER1) or three (EVER2) putative leucine-zipper motifs and two putative glycosylation sites. The terminal regions are predicted to be lumenal for EVER1 and cytoplasmic for EVER2 (Q7Z403 and Q8IU68, respectively; UniProtKB/Swiss-Prot database). Both proteins were found located in the endoplasmic reticulum when transiently expressed in human keratinocytes (HaCat cells) (Ramoz et al. 2002). All mutations identified so far eliminate the conserved TMC domain located immediately upstream of the ninth (EVER1/TMC6) or seventh (EVER2/TMC8) putative transmembrane domain (Fig. 3).

The functions of the related, membrane-spanning EVER1/TMC6 and EVER2/TMC8 proteins had remained unknown until recent work demonstrating that EVER proteins regulate cellular zinc balance (Lazarczyk et al. 2008). EVER1 and EVER2 proteins were shown to form a complex and to interact with the zinc transporter ZnT1. Neither EVER nor ZnT1proteins interacted with the E6 and E7 oncoproteins of HPV-5 and HPV-16, but they were found to bind the HPV-16 E5 protein, as already reported for ZnT1 (Nonnenmacher et al. 2006). When expressed in human keratinocytes (HaCat cells), EVER and Znt1 were found to downregulate transcription factors stimulated by zinc (MTF-1) or by cytokines (c-Jun and Elk), and this negative regulation was blocked by HPV-16 E5 (Lazarczyk et al. 2008).

The demonstration that the proteins encoded by the viral E5/E8 genes (missing in EV HPVs) and the cellular *EVER* genes share the same cellular partner, ZnT1, and are likely to modulate zinc homeostasis, provides exciting new insights into the pathogenesis of EV.

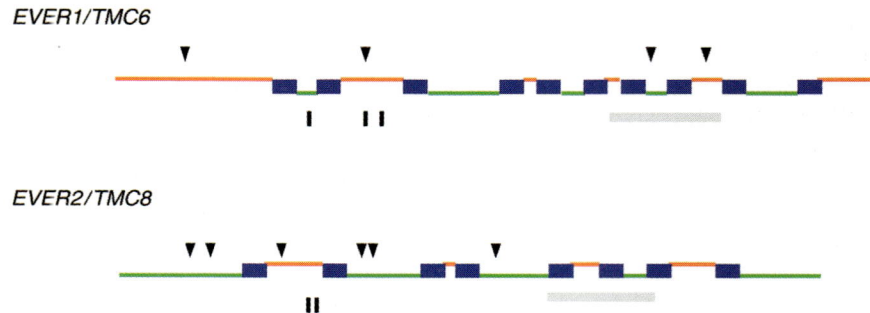

Fig. 3 Schematic representation of *EVER1* and *EVER2* genes showing location of mutations in EV patients. The transmembrane domains are represented by *blue boxes*, the putative cytoplasmic and lumenal regions by *red* and *green lines*, respectively, and the conserved TMC domain by a *gray box*. *Arrowheads* represent mutations identified in our study, and *vertical bars* indicate mutations reported in the literature for *EVER1* (Tate et al. 2004; Zuo et al. 2006; Gober et al. 2007) and *EVER2* (Sun et al. 2005; Berthelot et al. 2007)

EV as a Primary Immunodeficiency Disease

Two Nonmutually Exclusive Hypotheses for EV Pathogenesis

EV is one of the Mendelian conditions manifesting as a narrow susceptibility to infections in otherwise healthy patients (with no overt immunological phenotype), which constitute a newly recognized group of "nonconventional" human PIDs (Casanova et al. 2005). These Mendelian traits include both hematopoietic and nonhematopoietic PIDs, as host defenses not only involve immunological cells of hematopoietic origin but also other cells playing an important role in local immune responses, such as endothelial cells, enterocytes, and keratinocytes (Casanova and Abel 2007). Such diseases have proved to be valuable model systems to dissect the molecular mechanisms underlying immunity to infection in humans (Casanova and Abel 2004, 2007; Fischer 2004).

The strictly epitheliotropic, cutaneous human papillomaviruses most likely target the epidermal stem cells, and their life cycle is tightly linked to the biology of their host cells (Longworth and Laimins 2004; Orth 2008). Keratinocytes are not only responsible for the renewal, cohesion, and barrier function of the skin but also contribute to the skin immune system by secreting, and responding to, various cytokines, chemokines, and growth factors, allowing a cross-talk between keratinocytes and immunocytes (Kupper and Fuhlbrigge 2004; Bos 2005; Nickoloff 2007). Furthermore, keratinocytes express Toll-like receptors (TLRs), and immune responses are initiated after the activation of these receptors by their respective microbial ligands (Lebre et al. 2007; Miller and Modlin 2007). It has been shown that *EVER* genes are transcribed in the normal human skin (Ramoz et al. 2002), highly transcribed in CD4[+] and CD8[+] T lymphocytes, B lymphocytes, and NK cells, and, for *EVER1* at least, significantly transcribed in endothelial cells, bone marrow CD33[+] myeloid cells, and dendritic cells (Su et al. 2004; http://symatlas.gnf.org).

When discussing the role of *EVER* genes in the pathogenesis of EV, two hypotheses can thus be proposed that are not mutually exclusive: (1) EVER proteins act as restriction factors that hinder the complete expression of the EV HPV genomes in keratinocytes and the development of EV lesions (the EV phenotype), (2) EVER proteins play a specific role in the innate immune responses and the shaping of adaptive immunity against EV HPV-infected keratinocytes (Orth 2006).

A Primary Deficiency in Intrinsic Immunity

Intrinsic immunity is the front line of host defense against viral infections and does not require any virus-triggered signaling or intercellular communication (Bieniasz 2004). It can be assumed that, by modulating zinc homeostasis, EVER proteins contribute to a regulatory pathway controlling the division of epidermal stem cells. It is worth stressing recent studies indicating that the *Caenorhabditis elegans* homolog of ZnT1, the cation diffusion facilitator1, is a positive modulator of EGFR signaling in vulval development (Bruinsma et al. 2002), and that the zinc transporter LIV1/Zip6 controls epithelial–mesenchymal transition during gastrulation in zebrafish (Yamashita et al. 2004). Our hypothesis implies that EVER proteins act as dominant restriction factors for HPVs, and that the function of E5/E8 proteins is, at least in part, to overcome this restriction and to trigger the viral life cycle. It is thus tempting to speculate that the inactivation of *EVER1/TMC6* or *EVER2/TMC8* compensates for the missing EV HPV E5/E8 protein in the induction of EV lesions (Nonnenmacher et al. 2006; Orth 2006). According to this hypothesis, host restriction of betapapillomaviruses in patients harboring wildtype *EVER* genes should be overcome by co-infection of EV HPV-infected keratinocytes with a genotype expressing a functional E5/E8 protein. Notably, high levels of EV HPV DNA (easily detected by Southern blot hybridization) have been detected in warts induced by HPV-3 or related genotypes (alphapapillomaviruses) in some immunosuppressed patients (Obalek et al. 1992).

A Primary Defect in Innate Immunity

If one considers that a primary defect in intrinsic immunity may be responsible for the growth of EV lesions in genetically predisposed individuals, it remains to be understood why these lesions never regress. This is in contrast with cutaneous warts caused by alpha-, gamma-, or mupapillomaviruses, which usually retrogress in the general population under the influence of cell-mediated immune responses (Tagami et al. 1985; Stanley 2006). Typical HPV-5-associated scaly macules were reported to have regressed in a renal allograft recipient (phenocopy of EV) after withdrawal of azathioprine, an immunosuppressive drug (Lutzner et al. 1983). EV patients may thus present a specific immune defect, as suggested by early studies (Cooper et al. 1990; Majewski et al. 1990).

A Central Role for Keratinocytes?

Since *EVER* genes are expressed in the skin (Ramoz et al. 2002) and various hematopoietic immune cell types (Su et al. 2004; http://symatlas.gnf.org), *EVER* mutations might affect various arms of the immune response to EV HPVs. The phenotype resulting from inactivation of either *EVER* gene in the mouse is, unfortunately, still unknown. As the home cells of HPVs, and as important elements of the skin immune system (Kupper and Fuhlbrigge 2004; Bos 2005; Nickoloff 2007), keratinocytes are thought to play a central role in the innate and adaptive immune responses to papillomaviruses. The resident skin immature antigen-presenting cells, epidermal Langerhans cells and dermal dendritic cells, may also encounter viral particles during primary infection, following a microtrauma of the skin (Orth 2008). Generally speaking, antiviral responses are initiated after receptors expressed in different cell compartments, such as TLRs, recognize pathogen-associated molecular patterns (PAMPs). Pattern recognition results in (1) the production of type I interferons and proinflammatory cytokines and chemokines, (2) the activation of dendritic cells, and (3) the development of adaptive antiviral immune responses (Beutler et al. 2006; Kawai and Akira 2006). The only PAMP identified to date for HPVs is the viral capsid, a highly ordered structure. Papillomavirus-like particles (very similar to the capsids of native virions) have been shown to effectively activate human dendritic cells, but not Langerhans cells, and to directly activate B cells to induce CD4[+] T cell-independent humoral responses, both cell activations occurring via TLR4-MyD88-dependent signaling pathways (Fausch et al. 2002; Yang et al. 2004, 2005). Whether functional EVER proteins are required remains to be established. TLRs expressed by keratinocytes have been found to functionally respond to ligands mimicking viral PAMPs, synthetic double-stranded RNA (poly I:C), and CpG-oligodeoxynucleotides (Lebre et al. 2007). No data are yet available on the innate responses of keratinocytes to HPV capsids.

Zinc, EVER Proteins, and Immunity to HPVs

Since the EVER proteins have recently been shown to regulate cellular zinc balance by interacting with ZnT1 (Lazarczyk et al. 2008), it is conceivable that a modulation of the concentration or localization of intracellular free zinc ions is required for signaling pathways triggered by EV HPVs in keratinocytes or other immune cells. It is well known that zinc deficiency results in defects in innate and acquired immunity and in an increased susceptibility to infections (Wellinghausen et al. 1997; Fischer and Black 2004; Rink and Haase 2007). The link between zinc homeostasis and immunity is well illustrated by acrodermatitis enteropathica (MIM 201100), a rare, autosomal, recessively inherited disease caused by mutations in the gene encoding the zinc transporter Zip4 and a defect in zinc uptake by intestinal cells. This defect results in, among other symptoms, dermatitis and diarrhea, reflecting a dysfunction of the immune system (Wang et al. 2002; Rink and Haase 2007). Mutations in ZnT1 are unlikely to cause any disease, since this gene was found to be essential for early embryonic development in the mouse (Andrews et al. 2004). Interestingly, topical zinc oxide and oral zinc sulfate were reported to represent an efficacious therapeutic option for recalcitrant skin warts (Al-Gurairi et al. 2002; Khattar et al. 2007).

Recent studies have shown how variations in intracellular concentrations of free zinc influence signaling pathways mediating the cellular responses to various stimulations (Spahl et al. 2003; Zhou et al. 2004; Liuzzi et al. 2005; Cousins et al. 2006; Kitamura et al. 2006; Kröncke 2007; Yamasaki et al. 2007). For instance, variations in the concentration or localization of intracellular free Zn^{++} ions are involved in the maturation of murine dendritic cells induced by the TLR4 ligand lipopolysaccharide (LPS) (Kitamura et al. 2006), the activation of mast cells after cross-linking of the high affinity receptor FcεRI (Yamasaki et al. 2007), the response of endothelial cells to inflammatory cytokines (Spahl et al. 2003), and the production of inflammatory cytokines by monocytes (von Bülow et al. 2005). Coexpression of EVER and ZnT1 proteins in human keratinocytes has been shown to downregulate transcription factors stimulated by cytokines (Lazarczyk et al. 2008). How the EVER proteins could participate in the cross-talk between keratinocytes and immunocytes remains to be understood.

If modulations of zinc homeostasis are involved in innate immune defenses and the shaping of acquired immunity to HPVs, the signaling pathways mediated by the EVER proteins should be crucial for protection against betapapillomaviruses, but be redundant for immunity to other HPV genotypes. The other Mendelian traits characterized by a narrow vulnerability to microorganisms have taught us already that major pathways (such as the IL-12–IFN-γ, TIR–NF-κB, or TLR3–IFN-α/β pathways) may be critical for protective immunity against specific viruses or bacteria but redundant for immunity to most other pathogens (Casanova and Abel 2007).

Viral Proteins, Immune Evasion, and EV Persistence

The genital oncogenic alphapapillomaviruses (such as HPV-16 and HPV-18) have evolved strategies to evade host immunity. The multifunctional E6 and E7 oncoproteins are endowed with the capacity to interfere with the expression of, or the response to, type I interferons and inflammatory cytokines or chemokines, and this may contribute to the suppression of antiviral responses and to the persistence of infection (Frazer et al. 1999; Koromilas et al. 2001; Guess and McCance 2005; Stanley 2006). The whole spectrum of viral proteins is expressed in EV lesions, and similar viral mechanisms could contribute to the lifelong persistence of the disease. The overexpression of TNF-α and TGF-β may represent such a mechanism

(Majewski et al. 1991). A defect in local CMI revealed by an anergy to contact sensitizers, and other abnormalities in nonspecific CMI and have been observed in most, but not all, EV patients (Majewski and Jablonska 1995; Oliveira et al. 2003). Whether these abnormalities are linked to *EVER* mutations or are secondary to a longstanding massive infection remains to be understood.

Concluding Remarks

Little is known about the genetic factors controlling HPV infections, from latency to invasive carcinoma. As a Mendelian trait, EV represents an outstanding model for studying the part played by viral and host genetic factors in the outcome of these infections. New insights in the pathogenesis of EV have recently been gained from three major advances: (1) EV-specific HPVs are likely to be defective for an important growth-promoting function encoded by the E5/E8 gene present in other HPV genotypes (Nonnenmacher et al. 2006; Orth 2006); (2) most EV cases are caused by inactivating mutations within the related *EVER1* and *EVER2* genes (Ramoz et al. 2002; Orth 2006); (3) the transmembrane viral E5/E8 and cellular EVER proteins share the same cellular partner, the zinc transporter ZnT1, and both are likely to modulate zinc homeostasis (Nonnenmacher et al. 2006; Lazarczyk et al. 2008). Since zinc is an essential factor required for the structure and function of a great number of proteins, variations in zinc homeostasis may influence many aspects of cellular signaling in immune or nonimmune cells (Cousins et al. 2006; Rink and Haase 2007; Yamasaki et al. 2007). According to the two nonmutually exclusive hypotheses that can be proposed, EV may represent a primary deficiency in intrinsic (constitutive) immunity to betapapillomaviruses, a primary deficiency in innate immunity against these viruses, or both. The mechanisms for the control of EV HPV infections by EVER proteins in keratinocytes, which are likely to play a central role, and immune cells remain to be established. It must be stressed that only 75% of the patients studied so far harbor an *EVER* mutation. A second EV susceptibility locus (2p21-p24) with an autosomal recessive mode of transmission has been identified (Ramoz et al. 2000), and evidence for an X-linked recessive inheritance has been reported (Androphy et al. 1985). Identification of additional genes associated with EV should provide further clues for understanding host defenses against papillomaviruses.

It thus appears likely that, in the general population, susceptibility or resistance to HPV infections and HPV-associated diseases depends both on the diversity of HPV genotypes and on mutations in, or allelic polymorphisms of, host genes involved in intrinsic, innate, or adaptive immunity. We are just beginning to discover the nature of these genes. If EVER proteins play a part in host defenses against all HPVs, as suggested by the interaction between HPV-16 E5 and both ZnT1 and EVER proteins (Nonnenmacher et al. 2006; Lazarczyk et al. 2008), the pathways involved should be redundant for genotypes other than EV HPVs. SCID patients and patients suffering from WHIM syndrome have taught us that γc/JAK-3 and CXCR4 signaling pathways are crucial for immunity against HPVs (Hernandez et al. 2003; Laffort et al. 2004). Focal epithelial hyperplasia of the oral mucosa, or Heck's disease, is another HPV-associated Mendelian trait (MIM 229045) that could allow further advances. Heck's disease is specifically associated with two oral alphapapillomaviruses, HPV types 13 and 32, and is observed predominantly among Eskimos and American Indians (Archard et al. 1965; Beaudenon et al. 1987). No susceptibility locus has been identified so far for this disease.

Unraveling the genetic bases of the susceptibility to HPV infections and diseases represents a major issue. The challenge is to understand why and how genital alphapapillomaviruses, including potentially carcinogenic genotypes, often cause asymptomatic, transient infections, and why only a minority of the infected women will develop invasive anogenital cancers (Bosch et al. 2002; Schiffman and Kjaer 2003).

Acknowledgements This review is dedicated to Prof. Stefania Jablonska (Warsaw, Poland). I thank the patients and their families for their trust. I acknowledge our colleagues dermatologists B. Bouadjar, K. Fukai, S. Majewski, and L.-A. Rueda, and the members of the former Papillomavirus Unit for their contribution to the work discussed in this review. I would also like to thank F. Breitburd for stimulating discussions.

References

Akgül B, Köse O, Safali M, Purdie K, Cerio R, Proby C, Storey A (2007) A distinct variant of epidermodysplasia verruciformis in a Turkish family lacking EVER1 and EVER2 mutations. J Dermatol Sci 46:214–216

Al-Gurairi FT, Al-Waiz M, Sharquie KE (2002) Oral zinc sulfate in the treatment of recalcitrant viral warts: randomized placebo-controlled clinical trial. Br J Dermatol 146:423–431

Alonso I, Fuchs E (2003) Stem cells of the skin epithelium. Proc Natl Acad Sci USA 100:11830–11835

Andrews GK, Wang H, Dey SK, Palmiter RD (2004) Mouse zinc transporter 1 gene provides an essential function during early embryonic development. Genesis 40:74–81

Androphy EJ, Dvoretzky I, Lowy DR (1985) X-linked inheritance of epidermodysplasia verruciformis: genetic and virologic studies of a kindred. Arch Dermatol 121:864–868

Antonsson A, Forslund O, Ekberg H, Sterner G, Hansson BG (2000) The ubiquity and impressive genomic diversity of human skin papillomaviruses suggest a commensalic nature of these viruses. J Virol 74:11636–11641

Antonsson A, Karanfilovska S, Lindqvist PG, Hansson BG (2003) General acquisition of human papillomavirus infections of skin occurs in early infancy. J Clin Microbiol 4:2509–2514

Archard HO, Heck JW, Stanley HR (1965) Focal epithelial hyperplasia: an unusual oral mucosal lesion found in Indian children. Oral Surg Oral Med Oral Pathol 20:201–212

Astori G, Lavergne D, Benton C, Hockmayr B, Egawa K, Garbe C, de Villiers EM (1998) Human papillomaviruses are commonly found in normal skin of immunocompetent hosts. J Invest Dermatol 110:752–755

Barr BB, Benton EC, Mc Laren K, Bunney MH, Smith IW, Blessing K, Hunter JA (1989) Human papillomavirus infection and skin cancer in renal allograft recipients. Lancet 1:124–129

Beaudenon S, Praetorius F, Kremsdorf D, Lutzner M, Worsaae N, Pehau-Arnaudet G, Orth G (1987) A new type of human papillomavirus associated with oral focal epithelial hyperplasia. J Invest Dermatol 88:130–135

Berthelot C, Dickerson MC, Rady P, He Q, Niroomand F, Tyring SK, Pandya AG (2007) Treatment of a patient with epidermodysplasia verruciformis carrying a novel EVER2 mutation with imiquimod. J Am Acad Dermatol 56:882–886

Beutler B, Jiang Z, Georgel P, Crozat K, Croker B, Rutschmann S, Du X, Hoebe K (2006) Genetic analysis of host resistance: Toll-like receptor signaling and immunity at large. Annu Rev Immunol 24:353–389

Bieniasz PD (2004) Intrinsic immunity: a front-line defense against viral attack. Nat Immunol 5:1109–1115

Blanpain C, Horsley V, Fuchs E (2007) Epithelial stem cells: turning over new leaves. Cell 128:445–458

Bos JD (ed) (2005) Skin immune system. Cutaneous immunology and clinical immunodermatology. 3rd edition, Boca Raton, CRC Press

Bosch FX, Lorincz A, Munoz N, Meijer CJ, Shah KV (2002) The causal relation between human papillomavirus and cervical cancer. J Clin Pathol 55:244–265

Boxman ILA, Berkhout RJM, Mulder LHC, Wolkers MC, Bouwes Bavinck JN, Vermeer BJ, ter Schegget J (1997) Detection of human papillomavirus DNA in plucked hairs from renal transplant recipients and healthy volunteers. J Invest Dermatol 108:712–715

Brash DE (1997) Sunlight and the onset of skin cancer. Trends Genet 13:410–414

Bruinsma JJ, Jirakulaporn T, Muslin AJ, Kornfeld K (2002) Zinc ions and cation diffusion facilitator proteins regulate Ras-mediated signaling. Dev Cell 2:567–578

Bruton OC (1952) Agammaglobulinemia. Pediatrics 9:722–728

Carré D, Dompmartin A, Verdon R, Comoz F, Le Brun E, Freymuth F, Leroy D (2003) Epidermodysplasia verruciformis in a patient with HIV infection: no response to highly active antiretroviral therapy. Int J Dermatol 42:296–300

Casanova JL, Abel L (2004) The human model: a genetic dissection of immunity to infection in natural conditions. Nat Rev Immunol 4:55–66

Casanova JL, Abel L (2007) Primary immunodeficiencies: a field in its infancy. Science 317:617–619

Casanova JL, Fieschi C, Bustamante J, Reichenbach J, Remus N, von Bernuth H, Picard C (2005) From idiopathic infectious diseases to novel primary immunodeficiencies. J Allergy Clin Immunol 116:426–430

Cockayne EA (1933) Inherited abnormalities of the skin and its appendages. Oxford University Press, London, p 156

Coleman N, Birley HDL, Renton AM, Hanna NF, Ryait BK, Byrne M, Taylor-Robinson D, Stanley MA (1994) Immunological events in regressing genital warts. Am J Clin Pathol 102:768–774

Cooper KD, Androphy EJ, Lowy D, Katz SI (1990) Antigen presentation and T-cell activation in epidermodysplasia verruciformis. J Invest Dermatol 94:769–776

Cousins RJ, Liuzzi JP, Lichten LA (2006) Mammalian zinc transport, trafficking, and signals. J Biol Chem 281:24085–24089

de Villiers EM, Fauquet C, Broker TR, Bernard HU, zur Hausen H (2004) Classification of papillomaviruses. Virology 324:17–27

DiMaio D, Mattoon D (2001) Mechanisms of cell transformation by papillomavirus E5 proteins. Oncogene 20:7866–7873

Euvrard S, Kanitakis J, Claudy A (2003) Skin cancers after organ transplantation. N Engl J Med 348:1681–1691

Fausch SC, Da Silva DM, Rudolf MP, Kast WM (2002) Human papillomavirus virus-like particles do not activate Langerhans cells: a possible immune escape mechanism used by human papillomaviruses. J Immunol 169:3242–3249

Favre M, Orth G, Majewski S, Baloul S, Pura A, Jablonska S (1998) Psoriasis: a possible reservoir for human papillomavirus type 5, the virus associated with skin carcinomas of epidermodysplasia verruciformis. J Invest Dermatol 110:311–317

Favre M, Majewski S, Noszczyk B, Maienfisch F, Pura A, Orth G, Jablonska S (2000) Antibodies to human papillomavirus type 5 are generated in epidermal repair processes. J Invest Dermatol 114:403–407

Feltkamp MCW, Broer R, di Summa FM, Struijk L, van der Meijden E, Verlaan BPJ, Westendorp RGJ, ter Schegget J, Spaan WJM, Bouwes Bavinck JN (2003) Seroreactivity to epidermodysplasia verruciformis-related human papillomavirus types is associated with nonmelanoma skin cancer. Cancer Res 63:2695–2700

Fischer A (2004) Human primary immunodeficiency diseases: a perspective. Nat Immunol 5:23–30

Fischer WC, Black RE (2004) Zinc and the risk for infectious disease. Annu Rev Nutr 24:255–275

Frank M, Kemler R (2002) Protocadherins. Curr Opin Cell Biol 14:557–562

Frazer IH, Thomas R, Zhou J, Leggatt GR, Dunn L, McMillan N, Tindle RW, Filgueira L, Manders P, Barnard P, Sharkey M (1999) Potential strategies utilised by papillomavirus to evade host immunity. Immunol Rev 168:131–142

Friedewald WF (1944) Certain conditions determining enhanced infection with the rabbit papilloma virus. J Exp Med 80:65–76

Fuchs E, Tumbar T, Guasch G (2004) Socializing with the neighbors: stem cells and their niche. Cell 116:769–778

Fuchs PG, Pfister H (1996) Papillomaviruses in epidermodysplasia verruciformis. In: Lacey C (ed) Papillomavirus reviews: current research on papillomaviruses, vol 2 (The papillomaviruses). Leeds University Press, Leeds, pp 253–261

Garcia-Vallvé S, Alonso A, Bravo IG (2005) Papillomaviruses: different genes have different histories. Trends Microbiol 13:514–521

Genther Williams SM, Disbrow GL, Schlegel R, Lee D, Threadgill DW, Lambert PF (2005) Requirement of epidermal growth factor receptor for hyperplasia induced by E5, a high-risk human papillomavirus oncogene. Cancer Res 65:6534–6542

Glinski W, Jablonska S, Langner A, Obalek S, Haftek M, Proniewska M (1976) Cell-mediated immunity in epidermodysplasia verruciformis. Dermatologica 153:218–227

Glinski W, Obalek S, Jablonska S, Orth G (1981) T-cells defect in patients with epidermodysplasia verruciformis due to human papillomavirus types 3 and 5. Dermatologica 162:141–147

Gober MD, Rady PL, He Q, Turker SB, Tyring SK, Gaspari AA (2007) Novel homozygous frameshift mutation of *EVER1* gene in an epidermodysplasia verruciformis patient. J Invest Dermatol 127:817–820

Gorlin RJ, Gelb B, Diaz GA, Lofsness KG, Pittelkow MR, Fenyk JR (2000) WHIM syndrome, an autosomal dominant disorder: clinical, hematological, and molecular studies. Am J Med Genet 91:368–376

Guess JC, McCance DJ (2005) Decreased migration of Langerhans precursor-like cells in response to human keratinocytes expressing human papillomavirus type 16 E6/E7 is related to reduced macrophage inflammatory protein-3a production. J Virol 79:14852–14862

Harry JB, Wettstein FO (1996) Transforming properties of the cottontail rabbit papillomavirus oncoproteins LE6 and SE6 and the E8 protein. J Virol 70:3355–3362

Harwood CA, Proby CM (2002) Human papillomaviruses and non-melanoma skin cancer. Curr Opin Infect Dis 15:101–114

Hernandez PA, Gorlin RJ, Lukens JN, Taniuchi S, Bohinjec J, Francois F, Klotman ME, Diaz GA (2003) Mutations in the chemokine receptor gene *CXCR4* are associated with WHIM syndrome, a combined immunodeficiency disease. Nat Genet 34:70–74

Howley PM, Lowy DR (2007) Papillomaviruses. In: Knipe DM, Howley PM, Griffin DE, et al (eds) Fields virology, 5th edn. Wolters Kluwer/Lippincott Williams and Wilkins, Philadelphia, pp 2299–2354

Hu J, Han R, Cladel NM, Pickel MD, Christensen ND (2002) Intracutaneous DNA vaccination with the E8 gene of cottontail rabbit papillomavirus induces protective immunity against virus challenge in rabbits. J Virol 76:6453–6459

Jablonska S, Formas I (1959) Weitere positive Ergebnisse mit Auto- und Heteroinokulation bei Epidermodysplasia verruciformis Lewandowsky-Lutz. Dermatologica 118:86–93

Jablonska S, Orth G (1985) Epidermodysplasia verruciformis. Clin Dermatol 3(4):83–96

Jablonska S, Dabrowski J, Jakubowicz K (1972) Epidermodysplasia verruciformis as a model in studies on the role of papovaviruses in oncogenesis. Cancer Res 32:583–589

Jablonska S, Orth G, Jarzabek-Chorzelska M, Rzesa G, Obalek S, Glinski W, Favre M, Croissant O (1979) Epidermodysplasia verruciformis versus disseminated verrucae planae: is epidermodysplasia verruciformis a generalized infection with wart virus? J Invest Dermatol 72: 114–119

Karagas MR, Nelson HH, Sehr P, Waterboer T, Stukel TA, Andrew A, Green AC, Bouwes Bavinck JN, Perry A, Spencer S, Rees JR, Mott LA, Pawlita M (2006) Human papillomavirus infection and incidence of squamous cell and basal cell carcinomas of the skin. J Natl Cancer Inst 98:389–395

Kawai T, Akira S (2006) Innate immune recognition of viral infection. Nat Immunol 7:131–137

Kawashima M, Favre M, Obalek S, Jablonska S, Orth G (1990) Premalignant lesions and cancers of the skin in the general population: evaluation of the role of human papillomaviruses. J Invest Dermatol 95:537–542

Keresztes G, Mutai H, Heller S (2003) TMC and EVER genes belong to a larger novel family, the TMC gene family encoding transmembrane proteins. BMC Genomics 4:24–35

Khattar JA, Musharrafieh UM, Tamim H, Hamadeh GN (2007) Topical zinc oxide vs. salicylic acid-lactic acid combination in the treatment of warts. Int J Dermatol 46:427–430

Kitamura H, Morikawa H, Kamon H, Iguchi M, Hojyo S, Fukada T, Yamashita S, Kaisho T, Akira S, Murakami M, Hirano T (2006) Toll-like receptor-mediated regulation of zinc homeostasis influences dendritic cell function. Nat Immunol 7:971–977

Koranda FC, Dehmel EM, Kahn G, Penn I (1974) Cutaneous complications in immunosuppressed renal homograft recipients. J Am Med Assoc 229:419–424

Koromilas AE, Li S, Matlashewski G (2001) Control of interferon signaling in human papillomavirus infection. Cytokine Growth Factor Rev 12:157–170

Kröncke KD (2007) Cellular stress and intracellular zinc dyshomeostasis. Arch Biochem Biophys 463:183–187

Kupper TS, Fuhlbrigge RC (2004) Immune surveillance in the skin: mechanisms and clinical consequences. Nat Rev Immunol 4:211–212

Kurima K, Peters LM, Yang Y, Riazuddin S, Ahmed ZM, Naz S, Arnaud D, Drury S, Mo J, Makishima T, Ghosh M, Menon PSN, Deshmukh D, Oddoux C, Ostrer H, Khan S, Riazuddin S, Deininger PL, Hampton LL, Sullivan SL, Battey JF, Keats BJB, Wilcox ER, Friedman TB, Griffith AJ (2002) Dominant and recessive deafness caused by mutations of a novel gene TMC1 required for cochlear hair-cell function. Nat Genet 30:277–284

Kurima K, Yang Y, Sorber K, Griffith AJ (2003) Characterization of the transmembrane channel-like (TMC) gene family: functional clues from hearing loss and epidermodysplasia verruciformis. Genomics 82:300–308

Laffort C, Le Deist F, Favre M, Caillat-Zucman S, Radford-Weiss I, Debré M, Fraitag S, Blanche S, Cavazzana-Calvo M, de Saint Basile G, de Villartay P, Giliani S, Orth G, Casanova JL, Bodemer C, Fischer A (2004) Severe cutaneous papillomavirus disease after haemopoietic stem-cell transplantation in patients with severe combined immune deficiency caused by common gamma cytokine receptor subunit or JAK-3 deficiency. Lancet 363:2051–2054

Lazarczyk M, Pons C, Mendoza JA, Cassonnet P, Jacob Y, Favre M (2008) Regulation of cellular zinc balance as a potential mechanism of EVER-mediated protection against pathogenesis by cutaneous oncogenic human papillomaviruses. J Exp Med 205:35–42

Lebre MC, van der Aar AM, van Baarsen L, van Capel TMM, Schuitemaker JHN, Kapsenberg ML, de Jong EC (2007) Human keratinocytes express functional Toll-like receptor 3, 4, 5 and 9. J Invest Dermatol 127:331–341

Lewandowsky F, Lutz W (1922) Ein Fall einer bisher nicht beschriebenen Hauterkrankung (Epidermodysplasia verruciformis). AMA Arch Derm Syphilol 141:193–203

Liuzzi JP, Lichten LA, Rivera S, Blanchard RK, Aydemir TB, Knutson MD, Ganz T, Cousins RJ (2005) Interleukin-6 regulates the zinc transporter Zip14 in liver and contributes to the hypozincemia of the acute-phase response. Proc Natl Acad Sci USA 102:6843–6848

Longworth MS, Laimins LA (2004) Pathogenesis of human papillomaviruses in differentiating epithelia. Microbiol Mol Biol Rev 68:362–372

Lutz WA (1946) A propos de l'épidermodysplasie verruciforme. Dermatologica 92:30–43

Lutzner MA (1978) Epidermodysplasia verruciformis: an autosomal recessive disease character-ized by viral warts and skin cancer. A model for viral oncogenesis. Bull Cancer 65 169–182

Lutzner MA, Croissant O, Ducasse MF, Kreis H, Crosnier J, Orth G (1980) A potentially onco-genic human papillomavirus (HPV5) found in two renal allograft recipients. J Invest Dermatol 75:353–356

Lutzner MA, Orth G, Dutronquay V, Ducasse MF, Kreis H, Crosnier J (1983) Detection of human papillomavirus type 5 DNA in skin cancers of an immunosuppressed renal allograft recipient. Lancet 2:422–424

Lutzner MA, Blanchet-Bardon C, Orth G (1984) Clinical observations, virologic studies, and treatment trials in patients with epidermodysplasia verruciformis, a disease induced by specific human papillomaviruses. J Invest Dermatol 83:18s–25s

Majewski S, Jablonska S (1992) Epidermodysplasia verruciformis as a model of human papillomavirus-induced genetic cancers: the role of local immunosurveillance. Am J Med Sci 304:174–179

Majewski S, Jablonska S (1995) Epidermodysplasia verruciformis as a model of human papillomavirus-induced genetic cancer of the skin. Arch Dermatol 131:1312–1318

Majewski S, Skopinska-Rozewska E, Jablonska S, Wasik M, Misiewicz J, Orth G (1986) Partial defects of cell mediated immunity in patients with epidermodysplasia verruciformis. J Am Acad Dermatol 15:966–973

Majewski S, Malejczyk J, Jablonska S, Misiewicz J, Rudnicka L, Obalek S, Orth G (1990) Natural cell-mediated cytotoxicity against various target cells in patients with epidermodysplasia ver-ruciformis. J Am Acad Dermatol 22:423–427

Majewski S, Hunzelmann N, Nischt R, Eckes B, Rudnicka L, Orth G (1991) TGF beta-1 and TNF alpha expression in the epidermis of patients with epidermodysplasia verruciformis. J Invest Dermatol 97:862–867

Majewski S, Jablonska S, Orth G (1997) Epidermodysplasia verruciformis. Immunological and nonimmunological surveillance mechanisms: role in tumor progression. Clin Dermatol 15:321–334

Majewski S, Jablonska S, Favre M, Ramoz N, Orth G (1999) Papillomavirus and autoimmunity in psoriasis. Immunol Today 20:475–476

Marcotti W, Erven A, Johnson SL, Steel KP, Kros CJ (2006) Tmc1 is necessary for normal func-tional maturation and survival of inner and outer hair cells in the mouse cochlea. J Physiol 574:677–698

Maufort JP, Williams SM, Pitot HC, Lambert PF (2007) Human papillomavirus 16 E5 oncogene contributes to two stages of skin carcinogenesis. Cancer Res 67:6106–6112

Mendoza JA, Jacob Y, Cassonnet P, Favre M (2006) Human papillomavirus type 5 E6 oncoprotein represses the transforming growth factor β signaling pathway by binding to SMAD3. J Virol 80:12420–12424

Miller LS, Modlin RL (2007) Human keratinocyte Toll-like receptors promote distinct immune responses. J Invest Dermatol 127:262–263

Münger K, Baldwin A, Edwards KM, Hayakawa H, Nguyen CL, Owens M, Grace M, Huh KW (2004) Mechanisms of human papillomavirus-induced oncogenesis. J Virol 78:11451–11460

Nickoloff BJ (2007) Cracking the cytokine code in psoriasis. Nat Med 13:242–244

Nonnenmacher M, Salmon J, Jacob Y, Orth G, Breitburd F (2006) Cottontail rabbit papillomavirus E8 protein is essential for wart formation and provides new insights into viral pathogenesis. J Virol 80:4890–4900

Obalek S, Favre M, Szymanczyk J, Misiewicz J, Jablonska S, Orth G (1992) Human papillomavi-rus (HPV) types specific of epidermodysplasia verruciformis detected in warts induced by HPV3 or HPV3-related types in immunosuppressed patients. J Invest Dermatol 98:936–941

Oliveira WRP, Carrasco S, Neto CF, Rady P, Tyring SK (2003) Nonspecific cell-mediated immu-nity in patients with epidermodysplasia verruciformis. J Dermatol 30:203–209

Orth G (1987) Epidermodysplasia verruciformis. In: Howley PM, Salzman NP (eds) The papova-viridae. Vol 2 The papillomaviruses. Plenum Publishing, New York, pp 199–243

Orth G (2004) Human papillomaviruses and the skin: more to be learned. J Invest Dermatol 123: xi–xiii

Orth G (2005) Human papillomaviruses associated with epidermodysplasia verruciformis in non-melanoma skin cancers: guilty or innocent? J Invest Dermatol 125:xii–xiii

Orth G (2006) Genetics of epidermodysplasia verruciformis: insights into host defense against papillomaviruses. Semin Immunol 18:362–374

Orth G (2008) General features of human papillomaviruses. In: Mahy B, Van Regelmortel M (eds) Encyclopedia of virology, 3rd edn. Elsevier, Oxford (in press)

Orth G, Jablonska S, Favre M, Croissant O, Jarzabek-Chorzelska M, Rzesa G (1978) Characterization of two types of human papillomaviruses in lesions of epidermodysplasia verruciformis. Proc Natl Acad Sci USA 75:1537–1541

Orth G, Jablonska S, Jarzabek-Chorzelska M, Rzesa G, Obalek S, Favre M, Croissant O (1979) Characteristics of the lesions and risk of malignant conversion as related to the type of the human papillomavirus involved in epidermodysplasia verruciformis. Cancer Res 39:1074–1082

Orth C, Favre M, Breitburd F, Croissant O, Jablonska S, Obalek S,Jarzabek-Chorzelska M, Rzesa G (1980) Epidermodysplasia verruciformis: a model for the role of papillomaviruses in human cancer. Cold Spring Harbor Conf Cell Prolif 7:259–282

Orth G, Favre M, Majewski S, Jablonska S (2001) Epidermodysplasia verruciformis defines a subset of cutaneous human papillomaviruses. J Virol 75:4952–4953

Ostrow RS, Bender M, Niimura M, Seki T, Kawashima M, Pass F, Faras AJ (1982) Human papillomavirus DNA in cutaneous primary and metastasized squamous cell carcinomas from patients with epidermodysplasia verruciformis. Proc Natl Acad Sci USA 79:1634–1638

Palmiter RD, Findley SD (1995) Cloning and functional characterization of a mammalian zinc transporter that confers resistance to zinc. EMBO J 14:639–649

Pass F, Reissig M, Shah KV, Eisinger M, Orth G (1977) Identification of an immunologically distinct papillomavirus from lesions of epidermodysplasia verruciformis. J Natl Cancer Inst 59:1107–1112

Pfister H (2003) Human papillomavirus and skin cancer. J Natl Cancer Inst Monogr 31:52–56

Pfister H, Gassenmaier A, Nürnberger F, Stüttgen G (1983) Human papillomavirus 5-DNA in carcinoma of an epidermodysplasia verruciformis patient infected with various human papillomavirus types. Cancer Res 43:1436–1441

Prawer SE, Pass F, Vance JC, Greenberg LJ, Yunis EJ, Zelickson AS (1977) Depressed immune function in epidermodysplasia verruciformis. Arch Dermatol 113:495–499

Ramoz N, Rueda LA, Bouadjar B, Favre M, Orth G (1999) A susceptibility locus for epidermodysplasia verruciformis, an abnormal predisposition to infection with the oncogenic human papillomavirus type 5, maps to chromosome 17qter in a region containing a psoriasis locus. J Invest Dermatol 112:259–263

Ramoz N, Taieb A, Rueda LA, Montoya LS, Bouadjar B, Favre M, Orth G (2000) Evidence for a nonallelic heterogeneity of epidermodysplasia verruciformis with two susceptibility loci mapped to chromosome regions 2p21-p24 and 17q 25. J Invest Dermatol 114:1148–1153

Ramoz N, Rueda LA, Bouadjar B, Montoya LS, Orth G, Favre M (2002) Mutations in two adjacent novel genes are associated with epidermodysplasia verruciformis. Nat Genet 32:579–581

Rink L, Haase H (2007) Zinc homeostasis and immunity. Trends Immunol 28:1–4

Schiffman M, Kjaer SK (2003) Natural history of anogenital human papillomavirus infection and neoplasia. J Natl Cancer Inst Monogr 31:14–19

Spahl DU, Berendji-Grün D, Suschek CV, Kolb-Bachofen V, Kröncke KD (2003) Regulation of zinc homeostasis by inducible NO synthase-derived NO: nuclear metallothionein translocation and intranuclear Zn^{2+} release. Proc Natl Acad Sci USA 100:13952–13957

Stanley M (2006) Immune responses to human papillomavirus. Vaccine 24 [Suppl 1]:S16–S22

Stark S, Petridis AK, Ghim S, Jenson AB, Bavinck JNB, Gross G, Stockfleth E, Fuchs PG, Pfister H (1998) Prevalence of antibodies against virus-like particles of epidermodysplasia verruciformis-associated HPV8 in patients at risk of skin cancer. J Invest Dermatol 111:696–701

Storey A (2002) Papillomaviruses: death-defying acts in skin cancer. Mol Med 8:417–421

Su AI, Wiltshire T, Batalov S, Lapp H, Ching KA, Block D, Zhang J, Soden R, Hayakawa M, Kreiman G, Cooke MP, Walker JR, Hogenesch JB (2004) A gene atlas of the mouse and human protein-encoding transcriptomes. Proc Natl Acad Sci USA 101:6062–6067

Sun XK, Chen JF, Xu AE (2005) A homozygous nonsense mutation in the *EVER2* gene leads to epidermodysplasia verruciformis. Clin Exp Dermatol 30:573–574

Tagami H, Aiba S, Rokugo M (1985) Regression of flat warts and common warts. Clin Dermatol 3(4):170–178

Tate G, Suzuki T, Kishimoto K, Mitsuya T (2004) Novel mutations of *EVER1/TMC6* gene in a Japanese patient with epidermodysplasia verruciformis. J Hum Genet 49:223–225

Ullrich SE (2005) Mechanisms underlying UV-induced immune suppression. Mutat Res 571:185–205

von Bülow V, Rink L, Haase H (2005) Zinc-mediated inhibition of cyclic nucleotide phosphodi-esterase activity and expression suppresses TNF-alpha and IL-1beta production in monocytes by elevation of guanosine 3′, 5′-cyclic monophosphate1. J Immunol 175:4697–4705

Vreugde S, Erven A, Kros CJ, Marcotti W, Fuchs H, Kurima K, Wilcox ER, Friedman TB, Griffith AJ, Balling R, Hrabé de Angelis MH, Avraham KB, Steel KP (2002) Beethoven, a mouse model for dominant, progressive hearing loss DFNA36. Nat Genet 30:257–258

Wang K, Zhou B, Kuo YM, Zemansky J, Gitschier J (2002) A novel member of a zinc transporter family is defective in acrodermatitis enteropathica. Am J Hum Genet 71:66–73

Weissenborn SJ, Höptl R, Weber F, Smola H, Pfister HJ, Fuchs PG (1999) High prevalence of a variety of epidermodysplasia verruciformis-associated human papillomaviruses in psoriasis skin of patients treated or not treated with PUVA. J Invest Dermatol 113:122–126

Wellinghausen N, Kirchner H, Rink L (1997) The immunobiology of zinc. Immunol Today 18:519–521

Woodworth CD (2002) HPV innate immunity. Front Biosci 7:2058–2071

Yamasaki S, Sakata-Sogawa K, Hasegawa A, Suzuki T, Kabu K, Sato E, Kurosaki T, Yamashita S, Tokunaga M, Nishida K, Hirano T (2007) Zinc is a novel intracellular second messenger. J Cell Biol 177:637–645

Yamashita S, Miyagi C, Fukada T, Kagara N, Che YS, Hirano T (2004) Zinc transporter LIV1 controls epithelial-mesenchymal transition in zebrafish gastrula organizer. Nature 429:298–302

Yang R, Murillo FM, Cui H, Blosser R, Uematsu S, Takeda K, Akira S, Viscidi RP, Roden RB (2004) Papillomavirus-like particles stimulate murine bone marrow-derived dendritic cells to produce alpha interferon and Th1 immune responses via MyD88. J Virol 78:11152–11160

Yang R, Murillo FM, Delannoy MJ, Blosser LR, Yutzy WH, Uematsu S, Takeda K, Akira S, Viscidi R, Roden RB (2005) B lymphocyte activation by human papillomavirus-like particles directly induces Ig class switch recombination via TLR4-MyD88. J Immunol 174:7912–7929

Zhou Z, Wang L, Song Z, Saari JT, McClain CJ, Kang YJ (2004) Abrogation of nuclear factor-κB activation is involved in zinc inhibition of lipopolysaccharide-induced tumor necrosis factor-α production and liver injury. Am J Pathol 164:1547–1556

Zuo YG, Ma D, Zhang Y, Qiao J, Wang B (2006) Identification of a novel mutation and a genetic polymorphism of *EVER1* gene in two families with epidermodysplasia verruciformis. J Dermatol Sci 44:153–159

Innate Resistance to Flavivirus Infections and the Functions of 2´-5´ Oligoadenylate Synthetases

T. Mashimo, D. Simon-Chazottes, J.-L. Guénet(✉)

Contents

Abstract Mouse susceptibility to experimental infections with flaviviruses is significantly influenced by a cluster of genes on chromosome 5 encoding a family of proteins with enzymatic properties, the 2´-5´ oligoadenylate synthetases (OAS). Positional cloning of the locus in question has revealed that susceptibility of laboratory inbred strains to this class of virus is associated with a nonsense mutation in the gene encoding the OAS1B isoform. Analysis of the molecular structure of the cluster in different mammalian species including human indicates that the cluster is extremely polymorphic with a highly variable number of genes and pseudogenes whose functions are not yet completely established. Although still preliminary, a few recent observations also substantiate a possible role for OAS1 in human susceptibility to viral infections (West Nile virus, SARS, etc.) and its possible involvement in some other diseases such as type 1 diabetes and multiple sclerosis. Finally, convergent observations indicate that the molecules encoded by the 2´-5´OAS cluster might be involved in other fundamental cellular functions such as cell growth and differentiation, gene regulation, and apoptosis.

J.-L. Guénet
Département de Biologie du Développement, Institut Pasteur, 75724 Paris Cedex 15, France
guenet@pasteur.fr

B. Beutler (ed.), *Immunology, Phenotype First: How Mutations Have Established New Principles and Pathways in Immunology.* Current Topics in Microbiology and Immunology 321. © Springer-Verlag Berlin Heidelberg 2008

Introduction

The severity of the clinical manifestations of most infectious diseases is greatly influenced by environmental factors and by the physiological status and the immune competence of the infected organism. It is also strongly influenced by genetic factors controlling the virulence of the pathogen and the susceptibility of the host. For this reason, co-evolution of infectious organisms with their hosts has been often compared to the "battle of two genomes" leading in general to infections with less deleterious consequences, which is after all the best way (if not the only way?) to ensure the survival of both organisms in the long term (Lengeling et al. 2001).

Investigations made with the aim of better understanding the genetic mechanisms that operate during the initial steps of infection are of major interest because they can provide information that may, in turn, help in the development of better strategies for fighting infectious diseases. Experiments of that kind, however, are not easy to perform because many parameters interfere with the experimental protocols, often making difficult the unambiguous delineation of "resistant" and "susceptible" phenotypes in a population of experimentally infected animals. In most cases, resistance or susceptibility to a pathogen depends on the complex interactions of multiple genes that control the host response. In a few cases, however, the situation is greatly simplified by the observation of clear-cut phenotypic differences between various inbred strains of laboratory mice after experimental infection. In this review we describe the historical case of genetic resistance to flaviviruses, the experiments that led to its elucidation at the molecular level, and the consequences of these discoveries.

The Pathogenicity of Flaviviruses

Flaviviruses are positive-sense, single-stranded, RNA viruses that are generally transmitted to warm-blooded animals through mosquito or tick bites. Many individuals exhibit flavivirus-specific antibodies, suggesting that infections by these viruses are mild or even unapparent, and revealing that some degree of adaptation has occurred between the virus and its host. In some other cases, however, flaviviruses can cause epidemic outbreaks in humans, and infected patients may exhibit a wide range of symptoms ranging from transient febrile illness to life-threatening hemorrhagic fevers (dengue and yellow fever) and meningo-encephalitis syndromes [Japanese encephalitis and West Nile (WN) fever]. The reasons why some flaviviruses cause severe clinical manifestations only in a small percentage of infected individuals are probably numerous and accordingly they have not yet been completely elucidated, but recurrent epidemiological observations and recent scientific data indicate that host-dependent genetic factors might be important.

Variations in innate flavivirus susceptibility in mice were reported for the first time in the early 1930s, and investigations performed during the following decades have fully confirmed these differences. By and large, one can consider that all laboratory inbred strains of mice that have been tested so far, with the exception of strain PL/J, are susceptible to experimental infections while most wild mice or mice from inbred strains recently derived from wild progenitors are resistant. To mention just one example of this difference in susceptibility, we reported that a single intra-peritoneal inoculation, equivalent to 100 times the median lethal dose (LD_{50}) of the WN virus (strain IS-98-ST1), administered to adult mice of the classical laboratory inbred strains BALB/c or C57BL/6 was lethal for all the animals 9.5±1.5 days after inoculation, while mice from unrelated inbred strains recently derived from wild ancestors of either the *Mus musculus domesticus* (WMP/Pas), *Mus µ. musculus* (MAI/Pas, MBT/Pas, PWK/Pas), or *Mus spretus* (SEG/Pas, STF/Pas) species were totally resistant to the same treatment (Mashimo et al. 2002). During this experiment, infectious particles of WN virus could be detected in the brain of all infected mice after 5 days of infection, and the amounts of virus peaked at 10^9 focus forming units (FFU)/g of brain tissue by day 7 (Mashimo et al. 2002). High levels of anti-WN antibody could also be detected in surviving animals, indicating that the virus replicated in resistant strains. This experiment was just one of many experiments of the same kind performed over the past 40 years with a variety of flaviviruses, using several routes of inoculation and several doses and strains of virus. All these experiments yielded similar results, confirming that the phenotype of resistance/susceptibility is not WN-specific but, on the contrary, extends to other types of flaviviruses as well.

The resistance to flaviviruses was also demonstrated to be controlled by a major locus on chromosome (Chr) 5, designated flavivirus resistance (symbol *Flv*), with basically two alleles: *Flv^r*, which is dominant and induces resistance, and *Flv^s*, which is recessive and correlates with susceptibility. Most classical laboratory inbred strains are homozygous for the *Flv^s* allele. A third allele leading to "minor resistance" (*Flv^mr*) has also been found segregating in wild mice of the *M. m. molossinus* subspecies [for historical details on the discovery and genetics of the *Flv* locus, readers may refer to Brinton and Perelygin (2003)]. Congenic "resistant" strains have been produced by back-crossing for several generations the successive resistant offspring of an initial cross between resistant wild mice (any species) with a "susceptible" laboratory inbred strain. This classical breeding strategy allowed, at the same time, refinement of the genetic localization of the *Flv* locus on mouse Chr 5 and allowed the production of unlimited populations of "resistant" and "susceptible" mice with an otherwise similar genetic constitution, a very helpful material for experimentation.

Investigating the Molecular Basis of Susceptibility to West Nile Infection

Considering the relatively simple (monofactorial) genetic basis of WN resistance in the mouse and the "genomic" tools that became available after the genome sequencing effort in this species, we decided to embark on the positional cloning of the *Flv* locus. Readers who may be interested in reading our publication about the positional cloning of *Flv* (Mashimo et al. 2002), must know that, since we had no evidence that the gene we were cloning was identical to *Flv* itself, we provisionally gave it another name (*Wnv* for WN virus—with two alleles *Wnv^r* and *Wnv^s*) even though we had little doubt that the two genes were presumably one-and-the-same entity. We now have molecular proof of this identity.. A first difficulty in this project arose when we found that, among the offspring of an intersubspecific backcross of the type (BALB/c×MBT/Pas)F1×BALB/c, which we expected to be a mixed population with 50% of the individuals being *Flv^r/Flv^s* and the other 50% being *Flv^s/Flv^s*, all mice heterozygous for *Flv^r* survived while not all mice with a *Flv^s/Flv^s* genetic constitution died as we would have expected. This is a good illustration of a major pitfall in this kind of experiment, where it is always risky or even impossible to trust in a "dead-or-alive" phenotype after an experimental infection, even if the latter is performed in the same highly standardized conditions. To bypass this difficulty and be able to achieve a high-resolution genetic mapping of the *Flv* locus, an absolutely necessary step in the positional cloning process, we derived a set of subcongenic mice by selecting, with the help of microsatellite markers, those offspring where a crossover event occurred that reduced the critical genetic interval containing the *Flv* locus. Offspring from these mice (all of the same genetic constitution) were challenged with a standardized dose of virus and finally classified as "resistant" or "susceptible." This rather tedious procedure allowed us to localize, with a very high degree of confidence, the *Flv* locus within an interval flanked by markers *D5Mit408* and *D5Mit242*, which is roughly equivalent to 300 kb of DNA (Fig. 1).

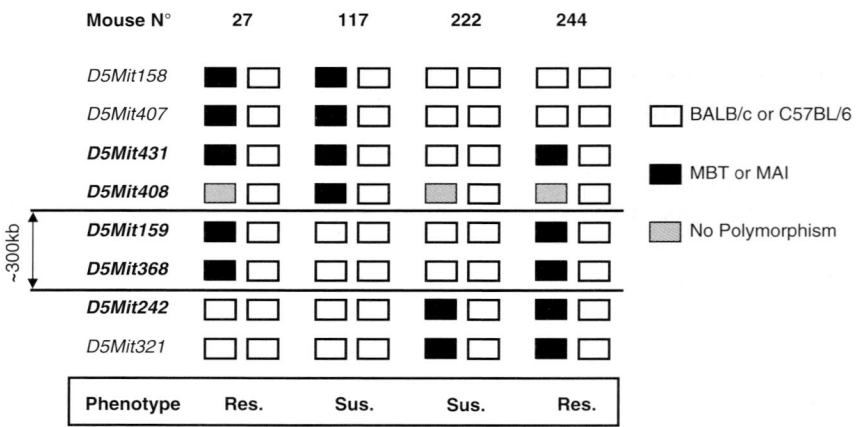

Fig. 1 Over 350 offspring from two intersubspecific backcrosses [(BALB/c×MBT)F1×BALB/c or (C57BL/6×MAI)F1×C57BL/6] were raised and genotyped for the region of Chr 5 flanking the locus for flavivirus resistance and four mice were found with a recombinant haplotype in the critical region (Nos. 27, 117, 222, and 244). These recombinant mice were then mated with either BALB/c or C57BL/6 susceptible partners, and around 30/50 progenies of these crosses were challenged with West Nile virus and classified as "susceptible" or "resistant." This protocol, because it involves a rather large sample of animals with exactly the same genotype, is highly reliable for the purpose phenotyping based on a dead-or-alive phenotype

This genetic interval contains about 30 genes whose sequence and expression pattern are well known (Fig. 2). Among these genes, the cluster encoding the interferon inducible oligoadenylate synthetases (*Oas1, Oas2, Oas3* etc.) appeared top-ranked in the list of candidates for reasons that will be explained later. We then decided to have a more careful look at the sequence of these genes in both "resistant" and "susceptible" mice. We observed several single nucleotide polymorphisms (SNPs) among the different strains or species studied, a finding that was not surprising considering the polyphyletic origins of the laboratory inbred strains of mice (Wade et al. 2002). We found it remarkable, however, that in one of the elements of the cluster, namely the *Oas1b* gene, all susceptible mice had a T→C transition in the fourth exon of this gene, replacing an arginine residue with a premature stop codon. The perfect and absolute correlation between susceptibility to viral infection and the occurrence of a stop codon was observed independently in two laboratories (Mashimo et al. 2002; Perelygin et al. 2002) and supported the hypothesis that a truncated, and presumably inactive form of 2'-5'OAS is indeed causative of the innate susceptibility to flavivirus infection. The presence of a stop codon is also compatible with susceptibility behaving as a fully recessive trait and fits perfectly with one of the known functions of the interferon inducible enzyme 2'-5'OAS. In addition to this absolute phenotype/genotype correlation, it has also been reported that a flavivirus-resistant phenotype could be restored in a susceptible mouse strain by replacing the 3' portion of the susceptible *Oas1b* sequence in 129/SvJ/RW4 ES cells, by homologous recombination with a 129/SvJ/ RW4 DNA sequence containing four substitutions characteristic of the *Oas1b* resistance allele, in particular a reversion from TGA to CGA (Scherbik et al. 2007).

The Molecular Organization and Evolution of the *OAS* Gene Family in Mammals

2'-5'OAS are a relatively homogeneous family of enzymatic proteins with a remote evolutionary origin, since molecules with a similar structure have been identified in a wide range of species including most mammals and birds, and even the marine sponge *Geodia cydonium* (Cayley et al. 1982; Wiens et al. 1999; Yamamoto et al. 1998). In the species where the molecular organization has been studied in detail, the genes encoding 2'-5'OAS have been found to be clustered, with variations in gene copy numbers (orthologs and paralogs) among the different species, indicating that rapid evolutionary changes occurred in these regions. In this section, we will summarize the most recent findings with reference to the corresponding publications.

The *human* cluster is the simplest with only three genes *OAS1, OAS2*, and *OAS3* within a 130-kb stretch of Chr 12 (12q24.13) (Hovnanian et al. 1998). These three genes share the same order of transcription and are arranged on the chromosome in the following order: centromere 5'–*OAS1*–*OAS3*–*OAS2*–3' (Hovanessian and Justesen 2007). The size of these genes is relatively short (~12 kb for *OAS1*; ~36 kb for both *OAS2* and *OAS3*) and analysis of their sequence reveals the presence of a conserved domain of five exons (the first 346-amino acid residues of *OAS1*), designated

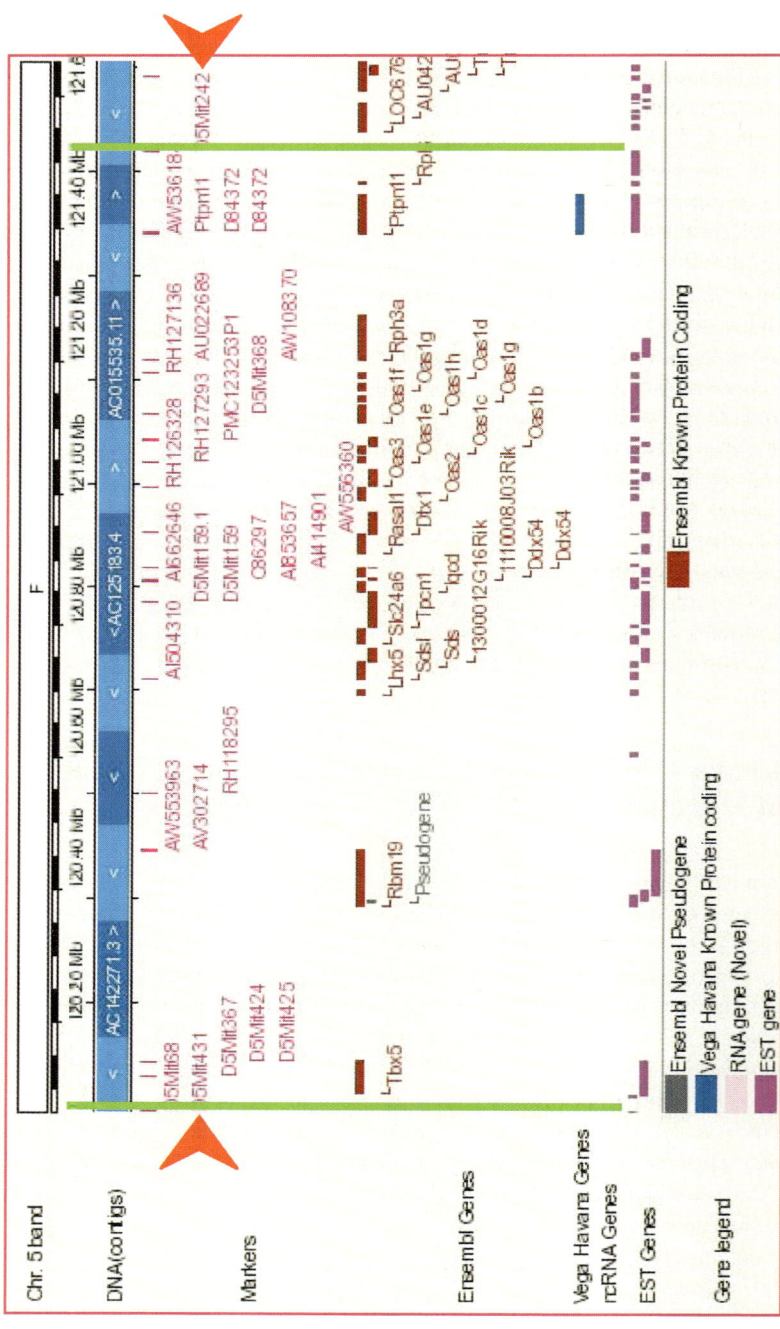

Fig. 2 This figure, from the *Ensembl* database, represents a segment of mouse Chr 5 in the critical region between markers *D5Mit431* and *D5Mit242* and shows the approx. 30 genes that are in the region. In this sequence (released after the positional cloning of *Flv*) the genes *Oas2*, *Oas3*, and the eight genes in the *Oas1* cluster are obvious. From the knowledge we have of their function, they appear as top-ranked candidates in the determinism of susceptibility to flaviviruses

the 2´-5´OAS unit, with one copy in *OAS1*, two copies in *OAS2*, and three copies in *OAS3*. This organization and sequence homology suggest that the *OAS1* gene is probably the ancestral gene, the other two genes being derived after duplication or triplication of this ancestral gene. The promoter region of the three genes contains an interferon-stimulated response element (ISRE), which is consistent with the fact that most of the 2´-5´OAS proteins are interferon (IFN)-inducible enzymes. *OAS1* is transcribed in four isoforms of 42, 44, 46, and 48 kDa respectively, depending on alternative splicing of exons 5 and 6. These isoforms, which have identical amino-termini but different carboxyl-termini, may have different functions. Formation of a human OAS1 tetramer is essential for the catalytic activity of the protein (Torshin 2005). *OAS2* is also spliced in two isoforms of 69 and 71 kDa that share a common amino-terminus of 683 residues, with extensions of 4 and 44 amino acids, respectively. *OAS3* encodes a unique protein of 100 kDa (Hovanessian and Justesen 2007; Justesen et al. 2000; Rebouillat and Hovanessian 1999; Fig. 3).

Aside from *OAS1*, *OAS2*, and *OAS3*, another gene—identified by screening a cDNA expression library with anti-OAS3 polyclonal antibodies (Rebouillat et al. 1998) and by screening an EST library (Hartmann et al. 1998)—with a sequence similar to the one of *OAS1*, although somewhat bigger, was discovered. This gene encodes a 56-kDa protein that differs from the other OAS proteins by an approx. 160-amino acid extension at its C-terminus, which has homology to the interferon-inducible protein ISG15 and also has a tandem repeat of two ubiquitin-like domains (Hartmann et al. 1998). This protein is devoid of 2´-5´OAS activity and accordingly was named OASL for "OAS like" protein. The human *OASL* gene exhibits a high degree of homology with the chicken *OAS* gene, but the latter encodes a highly active 2´-5´OAS (Torshin 2005).

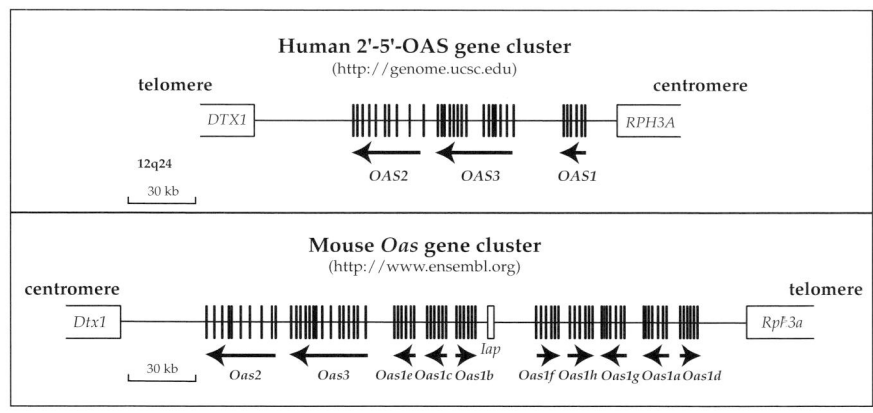

Fig. 3a A schematic organization of the OAS cluster in human and in mouse. Human *OAS1*, *OAS2*, and *OAS3* are paralogous copies of an ancestral gene. The mouse has at least eight orthologous copies of the human *OAS1*, some of them likely being nonfunctional pseudogenes (updated and modified from Mashimo et al. 2003)

Human OAS transcripts

[Sarker *et al.* 1998, Rebouillat *et al.* 1999, Justesen *et al.* 2000]

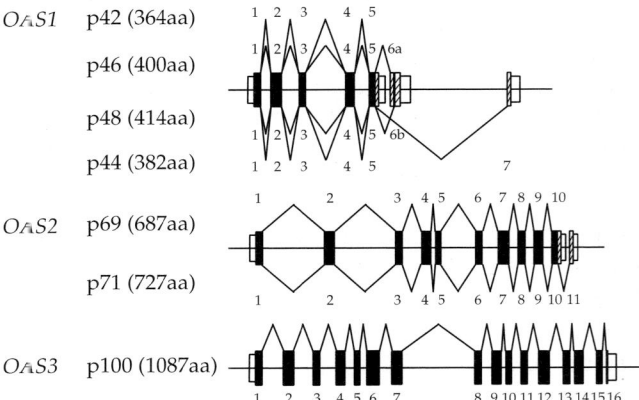

Mouse Oas transcripts

[Mashimo *et al.* 2003]

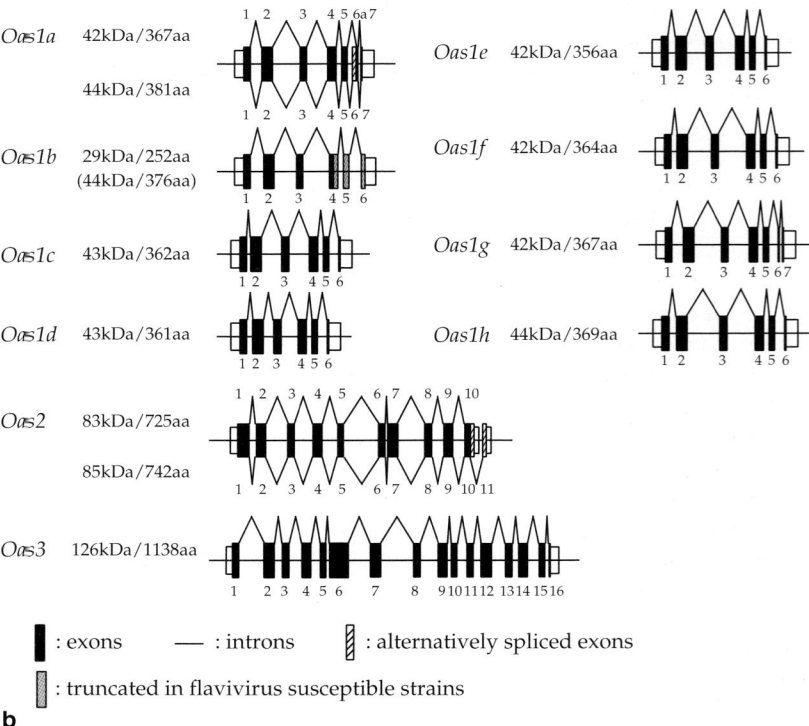

Fig. 3 b The transcription pattern of the different genes in the mouse *Oas* cluster. All these genes are transcribed, but with minor tissue-specific variations. Among the different genes of the mouse *Oas1* cluster, only *Oas1a* is alternatively transcribed. *Oas1a* and *Oas1g* have an extra seventh exon.

The *mouse Oas* cluster is the second most well known after human. It contains one *Oas2* and one *Oas3* gene, and ten *Oas1* genes (or pseudogenes?) designated *Oas1a* to *Oas1j* (Eskildsen et al. 2002; Kakuta et al. 2002; Mashimo et al. 2003; Perelygin et al. 2006; Figs. 2 and 3). These 12 genes are arranged in tandem within a stretch of DNA that spans approximately 230 kb of mouse Chr 5. The segment harboring the *Oas* cluster (and a few other flanking genes) is inverted when compared to the human configuration (Mashimo et al. 2003). Mouse *Oas2/Oas3* genes have a genomic structure very similar to the one of human, and a very similar pattern of transcription even if the transcription products are somewhat bigger in the mouse (725 and 742 amino acids compared to 687 and 727 for OAS2; 1,138 amino acids compared to 1,087 for OAS3). Here again, based on their sequences and orientation, one can guess that these 12 genes result from the duplication, in several steps, of an ancestral copy after divergence of the primates and rodents phyla. RT-PCR performed with a set of specific primers on RNA extracted from several adult and fetal tissues, either before or after induction with double-stranded RNA (dsRNA), indicated that nine genes of the *Oas1* family (*Oas1a* to *Oas1i*) are transcribed and some variations can be observed in the different patterns of expression. According to Mashimo and coworkers (2003) each of the nine *Oas1* genes exhibits a unique battery of transcriptional regulatory elements, suggesting that each of these units has the potential to be differentially regulated. So far only *Oas1a* has been found to be alternatively spliced yielding two transcripts each including different parts of exon 6 (Kakuta et al. 2002; Mashimo et al. 2003; Fig. 3). Two genes, homologous to the human *OASL*, have also been identified in the mouse: *Oasl1* and *Oasl2*. Analysis of their structure indicates that they are probably nonfunctional pseudogenes.

Twelve 2'-5'OAS (*Oas*) genes were identified in the *rat* genome (Chr 12) (Mashimo et al. 2003), including eight *Oas1* genes (the orthologs of mouse *Oas1a* and *Oas1e* are missing in this species, while two additional isoforms are present: *Oas1k* and *Oas1l*). Two *Oas1* pseudogenes, a single *Oas2* and a single *Oas3*, and two *Oas*-like genes, *Oasl1* and *Oasl2*, are also present. The structure and organization of the rat cluster is very similar to the one of the mouse, which is no surprise.

The structure of the 2'-5'OAS cluster has also been investigated in detail in four other mammalian species (pig, dog, cow, and horse) and in chicken (Perelygin et al. 2005, 2006). Four *OAS* genes (*OAS1X, OAS1Y, OAS1Z,* and *OAS2*) plus a single copy of *OASL1* were detected in the cow genome. The cluster in the pig genome is similar to the *OAS* cluster of cattle although *OAS1Z* is absent. Remarkably, the orthologous copy of mouse/human *OAS3* is not found in either the pig or the cow genomes. The dog and horse clusters are also similar and are more like the human cluster than either the mouse or rat clusters. Dog and horse have three copies of the

---

Fig. 3 b   (continued) Alignment of the predicted amino acid sequences for the proteins encoded by the eight *Oas1* genes indicates that *Oas1c, Oas1d, Oas1e, Oas1f,* and *Oas1h* are structurally similar and lack several functional domains. These observations suggest that these isoforms may actually be inactive pseudogenes rather than real isoforms. In contrast, *Oas1g* and *Oas1a* encode proteins that could be functional in the 2',5'OAS/RNase L cascade. Note that for both **a** and **b** the scale for exons is five times larger than for introns

human/mouse *OAS3* ortholog (*OAS3C*, *OAS3M*, and *OAS3N*), two copies of *OAS2* (*OAS2N* and *OAS2C*) and a single copy of the human *OAS1* ortholog. However, while the dog has two copies of the *OASL* orthologous gene (*OASL1* and *OASL2*), the horse has only one. Two tandemly duplicated OAS-like (*OASL*) genes were identified in the dog genome but only a single *OASL* ortholog was found in both the cattle and the pig genomes. The bovine and porcine *OASL* genes contain premature stop codons and encode truncated proteins, which lack the typical C-terminal double ubiquitin-like domains. Evidence of concerted evolution of all these paralogous *2′-5′OAS* genes was obtained in rodents (*Rodentia*) and even-toed ungulates (*Artiodactyla*) (Perelygin et al. 2006).

The Functions of the OAS Molecules

The Antiviral Functions of OAS1 Molecules

The best known molecules among those that are encoded by the 2′-5′OAS cluster are described as interferon-induced enzymes that polymerize ATP into 2′-5′ oligomers of adenosine with the general formula pppA $(2′p5′A)_n$. These enzymes are activated by binding to double-stranded RNA, and their products, the 2′-5′ oligoadenylates, activate the latent endoribonuclease RNase L that finally degrades viral or cellular RNA molecules (Hovanessian and Justesen 2007). This is how the antiviral activity of these enzymes is generally explained. Several experiments have confirmed this crucial function in the innate, antiflavivirus mechanism of defense in the mouse (Kajaste-Rudnitski et al. 2006; Lucas et al. 2003) although some experiments suggest that RNase L activation is not a major component of the OAS1B-mediated flavivirus resistance phenotype (Scherbik et al. 2006).

Sequence alignment of human OAS1, OAS2, and OAS3 reveals the presence of highly conserved stretches of 7–14 amino acids among which the pentapeptide D-F-L-K$_{199}$-Q has been reported to represent a part of the ATP binding site, while K$_{199}$ inside this pentapeptide seems to be essential for catalytic activity (Justesen et al. 2000; Rebouillat and Hovanessian 1999). In the mouse, interferon is also an inducer of the different OAS molecules, and alignment of the predicted amino acid sequences for the proteins encoded by *Oas1c*, *Oas1d*, *Oas1e*, *Oas1f*, *Oas1h*, *Oas1i*, and *Oas1j*—although structurally very similar—lack some essential functional domains, such as the LXXXPA motif (Ghosh et al. 1997), the highly conserved aspartic acid residues in exon 2 (Sarkar et al. 1999), and the CFK motif (Ghosh et al. 1997). These observations suggest that, although these isoforms have retained their binding activity to dsRNA, they have lost their Mg^{2+}-dependent catalytic activity and accordingly are most probably inactive pseudogenes rather than genes encoding a protein with 2′-5′OAS activity (Sarkar et al. 1999; Shibata et al. 2001). Another possibility that should be kept in mind would be that these isoforms, encoded in the above-mentioned genes, have acquired other functions. The three genes, *Oas1g*, *Oas1a*, and of course *Oas1b*, encode proteins that have been proved (or are likely) to be functional in the 2´-5´OAS/RNase L cascade.

The suspected role of the OAS1B isoform in the innate mechanisms of defense in the mouse, hypothesized after experimental infection of mice with flaviviruses and positional cloning of the *Flv* locus, has been confirmed by the production of a knock-in, as already mentioned. It has also been confirmed by experiments performed in vitro in which stable neuroblastoma cell clones overexpressing either the mutant or wild-type OAS1B were infected with WN virus. These experiments indicated that viral replication is less efficient in cells that produce the normal copy of OAS1B than in those expressing the mutant form of the protein (Lucas et al. 2003). The experiments have been confirmed and reinforced by other experiments performed on genetically engineered fibroblasts that could upregulate OAS1B protein expression under the control of the *Tet-Off* expression system (Kajaste-Rudnitski et al. 2006).

The role played by the OAS1B isoform of 2´-5´OAS in the innate mechanisms of defense of the mouse against flavivirus infection now seems firmly established. In human and other mammalian species, however, the role of 2´-5´OAS in viral pathogenesis is much less clear. According to Perelygin and colleagues, the flavivirus-specific activity of the mouse OAS1B isoform on flaviviral replication might be correlated with a 4-amino acid deletion in the P-loop motif that is unique to this isoform and does not appear to exist in human (Perelygin et al. 2002). This 4-amino acid deletion (12 bp) might be of special importance for the OAS1B protein to specifically interact with the ATP substrate if one considers recent data from the crystalline structure of the porcine OAS1 enzyme (Hartmann et al. 2003). Even if this hypothesis is supported by other experiments in vitro (Urosevic et al. 1999), an alternative explanation for the specific activity of OAS1B on flavivirus replication might be found in its promoter sequence, where several binding sites [for NF-κB, GAS, and interferon (IFN)-stimulated specific response element (ISRE)] exhibit a unique organization. In particular, it is noteworthy that OAS1B is the only gene where the NF-κB and ISRE binding sites are closely associated in tandem, producing a genomic structure that has previously been reported as capable of triggering gene expression upon viral induction (Cheng et al. 1998). Sequencing the promoter regions of the OAS1B isoform in remotely related mouse species did not provide evidence that some particular structural changes in this promoter might be associated with the phenotype of resistance or susceptibility after flavivirus infection. This supports the hypothesis that the stop codon found in the OAS1B coding sequence of most laboratory strains, which is the only obvious structural difference between susceptible and resistant genotypes, indeed is directly related to this phenotype. The 4-amino acid deletion in the P-loop motif has not been found in the orthologous region of the rat OAS1B isoform but does occur in rat OAS1F. The rat, like wild mice, seems to be naturally resistant when naturally infected (Eldadah et al. 1967).

Two recent observations arguing in favor of genetic control of human susceptibility to flavivirus infections have been published recently. The first, by Bonnevie-Nielsen and colleagues, reports a significant correlation between the basal activity of OAS1 and an A/G SNP at the exon 7 splice-acceptor site (AG or AA) of the OAS1 gene (Bonnevie-Nielsen et al. 2005). According to these authors, in a cohort of 83 families each containing two parents and two children, allele G had a higher frequency in people with high enzyme activity than in those with low enzyme activity, with the activity being related to this polymorphism in a dose-dependent manner across the GG, GA, and AA genotypes. Allele G generates the p46 enzyme isoform, whereas allele A ablates the splice site and generates a dual-function antiviral/ pro-apoptotic p48 isoform and a novel p52 isoform. The discovery of this genetic polymorphism and of its influence on host susceptibility to flavivirus infections clearly underlines the likely importance of OAS1 in the innate mechanisms of defense.

The second observation was made in a survey performed on 33 individuals hospitalized with WN virus infection. The survey was designed to assess whether a structural change could be detected in the *OAS* genes of patients with a clinically severe form of the disease. Sequence comparisons between case patients and control subjects identified 23 SNPs, including a synonymous SNP in *OASL* exon 2 in which the reference allele occurred at a higher frequency in case patients ($p<.004$). According to the authors, the RNA transcripts generated from this allele may undergo increased splicing, resulting in a dominant-negative OASL isozyme similar to the nonsense/truncation mutant form of *Oas1b* in mice (Yakub et al. 2005). These two reports, although preliminary, are indicative of a possible role for the OAS1 molecules in human mechanisms of defense.

Although the role of the OAS1 molecules in innate immunity against flavivirus infections is now established, at least in the mouse, several experiments indicate that this resistance, unlike resistance to myxovirus associated with the *Mx* locus (Haller et al. 1998), does not require induction by interferon (Brinton and Perelygin 2003). This observation is totally consistent with the observation that plants transgenic for 2´-5´OAS family and for the gene encoding RNase L, were found to be resistant to experimental infections with a number of viruses such as tobacco mosaic virus, cucumber mosaic virus, and potato virus Y (Honda et al. 2003; Mitra et al. 1996; Ogawa et al. 1996).

Finally, and again concerning the *Oas1b* gene of the mouse, a likely hypothesis to account for the presence of the same stop codon in virtually all laboratory strains is that all these strains inherited the same segment of Chr 5 from a common ancestor. Such a situation is not uncommon among mouse laboratory strains and was also observed by Staeheli and colleagues when they investigated the genetic basis of susceptibility to orthomyxovirus infection (Staeheli et al. 1986). However, whether this occurred by chance only or under some sort of selective pressure is an open question. Nonetheless, it is also clear that the use of inbred strains derived from wild specimens of different species might be a rich source of information for investigating the genetic basis of resistance/susceptibility to infectious diseases.

Aside from their well-established role in the pathology generated by flavivirus infections, 2´-5´OAS molecules (and more specifically those encoded by *OAS1*) may be involved in the outcome of diseases generated by coronaviruses or hepaciviruses. Two independent surveys indicated that SNPs in the *OAS1* gene (more precisely in exons 3, 6 or in the 3´-UTR region) were associated with severe acute respiratory syndrome (SARS) susceptibility in Vietnamese or Chinese Han populations (Hamano et al. 2005; He et al. 2006). Another study suggested that a polymorphism in the 3′-UTR of the *OAS1* gene was significantly associated with a higher frequency of self-limiting infection in patients with hepatitis C (Knapp et al. 2003). It is likely that with time, more associations between *OAS1* polymorphisms and resistance to viral infections will be discovered.

The Other Functions of OAS Molecules

Situations where different mammalian genomes harbor orthologous genes with a variable number of copies are not uncommon and it was suggested that such variations are the result of different selective environmental pressures experienced by the ancestors of modern rodents and primates. While infectious agents in natural environments certainly play an important role in natural selection (the "battle of two genomes"), however, the number and range of pathogens is not very different among the different mammalian species. It therefore makes sense to guess that the different OAS molecules have cellular functions other than the one made obvious by the accidental discovery of differential flavivirus resistance in the mouse species. In humans, for example, *OAS1*, *OAS2*, and *OAS3* appear to be differentially induced by interferon, induced in different types of cells, and for some of them expressed even in healthy individuals, which is indicative of an eventual role under physiological conditions and not only after infections. They are also characterized by different subcellular locations. Some OAS proteins might have as-yet-unidentified catalytic activities, suggesting that they may have distinct roles in the cell. In fact, 2′-5′OAS molecules have now been demonstrated to be involved in other cellular processes such as cell growth and differentiation, gene regulation, and apoptosis (Hovanessian and Justesen 2007).

Some polymorphisms at the *OAS1* locus have been reported to be associated with a variety of human pathologies. This is the case, for example, for a SNP generating an A/G splice-site in *OAS1*-exon 7, which was found to be associated with a protective effect against type 1 diabetes (Field et al. 2005). This observation was later disputed (Smyth et al. 2006) but another polymorphism in the same gene, generating a serine/glycine substitution resulting in a functional variant, was reported as a more likely cause for the observed association with type 1 diabetes (Tessier et al. 2006). Similarly, SNPs detected in exons 3 and 7 of *OAS1* demonstrated an association with risk for multiple sclerosis in 333 patients and 424 healthy controls, suggesting that OAS1 activity is involved in the etiology of this disease (Fedetz et al. 2006).

In the mouse species, with the unlimited possibilities of genetic engineering in embryonic stem (ES) cells in vitro, a comprehensive survey of the different functions of the OAS molecules should be undertaken in the forthcoming years, for example by knocking out each and every gene of the cluster. Although of importance, making alterations in the coding sequences of these genes in order to assess their function(s) would not necessarily require that the stop codon in *Oas1b* exon 4 be "repaired" in advance. Yan and colleagues, for example, demonstrated that mutant mice lacking OAS1D (*Oas1d*$^{-/-}$) displayed reduced fertility due to defects in ovarian follicle development, decreased efficiency of ovulation, and arrest at the one-cell stage of fertilized eggs (Yan et al. 2005). This was indeed a totally unexpected function for a protein exhibiting a very high degree of similarity with OAS1B.

As we already noted, the *2´-5´OAS* family of genes exhibits both an evolutionarily ancient origin and wide variations in the number of copies between species. Experimental data collected after experiments on mouse flavivirus susceptibility and preliminary observations made in humans suggest that the cluster in question is important for the maintenance of cellular homeostasis since evolutionary (environmental) forces contribute to its "shaping" (Godfrey et al. 2004). Since no sequences related to *2´-5´OAS* genes could be identified in either *Caenorhabditis elegans* or in *Drosophila melanogaster*, however, it seems that the OAS cluster is either not absolutely fundamental for cell physiology or that it is replaced by another structure with similar functions in other developed organisms.

References

Bonnevie-Nielsen V, Field LL, Lu S, Zheng DJ, Li M, Martensen PM, Nielsen TB, Beck-Nielsen H, Lau YL, Pociot F (2005) Variation in antiviral 2´,5´-oligoadenylate synthetase (2´5´AS) enzyme activity is controlled by a single-nucleotide polymorphism at a splice-acceptor site in the OAS1 gene. Am J Hum Genet 76:623–633

Brinton MA, Perelygin AA (2003) Genetic resistance to flaviviruses. Adv Virus Res 60:43–85

Cayley PJ, White RF, Antoniw JF, Walesby NJ, Kerr IM (1982) Distribution of the ppp(A2´p)nA-binding protein and interferon-related enzymes in animals, plants, and lower organisms. Biochem Biophys Res Commun 108:1243–1250

Cheng G, Nazar AS, Shin HS, Vanguri P, Shin ML (1998) IP-10 gene transcription by virus in astrocytes requires cooperation of ISRE with adjacent kappaB site but not IRF-1 or viral transcription. J Interferon Cytokine Res 18:987–997

Eldadah AH, Nathanson N, Sarsitis R (1967) Pathogenesis of West Nile virus encephalitis in mice and rats. 1. Influence of age and species on mortality and infection. Am J Epidemiol 86:765–775

Eskildsen S, Hartmann R, Kjeldgaard NO, Justesen J (2002) Gene structure of the murine 2´-5´-oligoadenylate synthetase family. Cell Mol Life Sci 59:1212–1222

Fedetz M, Matesanz F, Caro-Maldonado A, Fernandez O, Tamayo JA, Guerrero M, Delgado C, Lopez-Guerrero JA, Alcina A (2006) OAS1 gene haplotype confers susceptibility to multiple sclerosis. Tissue Antigens 68:446–449

Field LL, Bonnevie-Nielsen V, Pociot F, Lu S, Nielsen TB, Beck-Nielsen H (2005) OAS1 splice site polymorphism controlling antiviral enzyme activity influences susceptibility to type 1 diabetes. Diabetes 54:1588–1591

Ghosh A, Sarkar SN, Guo W, Bandyopadhyay S, Sen GC (1997) Enzymatic activity of 2´-5´-oligoadenylate synthetase is impaired by specific mutations that affect oligomerization of the protein. J Biol Chem 272:33220–33226

Godfrey PA, Malnic B, Buck LB (2004) The mouse olfactory receptor gene family. Proc Natl Acad Sci U S A 101:2156–2161

Haller O, Frese M, Kochs G (1998) Mx proteins: mediators of innate resistance to RNA viruses. Rev Sci Tech 17:220–230

Hamano E, Hijikata M, Itoyama S, Quy T, Phi NC, Long HT, Ha le D, Ban VV, Matsushita I, Yanai H, Kirikae F, Kirikae T, Kuratsuji T, Sasazuki T, Keicho N (2005) Polymorphisms of interferon-inducible genes OAS-1 and MxA associated with SARS in the Vietnamese population. Biochem Biophys Res Commun 329:1234–1239

Hartmann R, Olsen HS, Widder S, Jorgensen R, Justesen J (1998) p59OASL, a 2′-5′ oligoade-nylate synthetase like protein: a novel human gene related to the 2′-5′ oligoadenylate syn-thetase family. Nucleic Acids Res 26:4121–4128

Hartmann R, Justesen J, Sarkar SN, Sen GC, Yee VC (2003) Crystal structure of the 2′-specific and double-stranded RNA-activated interferon-induced antiviral protein 2′-5′-oligoadenylate synthetase. Mol Cell 12:1173–1185

He J, Feng D, de Vlas SJ, Wang H, Fontanet A, Zhang P, Plancoulaine S, Tang F, Zhan L, Yang H, Wang T, Richardus JH, Habbema JD, Cao W (2006) Association of SARS susceptibility with single nucleic acid polymorphisms of OAS1 and MxA genes: a case-control study. BMC Infect Dis 6:106

Honda A, Takahashi H, Toguri T, Ogawa T, Hase S, Ikegami M, Ehara Y (2003) Activation of defense-related gene expression and systemic acquired resistance in cucumber mosaic virus-infected tobacco plants expressing the mammalian 2′5′oligoadenylate system. Arch Virol 148:1017–1026

Hovanessian AG, Justesen J (2007) The human 2′-5′oligoadenylate synthetase family: unique interferon-inducible enzymes catalyzing 2′-5′ instead of 3′-5′ phosphodiester bond formation. Biochimie 89:779–788

Hovnanian A, Rebouillat D, Mattei MG, Levy ER, Marie I, Monaco AP, Hovanessian AG (1998) The human 2′,5′-oligoadenylate synthetase locus is composed of three distinct genes clustered on chromosome 12q24.2 encoding the 100-, 69-, and 40-kDa forms. Genomics 52:267–277

Justesen J, Hartmann R, Kjeldgaard NO (2000) Gene structure and function of the 2′-5′-oligoad-enylate synthetase family. Cell Mol Life Sci 57:1593–1612

Kajaste-Rudnitski A, Mashimo T, Frenkiel MP, Guenet JL, Lucas M, Despres P (2006) The 2′,5′-oligoadenylate synthetase 1b is a potent inhibitor of West Nile virus replication inside infected cells. J Biol Chem 281:4624–4637

Kakuta S, Shibata S, Iwakura Y (2002) Genomic structure of the mouse 2′,5′-oligoadenylate syn-thetase gene family. J Interferon Cytokine Res 22:981–993

Knapp S, Yee LJ, Frodsham AJ, Hennig BJ, Hellier S, Zhang L, Wright M, Chiaramonte M, Graves M, Thomas HC, Hill AV, Thursz MR (2003) Polymorphisms in interferon-induced genes and the outcome of hepatitis C virus infection: roles of MxA, OAS-1 and PKR. Genes Immun 4:411–419

Lengeling A, Pfeffer K, Balling R (2001) The battle of two genomes: genetics of bacterial host/pathogen interactions in mice. Mamm Genome 12:261–271

Lucas M, Mashimo T, Frenkiel MP, Simon-Chazottes D, Montagutelli X, Ceccaldi PE, Guenet JL, Despres P (2003) Infection of mouse neurones by West Nile virus is modulated by the inter-feron-inducible 2′-5′ oligoadenylate synthetase 1b protein. Immunol Cell Biol 81:230–236

Mashimo T, Lucas M, Simon-Chazottes D, Frenkiel MP, Montagutelli X, Ceccaldi PE, Deubel V, Guenet JL, Despres P (2002) A nonsense mutation in the gene encoding 2′-5′-oligoadenylate synthetase/L1 isoform is associated with West Nile virus susceptibility in laboratory mice. Proc Natl Acad Sci U S A 99:11311–11316

Mashimo T, Glaser P, Lucas M, Simon-Chazottes D, Ceccaldi PE, Montagutelli X, Despres P, Guenet JL (2003) Structural and functional genomics and evolutionary relationships in the cluster of genes encoding murine 2′,5′-oligoadenylate synthetases. Genomics 82:537–552

Mitra A, Higgins DW, Langenberg WG, Nie H, Sengupta DN, Silverman RH (1996) A mamma-lian 2–5A system functions as an antiviral pathway in transgenic plants. Proc Natl Acad Sci U S A 93:6780–6785

Ogawa T, Hori T, Ishida I (1996) Virus-induced cell death in plants expressing the mammalian 2′,5′ oligoadenylate system. Nat Biotechnol 14:1566–1569

Perelygin AA, Scherbik SV, Zhulin IB, Stockman BM, Li Y, Brinton MA (2002) Positional clon-ing of the murine flavivirus resistance gene. Proc Natl Acad Sci U S A 99:9322–9327

Perelygin AA, Lear TL, Zharkikh AA, Brinton MA (2005) Structure of equine 2′-5′oligoade-nylate synthetase (OAS) gene family and FISH mapping of OAS genes to ECA8p15→p14 and BTA17q24→q25. Cytogenet Genome Res 111:51–56

Perelygin AA, Zharkikh AA, Scherbik SV, Brinton MA (2006) The mammalian 2´-5´ oligoade-
    nylate synthetase gene family: evidence for concerted evolution of paralogous Oas1 genes in
    Rodentia and Artiodactyla. J Mol Evol 63:562–576
Rebouillat D, Hovanessian AG (1999) The human 2´,5´-oligoadenylate synthetase family:
    interferon-induced proteins with unique enzymatic properties. J Interferon Cytokine Res
    19:295–308
Rebouillat D, Marie I, Hovanessian AG (1998) Molecular cloning and characterization of two
    related and interferon-induced 56-kDa and 30-kDa proteins highly similar to 2´-5´ oligoade-
    nylate synthetase. Eur J Biochem 257:319–330
Sarkar SN, Ghosh A, Wang HW, Sung SS, Sen GC (1999) The nature of the catalytic domain of
    2´-5´-oligoadenylate synthetases. J Biol Chem 274:25535–25542
Scherbik SV, Paranjape JM, Stockman BM, Silverman RH, Brinton MA (2006) RNase L plays a
    role in the antiviral response to West Nile virus. J Virol 80:2987–2999
Scherbik SV, Kluetzman K, Perelygin AA, Brinton MA (2007) Knock-in of the Oas1br allele into
    a flavivirus-induced disease susceptible mouse generates the resistant phenotype. Virology
    368:232–237
Shibata S, Kakuta S, Hamada K, Sokawa Y, Iwakura Y (2001) Cloning of a novel 2´,5´-oligoade-
    nylate synthetase-like molecule, Oasl5 in mice. Gene 271:261–271
Smyth DJ, Cooper JD, Lowe CE, Nutland S, Walker NM, Clayton DG, Todd JA (2006) No evi-
    dence for association of OAS1 with type 1 diabetes in unaffected siblings or type 1 diabetic
    cases. Diabetes 55:1525–1528
Staeheli P, Danielson P, Haller O, Sutcliffe JG (1986) Transcriptional activation of the mouse Mx
    gene by type I interferon. Mol Cell Biol 6:4770–4774
Tessier MC, Qu HQ, Frechette R, Bacot F, Grabs R, Taback SP, Lawson ML, Kirsch SE, Hudson
    TJ, Polychronakos C (2006) Type 1 diabetes and the OAS gene cluster: association with splic-
    ing polymorphism or haplotype? J Med Genet 43:129–132
Torshin IY (2005) Three-dimensional models of human 2´-5´ oligoadenylate synthetases: a new
    computational method for reconstructing an enzyme assembly. Med Sci Monit 11:
    BR235–247
Urosevic N, Silvia OJ, Sangster MY, Mansfield JP, Hodgetts SI, Shellam GR (1999) Development
    and characterization of new flavivirus-resistant mouse strains bearing Flv(r)-like and Flv(mr)
    alleles from wild or wild-derived mice. J Gen Virol 80:897–906
Wade CM, Kulbokas EJ 3rd, Kirby AW, Zody MC, Mullikin JC, Lander ES, Lindblad-Toh K,
    Daly MJ (2002) The mosaic structure of variation in the laboratory mouse genome. Nature
    420:574–578
Wiens M, Kuusksalu A, Kelve M, Muller WE (1999) Origin of the interferon-inducible (2´-5´)oli-
    goadenylate synthetases: cloning of the (2´-5´)oligoadenylate synthetase from the marine
    sponge Geodia cydonium. FEBS Lett 462:12–18
Yakub I, Lillibridge KM, Moran A, Gonzalez OY, Belmont J, Gibbs RA, Tweardy DJ (2005)
    Single nucleotide polymorphisms in genes for 2´-5´-oligoadenylate synthetase and RNase L
    in patients hospitalized with West Nile virus infection. J Infect Dis 192:1741–1748
Yamamoto A, Iwata A, Koh Y, Kawai S, Murayama S, Hamada K, Maekawa S, Ueda S, Sokawa
    Y (1998) Two types of chicken 2´,5´-oligoadenylate synthetase mRNA derived from alleles at
    a single locus. Biochim Biophys Acta 1395:181–191
Yan W, Ma L, Stein P, Pangas SA, Burns KH, Bai Y, Schultz RM, Matzuk MM (2005) Mice defi-
    cient in oocyte-specific oligoadenylate synthetase-like protein OAS1D display reduced fertil-
    ity. Mol Cell Biol 25:4615–4624

Cmv1 and Natural Killer Cell Responses to Murine Cytomegalovirus Infection

A.A. Scalzo, W.M. Yokoyama(✉)

Contents

Abstract The dissection of genetic resistance to murine cytomegalovirus infection in inbred laboratory mouse strains led to the identification of a natural killer cell activation receptor that recognizes a virus-encoded protein. Herein, we summarize the genetic approach and findings that have provided novel insights into innate immune control of virus infections.

Abbreviations CMV: Cytomegalovirus; DAP12: DNAX activating protein of 12 kDa; Δm157: MCMV clone lacking m157 expression; ENU: *N*-Ethyl-*N*-nitrosourea; GFP: Green fluorescent protein; HCMV: Human CMV; Ig: Immunoglobulin;

W.M. Yokoyama

Howard Hughes Medical Institute, Division of Rheumatology, Campus Box 8045, Washington University School of Medicine, 660 South Euclid Avenue, St. Louis, MO 63110, USA

yokoyama@im.wustl.edu

B. Beutler (ed.), *Immunology, Phenotype First: How Mutations Have Established*   101
New Principles and Pathways in Immunology. Current Topics in Microbiology
and Immunology 321. © Springer-Verlag Berlin Heidelberg 2008

ILT: Ig-like transcripts; ITAM: Immunoreceptor tyrosine-based activation motif; ITIM: Immunoreceptor tyrosine-based inhibitory motif; KARAP:Killer associated receptor adapter protein; KIR: Killer Ig-like receptor; LCMV: Lymphocytic choriomeningitis virus; MCMV: Murine CMV; mAb: Monoclonal antibody; MHC: Major histocompatibility complex; NK: Natural killer; NKC: NK gene complex; ORF Open reading frame; RI: Recombinant inbred; SCID-MCMV: MCMV clones isolated from *scid* mice; TLR: Toll-like receptor

Introduction

Natural killer (NK) cells constitute the third major population of lymphocytes that can be distinguished from other lymphocytes by the absence of the T and B cell antigen receptor complexes (Yokoyama 2008). Although initially discovered because of their "natural" ability to kill tumor cells without prior sensitization, NK cells are now known to participate in the early, innate immune response to infection. This is best illustrated by case reports of human patients with selective NK cell deficiency. These patients have in common a propensity to severe, disseminated, and recurrent herpesvirus infections, including cytomegalovirus (CMV) (Biron et al. 1989; Jawahar et al. 1996), strongly suggesting that NK cells play important roles in host defense against pathogens, especially herpesviruses.

CMV are β-herpesviruses (Mocarski and Courcelle 2001), which are large-enveloped, double-stranded DNA viruses. Due to species tropism, each mammalian host has a characteristic CMV; human CMV does not replicate in mice. The β-herpesviruses have diverged somewhat but are most closely related in sequence to each other than to other herpesviruses. Murine CMV (MCMV) has a 230-kb genome, similar in structure to human CMV, and characteristically contains many open reading frames (ORFs) for viral molecules that interact with the host (Rawlinson et al. 1996). Moreover, MCMV has similar properties to human CMV during in vivo infections and thus is a particularly useful model pathogen for study of host-pathogen interactions. After systemic inoculation (typically via intraperitoneal route), MCMV causes an initial acute systemic infection phase with readily detectable viral replication, and is characterized by innate immune responses (Biron 1994, 1999) followed by viral latency during which infectious virus is below detection limits. As with other herpesviruses, the host then sheds the virus for its lifetime during periods of viral reactivation (Mocarski and Courcelle 2001).

As for mouse NK cell responses to MCMV, classic studies involved depletion of NK cells in vivo by administration of a monoclonal antibody (mAb) against NK1.1—the most specific serological marker on CD3⁻ NK cells in C57BL/6 mice—or other anti-NK cell antibodies (Bukowski et al. 1983; Bukowski et al. 1984; Welsh et al. 1990). When mice were then infected with MCMV, lethality and marked viral replication in internal organs was evident. Elevated viral titers were especially prominent in the spleen. If anti-NK cell antibody administration was delayed for a few days, there was no effect, indicating that NK cells are important in the early host immune response against viruses.

NK cells are activated by two major stimuli, cytokines and targets, and are capable of two major effector responses, cytokine production and target killing (Yokoyama 2008). In MCMV infections, NK cells can respond to interleukin (IL)-12 that is produced by macrophages and related cells, such as dendritic cells (DCs); IL-12 can stimulate NK cell production of interferon (IFN)-γ (Andoniou et al. 2005; Biron et al. 1999). In addition, through Jak/Stat pathways, other cytokines, such as IL-2, IFN-α, and IFN-β, stimulate NK cells to proliferate, produce IFN-γ and tumor necrosis factor (TNF)-α, and enhance their killing. Although cytokine-stimulated effector responses are important in MCMV infection (Orange et al. 1995; Orange and Biron 1996), most responses to cytokines are also seen in lymphocytic choriomeningitis virus (LCMV) infection even though NK cell depletion does not alter viral replication or survival (Biron et al. 1999; Bukowski et al. 1983, 1985). Thus, some of these effects may be bystander responses, suggesting that other effector mechanisms, especially killing, may be required for NK cell-mediated antiviral immunity.

Classically, NK cells kill their targets by the triggered release of preformed cytoplasmic granules containing perforin and granzymes, a process termed granule exocytosis (Henkart 1994), leading to target apoptosis. NK cells can kill certain targets through other means, including Fas and TNF-related apoptosis-inducing ligand (TRAIL), but the functional, especially in vivo, relevance of these pathways in antiviral innate defense is less clear (Zamai et al. 1998). In addition, resting NK cells apparently do not normally express Fas ligand, and must be triggered to mediate Fas-induced death (Bradley et al. 1998). Moreover, perforin-deficient mice have a defect in control of MCMV, implicating NK cell perforin-dependent killing (Loh et al. 2005; Tay and Welsh 1997). Thus, NK cell activation by their targets is a critical element, raising the issue that NK cell receptors specific for virus-infected cells may be important in infection control.

In this review, we will illustrate how a genetic approach was extremely valuable in elucidating the mechanisms by which NK cells recognize virus-infected cells.

Target Recognition by NK Cells

To further appreciate the possibility that NK cells may directly recognize virus-infected cells, it is useful to review the general topic of target recognition by NK cells that is regulated by target cell expression of major histocompatibility complex (MHC) class I molecules (Yokoyama 2008). Targets lacking MHC class I, occurring as a result of viral infection for example (Tortorella et al. 2000), are more susceptible to NK cell lysis than targets with normal levels of MHC class I molecules. This led Kärre to propose the "missing-self" hypothesis whereby NK cells survey tissues for normal expression of MHC class I that somehow prevents NK cell activation (Ljunggren and Kärre 1990). In the absence of MHC class I, NK cells are released to kill the target. This process is mediated through NK cell receptors that specifically bind MHC class I molecules and inhibit NK cell killing. There are two structural types of inhibitory receptors for MHC class I: (1) type I integral membrane proteins with immunoglobulin (Ig)-like domains, such as the human killer Ig-like receptors (KIR) and Ig-like transcripts (ILTs); and (2) type II integral membrane proteins with external lectin-like domains, including the mouse Ly49 family, and mouse and human NKG2/CD94 receptor. Regardless of structural type, inhibition occurs through motifs in the cytoplasmic domains of the inhibitory receptors, termed immunoreceptor tyrosine-based inhibitory motifs (ITIMs). When the ITIMs are tyrosine phosphorylated, they recruit and activate the cytoplasmic tyrosine phosphatase SHP-1, which then dephosphorylates molecules involved in NK cell activation. It is important to note, however, that the absence of MHC class I (and thus no inhibition) does not automatically lead to NK cell activation against cellular targets because activation requires engagement of activation receptors. Thus, NK cell responses to cellular targets are regulated by an interplay between inhibitory and activation receptors.

Transcripts for many receptors related to the inhibitory receptors were identified by cross-hybridization in cDNA library screenings (Yokoyama 2008). Whereas the deduced receptors were highly related to the inhibitory receptors in terms of amino acid sequence homology and domain structure, these receptors could not be inhibitory because they lack cytoplasmic ITIMs. Instead, many were found to be activation receptors that have charged transmembrane residues allowing association with transmembrane signaling chains, such as DAP12 (Lanier et al. 1998), also known as KARAP (killer cell-activating receptor-associated polypeptide) (Olcese et al. 1997). These signaling chains contain immunoreceptor tyrosine-based activation motifs (ITAMs) similar to those in the signaling chains of the T and B cell receptor complexes, allowing the putative ligand-binding activation receptors to deliver positive signals for NK cell activation. The physiological function of most putative activation receptors, however, remained elusive.

NK cell activation receptors were likely to be physiologically important in antiviral defense because several viruses, notably members of the herpesvirus family, encode proteins that interfere with natural killing (Cohen et al. 1999; Cosman et al. 1997; Farrell et al. 1997; Ishido et al. 2000; Reyburn et al. 1997; Tomasec et al. 2000; Ulbrecht et al. 2000). For example, human CMV (HCMV) encodes an MHC class I-like molecule (UL18) that interacts with ILT-2 (also known as LIR-1, leukocyte inhibitory receptor-1), an Ig-like inhibitory receptor on NK cells. HCMV also encodes a peptide (UL40) that binds HLA-E, an MHC class Ib molecule that typically binds only leader peptides derived from MHC class Ia molecules. The HCMV peptide enhances expression of HLA-E that in turn is recognized by CD94/NKG2A, a C-type lectin-like NK cell inhibitory receptor. Thus, HCMV produces molecules that bind both structural types of inhibitory receptors.

NK cell inhibitory receptors prevent in vitro killing by blocking signals from activation receptors (Long 1999; Ravetch and Lanier 2000), and the transfected expression of the HCMV molecules blocks killing of tumor targets (Cosman et al. 1997; Tomasec et al. 2000; Ulbrecht et al. 2000). The inhibitory receptors, however, should not block cytokine receptor signaling. These viral evasion strategies therefore strongly suggested that NK cells could mediate in vivo antiviral defense with activation receptors that are related to those involved in tumor killing, but it had been especially challenging to identify such activation receptors until a genetic approach was undertaken.

Early Studies of Genetically Determined Resistance to MCMV

Differences in mouse strain-dependent resistance to lethal MCMV infection were demonstrated in studies by Selgrade and Osborn (1974). More systematic investigations by Chalmer and colleagues (1977) using *H2* congenic mice on the BALB/c genetic background indicated that *H2* loci, and in particular the $H2^k$ haplotype, conferred resistance to MCMV. The conclusion that the $H2^k$ haplotype contributed a major resistance phenotype to MCMV was corroborated by follow-up studies using *H2* congenic mice on the BALB/c, C57BL/10, C3H and A backgrounds (Grundy et al. 1981). In this same study Grundy (Chalmer) and colleagues also observed, based on studies with (C57BL×BALB/c)F₁ hybrids, that non-*H2* loci on the C57BL genetic background conferred dominant resistance to MCMV. An assessment of MCMV replication in the spleens of the relatively resistant C57BL/6 strain and the susceptible $H2^b$-matched BALB.B strain revealed greater than 100-fold higher titers at days 2 and 3 after infection in the BALB.B strain (Allan and Shellam 1984). This provided the first clue that non-*H2* loci play an important role in regulating viral replication early after acute infection. Other studies provided evidence implicating a role for non-*H2* loci in the control of early interferon production (Allan and Shellam 1985; Grundy et al. 1982; Quinnan and Manischewitz 1987) and NK cell responses (Bancroft et al. 1981; Bukowski et al. 1984; Shellam et al. 1981, 1985) following MCMV infection, but did not define the number or chromosomal locations of the genes involved.

Cmv1 and NK Cell Resistance to MCMV

Defining the Cmv1 Locus

The observations that C57BL non-*H2* loci both provided dominant protection against lethal MCMV challenge (Grundy et al. 1981) and contributed to a greater than 100-fold reduction in viral replication in vivo relative to the BALB/c genetic background (Allan and Shellam 1984) provided a powerful phenotypic "window" through which to explore the genetic basis of this host-determined resistance. Using this information, we investigated viral replication in the spleens and livers of BALB/c, C57BL/6, and (BALB/c×C57BL/6)F₁ hybrids (Scalzo et al. 1990). Levels of viral replication in the spleen during the early acute phase of infection of the F₁ hybrids were as low as in the parental C57BL/6 strain. This pattern was observed for both male and female mice, but did not extend to the liver. This indicated that regulation of MCMV replication in the spleen was mediated in an autosomal-dominant manner (Scalzo et al. 1990). To enumerate the number of genes affecting this trait, viral replication in the spleens of (BALB/c×C57BL/6)F₁×BALB/c backcross and (BALB/c×C57BL/6)F₂ intercross mice was assessed, and it was found that ratios of 1:1 and 3:1 for low versus high titers were obtained for progeny from each cross, respectively. This indicated that control of MCMV replication was mediated by a single non-*H2* locus, which was named *Cmv1* (Scalzo et al. 1990). Resistant mouse strains, such as C57BL/6, are designated *Cmv1ʳ* and susceptible mouse strains, such as BALB/c, have the *Cmv1ˢ* allele. Mapping studies using the CXB set of recombinant inbred (RI) mouse strains derived from the BALB/c and C57BL/6 parental strains provided the first evidence that *Cmv1* mapped to the distal region of mouse chromosome 6 (Scalzo et al. 1990).

Distal Mouse Chromosome 6 Contains the NK Gene Complex

In the mouse, the majority of NK cell receptors are encoded in the NK gene complex (NKC) on distal chromosome 6. Initially described when the genes for the first puta-tive NK cell receptors (*Ly49, Nkrp1*) were localized (Yokoyama et al. 1990, 1991), the NKC is now known to consist of several multigene families, many of which are selectively expressed by NK cells but also may be expressed by other hematopoietic cells (Yokoyama and Plougastel 2003). These molecules are typically type II inte-gral membrane proteins with external C-type lectin-like domains. They are usually expressed as disulfide-linked dimers, either homo- or hetero-dimers. Both ITIM-containing inhibitory receptors and charged transmembrane residue-containing iso-forms without ITIMs are typically found within a family of highly related molecules (~80% amino acid identity). Between families there is limited homology (~25% amino acid identity), but there is preservation of the main features of these molecules (type II, C-type lectin-like domains), indicating superfamily relationships. The NKC is conserved in other mammals, including humans (chromosome 12p13) and rat (chromosome 4) where the syntenic regions have been most extensively studied (Hao et al. 2006; Kelley et al. 2005; Kveberg et al. 2006). Moreover, several loci involved in resistance to other large DNA viruses also map to the NKC, including *Rmp1* (mousepox, ectromelia virus) and *Rhs1* (herpes simplex virus) (Delano and Brownstein 1995; Pereira et al. 2001; Yokoyama and Plougastel 2003) as well as *Cmv1* and *Cmv4* (CMV) (Adam et al. 2006; Scalzo et al. 1990).

For the purposes of this review, it is especially important to highlight the role of the mouse Ly49 family of molecules which is encoded by a cluster of genes in the NKC (Smith et al. 1994; Wong et al. 1991; Yokoyama and Plougastel 2003). The first identified NK cell inhibitory receptor for MHC class I was Ly49 (now known as Ly49A) (Karlhofer et al. 1992). Several other Ly49 family members, such as Ly49C, Ly49G, and Ly49I, are also inhibitory receptors for MHC class I (Hanke et al. 1999). By contrast, Ly49D and Ly49H are activation receptors that couple to DAP12 (Bakker et al. 2000; Smith et al. 1998). The Ly49D receptor mediates the effect of the *Chok* locus, which was defined based on the genetic ability of C57BL/6-derived NK cells to kill a xenogeneic target cell, Chinese hamster ovary (CHO) cells (Idris et al. 1999; Nakamura et al. 1999). The ability of Ly49D to recognize CHO cells was determined by a genetic approach and verified by gene transfer of Ly49D and monoclonal antibody (mAb) blockade of Ly49D. Whereas Ly49D recognizes a hamster MHC class I molecule (Furukawa et al. 2002), Ly49H remained an orphan receptor, as are many other receptors encoded in the NKC.

Cmv1 Resistance Is Mediated via NK Cells

The very rapid regulation of MCMV replication suggested that the *Cmv1* effect must be mediated through effector functions that are elicited early after infection. While type I interferons and CD4[+] and CD8[+] T cells were excluded as playing roles in the *Cmv1* effect (Scalzo et al. 1992), NK cells were found to be critically important since the depletion of NK cells from C57BL/6 mice or *Cmv1[r]* CXB RI strains (CXBD, CXBE, and CXBJ), using an anti-NK1.1-depleting mAb (PK136), abrogated the early control of MCMV replication in the spleen, leading to levels of viral replication comparable to those seen in susceptible BALB/c mice (Scalzo et al. 1992). Coupled with the emerging concept of the NKC at that time (Yokoyama et al. 1991), these data strongly suggested that the *Cmv1* effect may be linked to the NKC itself.

By analyzing viral replication in the spleens of the larger set of BXD RI strains, derived from the susceptible DBA/2 and resistant C57BL/6 progenitor strains, we confirmed the chromosomal map location of *Cmv1* and refined it to a distal region of chromosome 6 (Scalzo et al. 1992). The strain distribution pattern of *Cmv1* phenotypes in the BXD RI set was identical to that for *Ly49* and *mNKR-P1*, i.e., the NKC, with one exception being that the phenotype in the BXD-8 strain was *Cmv1[s]*. Originally these data were interpreted as suggesting that *Cmv1* might be a distinct gene from *Ly49* and *mNKR-P1* (Scalzo et al. 1992), but subsequent genetic analysis of this strain indicated it had a C57BL/6-like genotype in the entire region of the NKC, suggesting it may harbor a germ-line mutation in the candidate gene for *Cmv1* (Scalzo et al. 1995a). Hence, the *Cmv1[s]* phenotype of the BXD-8 RI strain later became a critical factor in the successful identification of the gene encoding the protein that mediates the effects of the *Cmv1* locus.

High-Resolution Genetic and Physical Mapping of *Cmv1*

The initial localization of *Cmv1* to the NKC was confirmed by low-resolution mapping studies using (BALB/c×C57BL/6)F$_1$×BALB/c backcross mice and by the construction of a congenic mouse strain in which the *Cmv1[r]* allele and NKC alleles from the C57BL/6 mouse were introduced onto the BALB/c background to create the BALB.B6-*Cmv1[r]* strain (Scalzo et al. 1995a, b). Subsequent studies then focused on fine genetic mapping of the locus and its physical mapping. Two high-resolution genetic mapping studies were performed using large cohorts of over 1,000 backcross mice. In one study no segregation was found from the *Ly49a* locus, indicating very close linkage to the *Ly49* multigene family (Depatie et al. 1997). In the other study the map position of *Cmv1* was determined to be approximately 0.2 cM distal to *Ly49a* (Forbes et al. 1997). In the latter study, however, it should be noted that several mice that were critical for assignment of the map location of *Cmv1* possessed titers intermediate between those of the parental strains. Nonetheless, *Cmv1* was in close proximity to the NKC if not in the NKC itself.

Following determination of a low-resolution physical map of the NKC region (Brown et al. 1997), high-resolution mapping of the physical location of *Cmv1* on chromosome 6 was performed. One study localized *Cmv1* to an approximately 1.6 Mb region between the markers *D6Ott8* and *D6Ott115* that encompassed the entire *Ly49* multigene cluster (Depatie et al. 2000), whereas the other study provided evidence that the gene encoding *Cmv1* should physically reside between *Ly49t* and *Prp* (Brown et al. 1999). The reasons for differences in the fine positioning of *Cmv1* between these genetic and physical mapping studies may have been due to differences in the viral strain used (Smith versus K181), equivocal phenotyping of animals representing critical recombination events in the study by Forbes et al. (1997), or the contribution of modifying genes affecting the principal gene mediating the *Cmv1* effect (Scalzo et al. 2003). Nevertheless, abundant genetic mapping data from three different genetic approaches (RI, backcross panels, congenic strains) indicated that *Cmv1* is linked to the NKC, and subsequent investigations then focused on assessment of candidate genes in the distal NKC region.

Cmv1 Is Ly49h

The mapping of *Cmv1* in close proximity to the NKC and its dependence on NK cells for MCMV resistance strongly suggested that an NKC-encoded receptor on NK cells was responsible for its effect. However, identification of *Cmv1* remained challenging for several reasons including: (1) the high density of closely related genes in the NKC; (2) the already known allelic polymorphism for many of these genes and (3) a recombination "hotspot" with corresponding absence of additional informative recombination events in the NKC (discussed in Scalzo et al. 2003; Yokoyama and Plougastel 2003). Point Nos. 1 and 2 indicated that a direct sequencing approach would not be informative because it was unlikely to yield a specific candidate gene, and issue No. 3 made it difficult to narrow the genetic interval by further breeding experiments. Therefore, identification of *Cmv1* required clues from several other related lines of work.

In studies originally aimed at identifying NK cells in situ during MCMV, it became important to analyze the Ly49 repertoire on NK cells during the course of MCMV infection (Dokun et al. 2001a). In parallel, a mAb was generated that was specific for Ly49H, and it was used to demonstrate that Ly49H was an orphan activation receptor expressed only on a subset of NK cells from C57BL/6 mice (Smith et al. 2000). Subsequent studies revealed a marked and selective increase in the Ly49H subset during the latter stages (day 6) of infection (Dokun et al. 2001b), prompting an experiment to assess the effect of anti-Ly49H mAb administration on the course of MCMV infection (Brown et al. 2001). Interestingly, anti-Ly49H treatment adversely affected survival and led to increased viral titers, similar to depletion of all NK cells in C57BL/6 mice with mAb PK136 (anti-NK1.1). Similar results were obtained with an anti-Ly49 mAb with broader reactivity, including for

Ly49H, but these effects were not seen with other mAbs reactive with only Ly49 molecules other than Ly49H, such as anti-Ly49D (Brown et al. 2001; Daniels et al. 2001; Tay et al. 1999). Anti-Ly49H treatment did not appear to deplete the Ly49H subpopulation of NK cells and F(ab')$_2$ fragments of anti-Ly49H demonstrated similar effects, suggesting that anti-Ly49H was blocking recognition of MCMV infected cells.

Armed with a specific candidate gene (*Ly49h*) in mind for *Cmv1*, we obtained genetic evidence by analysis of susceptible BXD-8 mice which displayed an absence of Ly49H$^+$ NK cells even though they possess the C57BL/6 haplotype for the NKC (Brown et al. 2001). Other Ly49 receptors were normally expressed, the results being confirmed by specific absence of *Ly49h* transcripts (Brown et al. 2001; Lee et al. 2001). Southern blot analysis revealed a deletion in the 5' proximal portion of *Ly49h* in BXD-8 mice whereas other *Ly49* genes were intact. Finally, *Ly49h* was not present in *Cmv1^s* mice, such as BALB/c. These data firmly established that *Ly49h* is responsible for the *Cmv1* effect.

Subsequent corroborating evidence was provided by other laboratories examining transgenic and knockout mice. By transgenesis, a bacterial artificial chromosome containing the *Ly49h* gene from C57BL/6 genome was able to confer resistance to mouse strains that were otherwise susceptible to MCMV (Lee et al. 2003). Moreover, mice on the C57BL/6 background having a Tyr-to-Phe mutation in the ITAM of DAP12 displayed a nonfunctional Ly49H receptor (Tomasello et al. 2000). These mice were susceptible to MCMV infection (Sjolin et al. 2002). Taken together, these data firmly established that the Ly49H NK cell activation receptor is responsible for genetic resistance to MCMV infection.

Ly49H Recognizes m157 Encoded by MCMV

Identification of m157

The search for the ligand for Ly49H was aided by the generation of Ly49H reporter cells based on an approach pioneered by Nilabh Shastri (University of California, Berkeley) who produced a cell line (BWZ.36) by stably transfecting a derivative of the T cell hybridoma fusion partner, BW5147, with a reporter construct for nuclear factor of activated T cells (NFAT)-dependent expression of β-galactosidase in response to ITAM-dependent signaling (Sanderson and Shastri 1994). BWZ.36 was transfected with cDNAs for Ly49H and its ITAM-containing signaling chain DAP12 (Smith et al. 2002). The subsequent reporter cell line (HD12) produced β-gal when cross-linked with immobilized anti-Ly49H. Moreover, it responded to MCMV-infected but not uninfected cells and required cell–cell contact. Supernatants from infected cells did not stimulate nor did high doses of innate cytokines such as IFN-α/β. By contrast, stimulation occurred even when the infected cells were fixed. A wide variety of cells infected with MCMV stimulated HD12 cells, but when infected with other herpesviruses (HSV-1, γHV68) no stimulation occurred, suggesting that ligand expression was not due to herpesvirus infection per se. Thus, we concluded that the ligand for Ly49H was expressed on the cell surface, and was probably encoded by MCMV itself.

A bioinformatics approach was then undertaken for identification of ORFs in the MCMV genome encoding putative transmembrane proteins (Smith et al. 2002). Inasmuch as other Ly49 receptors recognize MHC class I molecules, MHC class I-like proteins were also considered, but only one ORF (m144) had basic local alignment search tool (BLAST) sequence homology to MHC class I. However, m144 is thought to be a ligand for an NK cell inhibitory receptor (Farrell et al. 1997; Kubota et al. 1999). Nonetheless, 11 other ORFs were identified with putative MHC class I folds with a structural prediction strategy (3D-PSSM, http://www.sbg.bio.ic.ac.uk/~3dpssm/index2.html) (Kelley et al. 2000). Most were also dispensable for in vitro viral replication as assessed by the study of MCMV mutants with large deletions covering these ORFs (Cavanaugh et al. 1996; Kleijnen et al. 1997; Thale et al. 1995). Thus, these ORFs are likely to interact with the host.

PCR primers were generated for all 40 ORFs encoding putative transmembrane proteins or MHC class I folds (Smith et al. 2002). Of them, 29 were readily amplifiable from a MCMV-infected cell cDNA library and were expressed in target cells with retroviral expression vectors. Only one, m157, stimulated HD12 reporter cells; m157 has a predicted MHC class I-like structure. Transduced expression of other ORFs did not stimulate and m157 did not stimulate another Ly49 activation receptor reporter cell. m157 transfectants also specifically and selectively stimulated primary Ly49H$^+$ NK cells to produce IFN-γ in vitro, and IFN-γ production was associated with downregulation of Ly49H expression. Finally, anti-Ly49H blocked m157 stimulation of Ly49H reporter cells and primary Ly49H$^+$ NK cells.

A related approach was undertaken by the Lanier laboratory (Arase et al. 2002) with a Ly49H transfectant with ITAM-dependent expression of green fluorescent protein (GFP). They refined their considerations to ORFs absent in MCMV deletion clones that failed to stimulate the Ly49H reporter cell. They further used an m157-Ig fusion protein to determine that m157 directly binds Ly49H-transfected cells and to the Ly49I inhibitory receptor on approx. 10% of NK cells from the 129/J strain mice. Thus, Ly49H recognizes m157 that may have originated as an MCMV ligand for an inhibitory receptor on NK cells.

Further validation that m157 is the ligand for Ly49H came from studies of an MCMV clone with a deletion in m157 (Δm157) (Bubic et al. 2004). This virus showed enhanced virulence in C57BL6 mice that was unchanged when NK cells were depleted. Furthermore, Δm157-infected cells did not stimulate Ly49H$^+$ NK cells in vitro and Ly49H expression was not downregulated. When m157 was ectopically replaced in the Δm157 clone, characteristics of wildtype (wt) MCMV infection were restored. Moreover, the Δm157 clone displayed a slight attenuation of virulence in BALB/c mice that lack any NK cell receptor for m157 (Arase et al. 2002). These studies provide in vivo evidence for the interaction between Ly49H and m157 and suggest m157 has another immune evasion role.

A mouse mAb was generated that is specific for m157, i.e., it bound m157 transfectants but not parental cells, and stains MCMV-infected cells but not Δm157-infected cells, indicating that it reacts exclusively with m157 on virus-infected cells (Tripathy et al. 2006). m157 is expressed with glycophosphatidylinositol linkage since a stop codon is present in the midst of its otherwise canonical transmembrane domain, and its expression is diminished with phosphatidylinositol phospholipase C treatment. m157 is readily expressed 12 h after infection, consistent with the expression of its transcript as an early gene. m157 is expressed upon in vitro MCMV infection of a wide variety of tumor and primary cells, including macrophages and hepatocytes, but is expressed much less on fibroblasts, suggesting that some infected cells may be better recognized by Ly49H$^+$ NK cells. Despite its putative MHC class I-like structure, m157 is expressed on β2m$^{-/-}$ and Tap1$^{-/-}$ bone marrow (BM)-derived macrophages infected with MCMV. Moreover, m157 is expressed equivalently on cells infected with an MCMV mutant lacking all ORFs (m04, m06, m152) that downregulate host cell MHC class I molecules. Finally, anti-m157 blocks recognition by Ly49H$^+$ NK cells and Ly49H-reporter cells. Thus, m157 is not subject to viral regulation of MHC class I and is specifically recognized by Ly49H.

MCMV Escape Mutants

Interestingly, the K181 strain of MCMV (containing *m157*) is typically passaged through BALB/c mice that lack *Ly49h*. When K181 was passaged through a BALB/c mouse strain congenic for the C57BL/6 allele of *Ly49h*, mutant MCMV clones arose with mutations in *m157* that affect m157 expression (Voigt et al. 2003). These clones essentially replaced viruses containing intact *m157* and evidence was obtained for *m157* mutation occurring by the third passage. Thus, selection pressure in immunocompetent C57BL/6 mice is sufficient to result in the emergence of MCMV clones that can escape Ly49H-mediated control.

Meanwhile, the early innate control of MCMV by Ly49H-dependent NK cell responses suggested that mice deficient in B and T cells should control the virus initially. Indeed, severe combined immunodeficiency (SCID) and recombination activation gene (RAG)-deficient mice initially survived infection, unlike early lethality in mice lacking NK cells or injected with anti-Ly49H, all of which die within 7 days post-infection (Brown et al. 2001). Immunodeficient mice succumbed, however, about 3–4 weeks after infection. There was early control of viral replication in SCID mice but subsequently viral titers increased. When viruses emerging from SCID mice at 3 weeks were cloned (termed SCID-MCMV), they produced early lethality in naïve SCID and wt mice, mostly occurring by day 7 post-infection. Also, SCID-MCMV isolates showed higher viral titers at day 3 compared to wt MCMV. Thus, these data indicated that MCMV clones with enhanced virulence emerge rapidly during infection of mice deficient in adaptive immunity.

The SCID-MCMV clones had similar properties to the Δm157 clone, i.e., SCID-MCMV-infected cells failed to stimulate Ly49H⁺ NK cells (French et al. 2004) and Ly49H reporter cells (French et al. 2005) in vitro, suggesting that the SCID-MCMV isolates had mutations in *m157*. Indeed, sequence analysis revealed mutations in m157 in more than 95% of isolates; most should disrupt expression. By contrast, no mutations were identified in the other ORFs tested. Furthermore, the original MCMV preparation was re-cloned and all clones contained intact m157. When one of these MCMV clones with verified intact m157 was expanded only in tissue culture and then inoculated into SCID mice, there was again late emergence of viruses that were cloned. Of them, 100% had m157 mutations. Thus, the innate immune system provides selection pressure on MCMV resulting in emergence of escape viruses.

Host-Pathogen Lessons from Ly49H and m157

The interaction of Ly49H with m157 is likely to reflect an ongoing "arms" race between the pathogen and the host, but this co-evolution story is likely to be complex. While more work is certainly required, the available data suggest that m157 may be an immune evasion molecule, allowing MCMV to avoid detection from NK or other immune cells. For example, m157 can be recognized by the 129 (mouse strain) allele of the Ly49I inhibitory receptor (Arase et al. 2002). Inasmuch as Ly49I is expressed on only a small fraction of NK cells, and there is no known activation receptor in 129 mice for recognition of MCMV, the significance of this finding is unclear, but it may provide a clue to further analysis. [There is abundant evidence that MCMV devotes several ORFs to target ligands for the NKG2D activation receptor, which is expressed in 129 mice (Hasan et al. 2005; Ho et al. 2002; Krmpotic et al. 2002, 2005; Lenac et al. 2006; Lodoen et al. 2004), suggesting that producing an inhibitory receptor ligand, i.e., m157, could be another means to affect NK cell activation through NKG2D.] In addition, the Δm157 clone replicates less well in BALB/c mice that do not have an NK cell receptor that binds m157, suggesting that m157 may be involved in evasion of other immune cells (Bubic et al. 2004).

On the other hand, Ly49H may be the host evolutionary response to the inhibitory effects of m157 (Arase et al. 2002). Moreover, it is important to recall that MCMV undergoes an acute replication phase during which NK cell control operates, followed by the establishment of latency (Biron et al. 1999). It is possible that an MCMV clone that is too virulent during this phase will kill the host, and not allow latency to be established. This might be detrimental to long-term survival of the virus at the population level, as noted in the co-evolution of hosts and poxvirus (rabbits and myxoma virus) (Fenner 1983). Thus, viruses can evolve mechanisms to attenuate their virulence, including addition of ORFs to enhance host responses with another example being the soluble IL1-R in poxviruses (Alcami and Smith 1992).

The rapid loss of m157 in *Ly49h* hosts (French et al. 2004; Voigt et al. 2003) nonetheless suggests that an NK cell activation receptor response can exert enough selection pressure to result in m157-deleted escape mutants, suggesting that m157 will become eventually absent in MCMV. So why is it still present in K181? It should be noted that C57BL/6 mice represent the minority of inbred mouse strains that demonstrate early innate resistance to MCMV (day 3 viral titers, for example) (Scalzo et al. 2005). The MA/My strain also shows early resistance but this is not due to *Ly49h* (Desrosiers et al. 2005; Dighe et al. 2005). Indeed, most inbred mouse strains lack *Ly49h*. Furthermore, early results indicate significant variability in wild mice with respect to control of MCMV (Scalzo et al. 2005). Most strains are unable to show resistance to the K181 strain of MCMV, suggesting that they lack *Ly49h*. Microsatellite marker data also suggest that they have different NKC haplotypes. It will therefore be informative to survey wild strains of mice, the majority of which are typically infected with MCMV, and determine the relationship between *Ly49h* and *m157* in these host-pathogen pairs.

Role of Ly49H in Host Resistance to MCMV: The Bigger Picture

The critical role of Ly49H in MCMV resistance strongly suggested that Ly49H⁺ NK cells are specifically triggered during MCMV infection. During an early phase of infection, however, nonspecific NK cell activation occurs without regard to Ly49H expression (Dokun et al. 2001b). This was manifested in two ways, IFN-γ production at 36 h (time of maximal production) as detected by intracellular staining, and proliferation at 2 days. Subsequently, there was preferential proliferation of Ly49H⁺ NK cells peaking in days 4–6. Ly49H-specific proliferation was virus-specific and inhibited by anti-Ly49H treatment, indicating that Ly49H itself is specifically stimulated in MCMV infection, and providing an explanation for the early clue to Ly49H involvement in the *Cmv1* effect. These studies indicate that NK cells undergo two distinct phases of activation during MCMV infection, an early generic response, presumably to cytokines, and a later specific response triggered through a virus-specific NK cell receptor.

Ly49H ligation by m157 on transfected cells also results in coordinated release of five cytokines/chemokines, [IFNγ, ATAC (lymphotactin), MIP-1α, MIP-1β, RANTES] from Ly49H⁺ NK cells (Dorner et al. 2004). Whereas other cytokines (IL-2, IL-12, IL-15, IL-18) also triggered release of the five cytokines/chemokines, stimulation was not confined to Ly49H⁺ cells. At the single cell level, production of all five mediators showed strong positive correlation with each other. NK cells were a major source of the five cytokines/chemokines in vitro and in vivo, whereas infected macrophages produced only limited amounts of MIP-1α, MIP-1β, and RANTES. These findings suggest that both virus-specific and nonspecific NK cells play crucial roles in activating other inflammatory cells during MCMV infection.

Ly49H engagement by itself does not lead to NK cell proliferation (French et al. 2006). NK cells require IL-15 and IL-15Rα for in vivo growth and survival. For example, mice deficient in IL-15 or the IL-15 receptor complex [IL15Rα, IL2/15Rβ (CD122), or common γ chain (γc)] fail to develop NK cells. Although IL15Rα is expressed by NK cells, IL15Rα can present IL-15 in *trans* (from another cell) to the NK cell (Dubois et al. 2002; Koka et al. 2003; Prlic et al. 2003). Regardless, IL-15 can supply the necessary growth factor to allow specific proliferation of Ly49H⁺ NK cells after Ly49H engagement whereas IL-18 is not required in contrast to early reports (French et al. 2006).

Recent studies indicate that other molecules are required for Ly49H-dependent MCMV control. For example, the *Unc13d* gene encodes a molecule that is required for efficient granule exocytosis (Crozat et al. 2007). *Jinx* mice, with an abnormal splice donor site in *Unc13d*, are extremely susceptible to MCMV. Moreover, it is intuitive that other molecules involved in Ly49H-dependent responses, such as DAP12, perforin, and granzymes, should also affect MCMV control, as has been shown, though it is sometimes difficult to isolate these effects to Ly49H and NK cells (Loh et al. 2005; Sjolin et al. 2002; Tay and Welsh 1997; van Dommelen et al. 2006).

On the other hand, the Ly49H-dependent responses alone are insufficient to control MCMV infection. The early nonspecific stimulus involves, at least in part, virus-induced activation of plasmacytoid DCs (pDCs, also known as interferon-producing cells, IPCs) via Toll-like receptor 9 (TLR9) whereas NK cells are not triggered through TLR9. This results in signaling through MyD88 leading to type I interferon responses that are critical in innate immune responses. In TLR9-deficient mice resulting from deliberate targeting of TLR9 or *N*-ethyl-*N*-nitrosourea (ENU)-mutagenesis, MCMV replication is poorly controlled (Krug et al. 2004; Tabeta et al. 2004). Interestingly, these responses are required even when the Ly49H pathway is intact and they affect nonspecific activation of NK cells, indicating that TLR9/MyD88 activation of pDCs is upstream of NK cell responses.

These studies highlight the complexities of the immune response to MCMV. Although preexisting genetic variation was related to only a relatively small number of polymorphic loci (~2, i.e., H-2 and *Cmv1* as discussed previously) (Grundy et al. 1981; Scalzo et al. 1990), this was limited by the numbers of inbred laboratory mouse strains that were compared and analyzed, as well as the inherent relatedness of inbred strains of the same species (Tsang et al. 2005). On the other hand, ENU mutagenesis of a single inbred strain (C57BL/6) and subsequent analysis of MCMV resistance suggest that nearly 300 genes play nonredundant roles in control of MCMV (Beutler et al. 2005). Thus, how these genes relate to Ly49H-mediated resistance will be of major interest in the near future.

Emerging Role of Other NK Cell Activation Receptors in Recognition of Virus-Infected Cells

The identity of Ly49H as an activation receptor that recognizes virus-infected cells prompted a broader search for other NK cell activation receptors involved in recognition of virus-infected cells. Some mouse strains resist MCMV in a Ly49H-independent manner. In genetic analysis, Ly49P from MA/My mice appears to recognize MCMV infection (Desrosiers et al. 2005; Dighe et al. 2005; Xie et al. 2007). In contrast to Ly49H and m157, however, a specific MHC allele, H2D^k is required, suggesting that Ly49P may recognize either altered H2D^k or peptides presented by H2D^k in the context of MCMV infection.

In humans, a notable example is the recognition of influenza hemagglutinin by human NKp46, an Ig-like receptor coupled to DAP12 (Mandelboim et al. 2001; Sivori et al. 1997). Although it has been difficult to define the basis for specificity since hemagglutinin recognition apparently requires sialic acid residues on NKp46 (sialic acid residues are ubiquitous), recent studies in NKp46-deficient mice indicate that mouse NKp46 is required for resistance to influenza (Gazit et al. 2006). Thus, these data indicate that NKp46 is important in control of influenza virus.

Finally, with respect to human NK cell recognition of HCMV, emerging data indicate a role for the lectin-like heterodimer CD94/NKG2C (Guma et al. 2006a, b). Whereas CD94 can partner with NKG2 family members (except NKG2D, which forms homodimers and probably should not be considered as a member of the NKG2 family despite its name), the NKG2 partner chain dictates the function of the heterodimer. NKG2A has a cytoplasmic ITIM and is inhibitory whereas NKG2C lacks an ITIM and has a charged transmembrane residue for association with DAP12 for signaling. Both CD94/NKG2 heterodimers recognize the nonclassical MHC class I molecule HLA-E (Qa1 in mouse) that binds peptides derived from the signal peptides of classical MHC class I molecules (Braud et al. 1998; Lee et al. 1998; Vance et al. 1998). The apparent preferential expansion of NK cells expressing CD94/NKG2C both in vitro and in vivo strongly suggests that activation through CD94/NKG2C itself is responsible (Guma et al. 2006a, b). Thus, it will be of interest to determine if human CD94/NKG2C molecules on NK cells recognize HLA-E molecules that have been altered during CMV infections.

Emerging data therefore strongly support a direct role for additional NK cell activation receptors in recognition of virus-infected cells.

Summary

The genetic dissection of mouse resistance to MCMV provided our first detailed insights into a physiologically important way by which NK cells recognize virus-infected cells. This approach was challenging at several levels, but the advances derived from it have continued to impact our understanding of NK cell activation receptors, recognition of virus-infected cells, and, more broadly, innate immunity, host-pathogen interactions, and pathogen evolution.

Acknowledgements The authors thank members of their laboratories, past and present, for their efforts and success in understanding the genetic basis for MCMV resistance. Work in the Scalzo laboratory is supported by grants from the National Health and Medical Research Council (NH and MRC) and A.A.S. is supported by an NH and MRC Senior Research Fellowship. The Yokoyama laboratory is supported by the Barnes-Jewish Hospital Foundation, and grants from the National Institutes of Health. W.M.Y is an investigator of the Howard Hughes Medical Institute.

References

Adam SG, Caraux A, Fodil-Cornu N, Loredo-Osti JC, Lesjean-Pottier S, Jaubert J, Bubic I, Jonjic S, Guenet JL, Vidal SM, Colucci F (2006) Cmv4, a new locus linked to the NK cell gene complex, controls innate resistance to cytomegalovirus in wild-derived mice. J Immunol 176:5478–5485

Alcami A, Smith GL (1992) A soluble receptor for interleukin-1 beta encoded by vaccinia virus: a novel mechanism of virus modulation of the host response to infection. Cell 71:153–167

Allan JE, Shellam GR (1984) Genetic control of murine cytomegalovirus infection: virus titres in resistant and susceptible strains of mice. Arch Virol 81:139–150

Allan JE, Shellam GR (1985) Characterization of interferon induction in mice of resistant and susceptible strains during murine cytomegalovirus infection. J Gen Virol 66:1105–1112

Andoniou CE, van Dommelen SL, Voigt V, Andrews DM, Brizard G, Asselin-Paturel C, Delale T, Stacey KJ, Trinchieri G, Degli-Esposti MA (2005) Interaction between conventional dendritic cells and natural killer cells is integral to the activation of effective antiviral immunity. Nat Immunol 6:1011–1019

Arase H, Mocarski ES, Campbell AE, Hill AB, Lanier LL (2002) Direct recognition of cytomegalovirus by activating and inhibitory NK cell receptors. Science 296:1323–1326

Bakker AB, Hoek RM, Cerwenka A, Blom B, Lucian L, McNeil T, Murray R, Phillips LH, Sedgwick JD, Lanier LL (2000) DAP12-deficient mice fail to develop autoimmunity due to impaired antigen priming. Immunity 13:345–353

Bancroft GJ, Shellam GR, Chalmer JE (1981) Genetic influences on the augmentation of natural killer (NK) cells during murine cytomegalovirus infection: correlation with patterns of resistance. J Immunol 126:988–994

Beutler B, Crozat K, Koziol JA, Georgel P (2005) Genetic dissection of innate immunity to infection the mouse cytomegalovirus model. Curr Opin Immunol 17:36–43

Biron CA, Byron KS, Sullivan JL (1989) Severe herpesvirus infections in an adolescent without natural killer cells. N Engl J Med 320:1731–1735

Biron CA (1994) Cytokines in the generation of immune responses to, and resolution of, virus infection. Curr Opin Immunol 6:530–538

Biron CA (1999) Initial and innate responses to viral infections—pattern setting in immunity or disease. Curr Opin Microbiol 2:374–381

Biron CA, Nguyen KB, Pien GC, Cousens LP, Salazar-Mather TP (1999) Natural killer cells in antiviral defense: function and regulation by innate cytokines. Annu Rev Immunol 17:189–220

Bradley M, Zeytun A, Rafi-Janajreh A, Nagarkatti PS, Nagarkatti M (1998) Role of spontaneous and interleukin-2-induced natural killer cell activity in the cytotoxicity and rejection of Fas+ and Fas− tumor cells. Blood 92:4248–4255

Braud VM, Allen DSJ, O'Callaghan CA, Söderström K, D'Andrea A, Ogg GS, Lazetic S, Young NT, Bell JI, Phillips JH, McMichael AJ (1998) HLA-E binds to natural-killer-cell receptors CD94/NKG2A, B and C. Nature 391:795–799

Brown MG, Fulmek S, Matsumoto K, Cho R, Lyons PA, Levy ER, Scalzo AA, Yokoyama WM (1997) A 2-Mb YAC contig and physical map of the natural killer gene complex on mouse chromosome 6. Genomics 42:16–25

Brown MG, Zhang J, Du Y, Stoll J, Yokoyama WM, Scalzo AA (1999) Localization on a physical map of the NKC-linked Cmv1 locus between Ly49b and the Prp gene cluster on mouse chromosome 6. J Immunol 163:1991–1999

Brown MG, Dokun AO, Heusel JW, Smith HR, Beckman DL, Blattenberger EA, Dubbelde CE, Stone LR, Scalzo AA, Yokoyama WM (2001) Vital involvement of a natural killer cell activation receptor in resistance to viral infection. Science 292:934–937

Bubic I, Wagner M, Krmpotic A, Saulig T, Kim S, Yokoyama WM, Jonjic S, Koszinowski UH (2004) Gain of virulence caused by loss of a gene in murine cytomegalovirus. J Virol 78:7536–7544

Bukowski JF, Woda BA, Habu S, Okumura K, Welsh RM (1983) Natural killer cell depletion enhances virus synthesis and virus-induced hepatitis in vivo. J Immunol 131:1531–1538

Bukowski JF, Woda BA, Welsh RM (1984) Pathogenesis of murine cytomegalovirus infection in natural killer cell-depleted mice. J Virol 52:119–128

Bukowski JF, Warner JF, Dennert G, Welsh RM (1985) Adoptive transfer studies demonstrating the antiviral effect of natural killer cells in vivo. J Exp Med 161:40–52

Cavanaugh VJ, Stenberg RM, Staley TL, Virgin HWt, MacDonald MR, Paetzold S, Farrell HE, Rawlinson WD, Campbell AE (1996) Murine cytomegalovirus with a deletion of genes spanning HindIII-J and -I displays altered cell and tissue tropism. J Virol 70:1365–1374

Chalmer JE, Mackenzie JS, Stanley NF (1977) Resistance to murine cytomegalovirus linked to the major histocompatibility complex of the mouse. J Gen Virol 37:107–114

Cohen GB, Gandhi RT, Davis DM, Mandelboim O, Chen BK, Strominger JL, Baltimore D (1999) The selective downregulation of class I major histocompatibility complex proteins by HIV-1 protects HIV-infected cells from NK cells. Immunity 10:661–671

Cosman D, Fanger N, Borges L, Kubin M, Chin W, Peterson L, Hsu ML (1997) A novel immunoglobulin superfamily receptor for cellular and viral MHC class I molecules. Immunity 7:273–282

Crozat K, Hoebe K, Ugolini S, Hong NA, Janssen E, Rutschmann S, Mudd S, Sovath S, Vivier E, Beutler B (2007) Jinx, an MCMV susceptibility phenotype caused by disruption of Unc13d: a mouse model of type 3 familial hemophagocytic lymphohistiocytosis. J Exp Med 204:853–863

Daniels KA, Devora G, Lai WC, O'Donnell CL, Bennett M, Welsh RM (2001) Murine cytomegalovirus is regulated by a discrete subset of natural killer cells reactive with monoclonal antibody to ly49 h. J Exp Med 194:29–44

Delano ML, Brownstein DG (1995) Innate resistance to lethal mousepox is genetically linked to the NK gene complex on chromosome 6 and correlates with early restriction of virus replication by cells with an NK phenotype. J Virol 69:5875–5877

Depatie C, Muise E, Lepage P, Gros P, Vidal SM (1997) High-resolution linkage map in the proximity of the host resistance locus CMV1. Genomics 39:154–163

Depatie C, Lee SH, Stafford A, Avner P, Belouchi A, Gros P, Vidal SM (2000) Sequence-ready BAC contig, physical, and transcriptional map of a 2-Mb region overlapping the mouse chromosome 6 host-resistance locus Cmv1. Genomics 66:161–174

Desrosiers MP, Kielczewska A, Loredo-Osti JC, Adam SG, Makrigiannis AP, Lemieux S, Pham T, Lodoen MB, Morgan K, Lanier LL, Vidal SM (2005) Epistasis between mouse Klra and major histocompatibility complex class I loci is associated with a new mechanism of natural killer cell-mediated innate resistance to cytomegalovirus infection. Nat Genet 37: 593–599

Dighe A, Rodriguez M, Sabastian P, Xie X, McVoy M, Brown MG (2005) Requisite H2k role in NK cell-mediated resistance in acute murine cytomegalovirus-infected MA/My mice. J Immunol 175:6820–6828

Dokun AO, Chu DT, Yang L, Bendelac AS, Yokoyama WM (2001a) Analysis of in situ NK cell responses during viral infection. J Immunol 167:5286–5293

Dokun AO, Kim S, Smith HR, Kang HS, Chu DT, Yokoyama WM (2001b) Specific and nonspecific NK cell activation during virus infection. Nat Immunol 2:951–956

Dorner BG, Smith HRC, French AR, Kim S, Poursine-Laurent J, Beckman DL, Pingel JT, Kroczek RA, Yokoyama WM (2004) Coordinate expression of cytokines and chemokines by natural killer cells during murine cytomegalovirus infection. J Immunol 172:3119–3131

Dubois S, Mariner J, Waldmann TA, Tagaya Y (2002) IL-15Ralpha recycles and presents IL-15 In trans to neighboring cells. Immunity 17:537–547

Farrell HE, Vally H, Lynch DM, Fleming P, Shellam GR, Scalzo AA, Davis-Poynter NJ (1997) Inhibition of natural killer cells by a cytomegalovirus MHC class I homologue in vivo. Nature 386:510–514

Fenner F (1983) The Florey lecture, 1983. Biological control, as exemplified by smallpox eradication and myxomatosis. Proc R Soc Lond B Biol Sci 218:259–285

Forbes CA, Brown MG, Cho R, Shellam GR, Yokoyama WM, Scalzo AA (1997) The Cmv1 host resistance locus is closely linked to the Ly49 multigene family within the natural killer cell gene complex on mouse chromosome 6. Genomics 41:406–413

French AR, Pingel JT, Wagner M, Bubic I, Yang L, Kim S, Koszinowski U, Jonjic S, Yokoyama WM (2004) Escape of mutant double-stranded DNA virus from innate immune control. Immunity 20:747–756

French AR, Pingel JT, Kim S, Yang L, Yokoyama WM (2005) Rapid emergence of escape mutants following infection with murine cytomegalovirus in immunodeficient mice. Clin Immunol 115:61–69

French AR, Sjolin H, Kim S, Koka R, Yang L, Young DA, Cerboni C, Tomasello E, Ma A, Vivier E, Kärre K, Yokoyama WM (2006) DAP12 signaling directly augments proproliferative cytokine stimulation of NK Cells during viral infections. J Immunol 177:4981–4990

Furukawa H, Iizuka K, Poursine-Laurent J, Shastri N, Yokoyama WM (2002) A ligand for the murine NK activation receptor Ly-49D: activation of tolerized NK cells from beta(2)-microglobulin-deficient mice. J Immunol 169:126–136

Gazit R, Gruda R, Elboim M, Arnon TI, Katz G, Achdout H, Hanna J, Qimron U, Landau G, Greenbaum E, Zakay-Rones Z, Porgador A, Mandelboim O (2006) Lethal influenza infection in the absence of the natural killer cell receptor gene Ncr1. Nat Immunol 7:517–523

Grundy JE, Mackenzie JS, Stanley NF (1981) Influence of H-2 and non-H-2 genes on resistance to murine cytomegalovirus infection. Infect Immun 32:277–286

Grundy JE, Trapman J, Allan JE, Shellam GR, Melief CJ (1982) Evidence for a protective role of interferon in resistance to murine cytomegalovirus and its control by non-H-2-linked genes. Infect Immun 37:143–150

Guma M, Budt M, Saez A, Brckalo T, Hengel H, Angulo A, Lopez-Botet M (2006a) Expansion of CD94/NKG2C+ NK cells in response to human cytomegalovirus-infected fibroblasts. Blood 107:3624–3631

Guma M, Cabrera C, Erkizia I, Bofill M, Clotet B, Ruiz L, Lopez-Botet M (2006b) Human cytomegalovirus infection is associated with increased proportions of NK cells that express the CD94/NKG2C receptor in aviremic HIV-1-positive patients. J Infect Dis 194:38–41

Hanke T, Takizawa H, McMahon CW, Busch DH, Pamer EG, Miller JD, Altman JD, Liu Y, Cado D, Lemonnier FA, Bjorkman PJ, Raulet DH (1999) Direct assessment of MHC class I binding by seven Ly49 inhibitory NK cell receptors. Immunity 11:67–77

Hao L, Klein J, Nei M (2006) Heterogeneous but conserved natural killer receptor gene complexes in four major orders of mammals. Proc Natl Acad Sci U S A 103:3192–3197

Hasan M, Krmpotic A, Ruzsics Z, Bubic I, Lenac T, Halenius A, Loewendorf A, Messerle M, Hengel H, Jonjic S, Koszinowski UH (2005) Selective down-regulation of the NKG2D ligand H60 by mouse cytomegalovirus m155 glycoprotein. J Virol 79:2920–2930

Henkart PA (1994) Lymphocyte-mediated cytotoxicity: two pathways and multiple effector molecules. Immunity 1:343–346

Ho EL, Carayannopoulos LN, Poursine-Laurent J, Kinder J, Plougastel B, Smith HRC, Yokoyama WM (2002) Co-stimulation of multiple NK cell activation receptors by NKG2D. J Immunol 169:3667–3675

Idris AH, Smith HRC, Mason LH, Ortaldo JH, Scalzo AA, Yokoyama WM (1999) The natural killer cell complex genetic locus, Chok, encodes Ly49D, a target recognition receptor that activates natural killing. Proc Natl Acad Sci U S A 96:6330–6335

Ishido S, Choi JK, Lee BS, Wang C, DeMaria M, Johnson RP, Cohen GB, Jung JU (2000) Inhibition of natural killer cell-mediated cytotoxicity by Kaposi's sarcoma-associated herpesvirus K5 protein. Immunity 13:365–374

Jawahar S, Moody C, Chan M, Finberg R, Geha R, Chatila T (1996) Natural Killer (NK) cell deficiency associated with an epitope-deficient Fc receptor type IIIA (CD16-II). Clin Exp Immunol 103:408–413

Karlhofer FM, Ribaudo RK, Yokoyama WM (1992) MHC class I alloantigen specificity of Ly-49+ IL-2-activated natural killer cells. Nature 358:66–70

Kelley J, Walter L, Trowsdale J (2005) Comparative genomics of natural killer cell receptor gene clusters. PLoS Genet 1:129–139

Kelley LA, MacCallum RM, Sternberg MJ (2000) Enhanced genome annotation using structural profiles in the program 3D-PSSM. J Mol Biol 299:499–520

Kleijnen MF, Huppa JB, Lucin P, Mukherjee S, Farrell H, Campbell AE, Koszinowski UH, Hill AB, Ploegh HL (1997) A mouse cytomegalovirus glycoprotein, gp34, forms a complex with folded class I MHC molecules in the ER which is not retained but is transported to the cell surface. EMBO J 16:685–694

Koka R, Burkett PR, Chien M, Chai S, Chan F, Lodolce JP, Boone DL, Ma A (2003) Interleukin (IL)-15R[alpha]-deficient natural killer cells survive in normal but not IL-15R[alpha]-deficient mice. J Exp Med 197:977–984

Krmpotic A, Busch DH, Bubic I, Gebhardt F, Hengel H, Hasan M, Scalzo AA, Koszinowski UH, Jonjic S (2002) MCMV glycoprotein gp40 confers virus resistance to CD8+ T cells and NK cells in vivo. Nat Immunol 3:529–535

Krmpotic A, Hasan M, Loewendorf A, Saulig T, Halenius A, Lenac T, Polic B, Bubic I, Kriegeskorte A, Pernjak-Pugel E, Messerle M, Hengel H, Busch DH, Koszinowski UH, Jonjic S (2005) NK cell activation through the NKG2D ligand MULT-1 is selectively prevented by the glycoprotein encoded by mouse cytomegalovirus gene m145. J Exp Med 201:211–220

Krug A, French AR, Barchet W, Fischer JAA, Dzionek A, Pingel JT, Orihuela MM, Akira S, Yokoyama WM, Colonna M (2004) TLR9-dependent recognition of MCMV by IPC and DC generates coordinated cytokine responses that activate antiviral NK cell function. Immunity 21:107–119

Kubota A, Kubota S, Farrell HE, Davis-Poynter N, Takei F (1999) Inhibition of NK cells by murine CMV-encoded class I MHC homologue m144. Cell Immunol 191:145–151

Kveberg L, Back CJ, Dai KZ, Inngjerdingen M, Rolstad B, Ryan JC, Vaage JT, Naper C (2006) The novel inhibitory NKR-P1C receptor and Ly49s3 identify two complementary, functionally distinct NK cell subsets in rats. J Immunol 176:4133–4140

Lanier LL, Cortiss BC, Wu J, Leong C, Phillips JH (1998) Immunoreceptor DAP12 bearing a tyrosine-based activation motif is involved in activating NK cells. Nature 391:703–707

Lee N, Llano M, Carretero M, Ishitani A, Navarro F, Lopez-Botet M, Geraghty DE (1998) HLA-E is a major ligand for the natural killer inhibitory receptor CD94/NKG2A. Proc Natl Acad Sci U S A 95:5199*5204

Lee SH, Girard S, Macina D, Busa M, Zafer A, Belouchi A, Gros P, Vidal SM (2001) Susceptibility to mouse cytomegalovirus is associated with deletion of an activating natural killer cell receptor of the C-type lectin superfamily. Nat Genet 28:42–45

Lee SH, Zafer A, de Repentigny Y, Kothary R, Tremblay ML, Gros P, Duplay P, Webb JR, Vidal SM (2003) Transgenic expression of the activating natural killer receptor Ly49H confers resistance to cytomegalovirus in genetically susceptible mice. J Exp Med 197:515–526

Lenac T, Budt M, Arapovic J, Hasan M, Zimmermann A, Simic H, Krmpotic A, Messerle M, Ruzsics Z, Koszinowski UH, Hengel H, Jonjic S (2006) The herpesviral Fc receptor fcr-1 down-regulates the NKG2D ligands MULT-1 and H60. J Exp Med 203:1843–1850

Ljunggren HG, Kärre K (1990) In search of the 'missing self': MHC molecules and NK cell recognition. Immunol Today 11:237–244

Lodoen MB, Abenes G, Umamoto S, Houchins JP, Liu F, Lanier LL (2004) The cytomegalovirus m155 gene product subverts natural killer cell antiviral protection by disruption of H60-NKG2D interactions. J Exp Med 200:1075–1081

Loh J, Chu DT, O'Guin AK, Yokoyama WM, Virgin HWt (2005) Natural killer cells utilize both perforin and gamma interferon to regulate murine cytomegalovirus infection in the spleen and liver. J Virol 79:661–667

Long EO (1999) Regulation of immune responses through inhibitory receptors. Annu Rev Immunol 17:875–904

Mandelboim O, Lieberman N, Lev M, Paul L, Arnon TI, Bushkin Y, Davis DM, Strominger JL, Yewdell JW, Porgador A (2001) Recognition of haemagglutinins on virus-infected cells by NKp46 activates lysis by human NK cells. Nature 409:1055–1060

Mocarski ES, Courcelle CT (2001) Cytomegalovirus and their replication. In: Knipe DM, Howley PM (eds) Fields virology. Lippincott Williams and Wilkins, Philadelphia, pp 2626–2673

Nakamura MC, Naper C, Niemi EC, Spusta SC, Rolstad B, Butcher GW, Seaman WE, Ryan JC (1999) Natural killing of xenogeneic cells mediated by the mouse Ly-49D receptor. J Immunol 163:4694–4700

Olcese L, Cambiaggi A, Semenzato G, Bottino C, Moretta A, Vivier E (1997) Human killer cell activatory receptors for MHC class I molecules are included in a multimeric complex expressed by natural killer cells. J Immunol 158:5083–5086

Orange JS, Wang B, Terhorst C, Biron CA (1995) Requirement for natural killer cell-produced interferon gamma in defense against murine cytomegalovirus infection and enhancement of this defense pathway by interleukin 12 administration. J Exp Med 182:1045–1056

Orange JS, Biron CA (1996) An absolute and restricted requirement for IL-12 in natural killer cell IFN-gamma production and antiviral defense. Studies of natural killer and T cell responses in contrasting viral infections. J Immunol 156:1138–1142

Pereira RA, Scalzo A, Simmons A (2001) Cutting edge: a NK complex-linked locus governs acute versus latent herpes simplex virus infection of neurons. J Immunol 166:5869–5873

Prlic M, Blazar BR, Farrar MA, Jameson SC (2003) In vivo survival and homeostatic proliferation of natural killer cells. J Exp Med 197:967–976

Quinnan GV Jr, Manischewitz JF (1987) Genetically determined resistance to lethal murine cytomegalovirus infection is mediated by interferon-dependent and -independent restriction of virus replication. J Virol 61:1875–1881

Ravetch JV, Lanier LL (2000) Immune inhibitory receptors. Science 290:84–89

Rawlinson WD, Farrell HE, Barrell BG (1996) Analysis of the complete DNA sequence of murine cytomegalovirus. J Virol 70:8833–8849

Reyburn HT, Mandelboim O, Vales-Gomez M, Davis DM, Pazmany L, Strominger JL (1997) The class I MHC homologue of human cytomegalovirus inhibits attack by natural killer cells. Nature 386:514–517

Sanderson S, Shastri N (1994) LacZ inducible, antigen/MHC-specific T cell hybrids. Int Immunol 6:369–376

Scalzo AA, Fitzgerald NA, Simmons A, La Vista AB, Shellam GR (1990) Cmv-1, a genetic locus that controls murine cytomegalovirus replication in the spleen. J Exp Med 171:1469–1483

Scalzo AA, Fitzgerald NA, Wallace CR, Gibbons AE, Smart YC, Burton RC, Shellam GR (1992) The effect of the Cmv-1 resistance gene, which is linked to the natural killer cell gene complex, is mediated by natural killer cells. J Immunol 149:581–589

Scalzo AA, Lyons PA, Fitzgerald NA, Forbes CA, Yokoyama WM, Shellam GR (1995a) Genetic mapping of Cmv1 in the region of mouse chromosome 6 encoding the NK gene complex-associated loci Ly49 and musNKR-P1. Genomics 27:435–441

Scalzo AA, Lyons PA, Fitzgerald NA, Forbes CA, Shellam GR (1995b) The BALB.B6-Cmv1r mouse: a strain congenic for Cmv1 and the NK gene complex. Immunogenetics 41:148–151

Scalzo AA, Wheat R, Dubbelde C, Stone L, Clark P, Du Y, Dong N, Stoll J, Yokoyama WM, Brown MG (2003) Molecular genetic characterization of the distal NKC recombination hotspot and putative murine CMV resistance control locus. Immunogenetics 55:370–378

Scalzo AA, Manzur M, Forbes CA, Brown MG, Shellam GR (2005) NK gene complex haplotype variability and host resistance alleles to murine cytomegalovirus in wild mouse populations. Immunol Cell Biol 83:144–149

Selgrade MK, Osborn JE (1974) Role of macrophages in resistance to murine cytomegalovirus. Infect Immun 10:1383–1390

Shellam GR, Allan JE, Papadimitriou JM, Bancroft GJ (1981) Increased susceptibility to cytomegalovirus infection in beige mutant mice. Proc Natl Acad Sci USA 78:5104–5108

Shellam GR, Flexman JP, Farrell HE, Papadimitriou JM (1985) The genetic background modulates the effect of the beige gene on susceptibility to cytomegalovirus infection in mice. Scand J Immunol 22:147–155

Sivori S, Vitale M, Morelli L, Sanseverino L, Augugliaro R, Bottino C, Moretta L, Moretta A (1997) p46, a novel natural killer cell-specific surface molecule that mediates cell activation. J Exp Med 186:1129–1136

Sjolin H, Tomasello E, Mousavi-Jazi M, Bartolazzi A, Kärre K, Vivier E, Cerboni C (2002) Pivotal role of KARAP/DAP12 adaptor molecule in the natural killer cell-mediated resistance to murine cytomegalovirus infection. J Exp Med 195:825–834

Smith HR, Chuang HH, Wang LL, Salcedo M, Heusel JW, Yokoyama WM (2000) Nonstochastic coexpression of activation receptors on murine natural killer cells. J Exp Med 191:1341–1354

Smith HR, Heusel JW, Mehta IK, Kim S, Dorner BG, Naidenko OV, Iizuka K, Furukawa H, Beckman DL, Pingel JT, Scalzo AA, Fremont DH, Yokoyama WM (2002) Recognition of a virus-encoded ligand by a natural killer cell activation receptor. Proc Natl Acad Sci U S A 99:8826–8831

Smith HRC, Karlhofer FM, Yokoyama WM (1994) Ly-49 multigene family expressed by IL-2-activated NK cells. J Immunol 153:1068–1079

Smith KM, Wu J, Bakker AB, Phillips JH, Lanier LL (1998) Cutting edge: Ly-49D and Ly-49H associate with mouse DAP12 and form activating receptors. J Immunol 161:7–10

Tabeta K, Georgel P, Janssen E, Du X, Hoebe K, Crozat K, Mudd S, Shamel L, Sovath S, Goode J, Alexopoulou L, Flavell RA, Beutler B (2004) Toll-like receptors 9 and 3 as essential components of innate immune defense against mouse cytomegalovirus infection. Proc Natl Acad Sci U S A 101:3516–3521

Tay CH, Welsh RM (1997) Distinct organ-dependent mechanisms for the control of murine cytomegalovirus infection by natural killer cells. J Virol 71:267–275

Tay CH, Yu LY, Kumar V, Mason L, Ortaldo JR, Welsh RM (1999) The role of LY49 NK cell subsets in the regulation of murine cytomegalovirus infections. J Immunol 162:718–726

Thale R, Szepan U, Hengel H, Geginat G, Lucin P, Koszinowski UH (1995) Identification of the mouse cytomegalovirus genomic region affecting major histocompatibility complex class I molecule transport. J Virol 69:6098–6105

Tomasec P, Braud VM, Rickards C, Powell MB, McSharry BP, Gadola S, Cerundolo V, Borysiewicz LK, McMichael AJ, Wilkinson GW (2000) Surface expression of HLA-E, an inhibitor of natural killer cells, enhanced by human cytomegalovirus gpUL40. Science 287:1031

Tomasello E, Desmoulins PO, Chemin K, Guia S, Cremer H, Ortaldo J, Love P, Kaiserlian D, Vivier E (2000) Combined natural killer cell and dendritic cell functional deficiency in KARAP/DAP12 loss-of-function mutant mice. Immunity 13:355–364

Tortorella D, Gewurz BE, Furman MH, Schust DJ, Ploegh HL (2000) Viral subversion of the immune system. Annu Rev Immunol 18:861–926

Tripathy SK, Smith HRC, Holroyd EA, Pingel JT, Yokoyama WM (2006) Expression of m157, a murine cytomegalovirus-encoded putative major histocompatibility class I (MHC-I)-like protein, is independent of viral regulation of host MHC-I. J Virol 80:545–550

Tsang S, Sun Z, Luke B, Stewart C, Lum N, Gregory M, Wu X, Subleski M, Jenkins NA, Copeland NG, Munroe DJ (2005) A comprehensive SNP-based genetic analysis of inbred mouse strains. Mamm Genome 16:476–480

Ulbrecht M, Martinozzi S, Grzeschik M, Hengel H, Ellwart JW, Pla M, Weiss EH (2000) Cutting edge: the human cytomegalovirus UL40 gene product contains a ligand for HLA-E and prevents NK cell-mediated lysis. J Immunol 164:5019–5022

van Dommelen SL, Sumaria N, Schreiber RD, Scalzo AA, Smyth MJ, Degli-Esposti MA (2006) Perforin and granzymes have distinct roles in defensive immunity and immunopathology. Immunity 25:835–848

Vance RE, Kraft JR, Altman JD, Jensen PE, Raulet DH (1998) Mouse CD94/NKG2A is a natural killer cell receptor for the nonclassical major histocompatibility complex (MHC) class I molecule Qa-1(b). J Exp Med 188:1841–1848

Voigt V, Forbes CA, Tonkin JN, Degli-Esposti MA, Smith HR, Yokoyama WM, Scalzo AA (2003) Murine cytomegalovirus m157 mutation and variation leads to immune evasion of natural killer cells. Proc Natl Acad Sci U S A 100:13483–13488

Welsh RM, Dundon PL, Eynon EE, Brubaker JO, Koo GC, O'Donnell CL (1990) Demonstration of the antiviral role of natural killer cells in vivo with a natural killer cell-specific monoclonal antibody (NK1.1). Nat Immun Cell Growth Regul 9:112–120

Wong S, Freeman JD, Kelleher C, Mager D, Takei F (1991) Ly-49 multigene family. New members of a superfamily of type II membrane proteins with lectin-like domains. J Immunol 147:1417–1423

Xie X, Dighe A, Clark P, Sabastian P, Buss S, Brown MG (2007) Deficient major histocompatibility complex-linked innate murine cytomegalovirus immunity in MA/My.L-H2b mice and viral downregulation of H-2k class I proteins. J Virol 81:229–236

Yokoyama WM, Kehn PJ, Cohen DI, Shevach EM (1990) Chromosomal location of the Ly-49 (A1, YE1/48) multigene family. Genetic association with the NK1.1 antigen. J Immunol 145:2353–2358

Yokoyama WM, Ryan JC, Hunter JJ, Smith HR, Stark M, Seaman WE (1991) cDNA cloning of mouse NKR-P1 and genetic linkage with Ly-49. Identification of a natural killer cell gene complex on mouse chromosome 6. J Immunol 147:3229–3236

Yokoyama WM, Plougastel BF (2003) Immune functions encoded by the natural killer gene complex. Nat Rev Immunol 3:304–316

Yokoyama WM (2008) Natural killer cells. In: Paul WE (ed) Fundamental immunology. Lippincott-Raven, New York, pp 575–603

Zamai L, Ahmad M, Bennett IM, Azzoni L, Alnemri ES, Perussia B (1998) Natural killer (NK) cell-mediated cytotoxicity: differential use of TRAIL and Fas ligand by immature and mature primary human NK cells. J Exp Med 188:2375–2380

Genetic Dissection of Host Resistance
to *Mycobacterium tuberculosis*: The *sst1* Locus
and the *Ipr1* Gene

I. Kramnik

Contents

Abstract Genetic variation of the host significantly contributes to dramatic differences in the outcomes of natural infection with virulent *Mycobacterium tuberculosis* (MTB) in humans, as well as in experimental animal models. Host resistance to tuberculosis is a complex multifactorial genetic trait in which many genetic polymorphisms contribute to the phenotype, while their individual contributions are influenced by gene–gene and gene–environment interactions. The most epidemiologically significant form of tuberculosis infection in humans is pulmonary tuberculosis. Factors that predispose immunocompetent individuals to this outcome, however, are largely unknown. Using an experimental mouse model of infection with virulent MTB for the genetic analysis of host resistance to this pathogen, we have identified several tuberculosis susceptibility loci in otherwise immunocompetent mice. The *sst1* locus has been mapped to mouse chromosome 1 and shown to be especially important for control of pulmonary tuberculosis. Rampant progression of tuberculosis infection in the lungs of the *sst1*-susceptible mouse was associated with the development of necrotic lung lesions, which was

I. Kramnik
Department of Immunology and Infectious Diseases, Harvard School of Public Health,
677 Huntington Avenue, Boston, MA 02115, USA
ikramnik@hsph.harvard.edu

B. Beutler (ed.), *Immunology, Phenotype First: How Mutations Have Established
New Principles and Pathways in Immunology.* Current Topics in Microbiology
and Immunology 321. © Springer-Verlag Berlin Heidelberg 2008

prevented by the *sst1*-resistant allele. Using a positional cloning approach, we have identified a novel host resistance gene, *Ipr1*, which is encoded within the *sst1* locus and mediates innate immunity to the intracellular bacterial pathogens MTB and *Listeria monocytogenes*. The *sst1* locus and the *Ipr1* gene participate in control of intracellular multiplication of virulent MTB and have an effect on the infected macrophages' mechanism of cell death. The Ipr1 is an interferon-inducible nuclear protein that dynamically associates with other nuclear proteins in macrophages primed with interferons or infected with MTB. Several of the Ipr1-interacting proteins are known to participate in regulation of transcription, RNA processing, and apoptosis. Further biochemical analysis of the Ipr1-mediated pathway will help delineate a mechanism of innate immunity that is especially important for control of tuberculosis progression in the lungs.

Pathogenesis of MTB Infection and Heterogeneity of Host Populations

The year 2007 marked the 125th anniversary of Robert Koch's discovery of *Mycobacterium tuberculosis* (MTB) and his demonstration of its causative role in human tuberculosis, for which he received the Nobel Prize in Physiology or Medicine in 1905. Koch's studies of tuberculosis became a cornerstone for the studies of pathogenic microorganisms (Kaufmann and Schaible 2005). In his classical work Koch firmly established the infectious nature of tuberculosis, and formulated postulates that defined how disease causality could be established for any microbial pathogen. Not only did he demonstrate the association of the acid-fast bacillus, MTB, with tuberculous lesions, but also proved that it was the causative agent of the disease by demonstrating that pure bacterial culture isolated from the tuberculosis patients caused similar disease in experimentally infected animals and that the bacilli could be re-isolated from their organs. Since Koch's truly pioneering work, animal models have played a pivotal role in tuberculosis research.

In the nineteenth century about 12% of all deaths were due to tuberculosis and Koch's discovery of its infectious nature and identification of the etiological agent was hailed as a major medical discovery of the century and was anticipated to bring about rapid victory over the "white plague" (Gradmann 2006). Indeed, within 100 years after Koch's discovery, lethality from tuberculosis was tremendously reduced, achieved through the development of specific antibacterial drugs, diagnostic tests, and a live attenuated vaccine, all made possible by Koch's discovery. Despite global efforts to control tuberculosis, however, it remains the second leading cause of death from any infectious disease, with approximately 8.9 million new cases and 1.7 million deaths in the year 2004 (WHO 2006). The number of new cases and deaths from this infection worldwide has not decreased globally for over a decade (Bleed et al. 2000). This alarming trend suggests that existing methods of prevention and treatment of the disease are reaching their limits and that novel strategies are urgently needed (Kaufmann et al. 2005; Orme 2006). Rational design of those strategies, however, requires new insights into the pathogen's virulence strategy, which it has developed over thousands of years of co-evolution with the human host (Gagneux et al. 2006).

What makes tuberculosis an especially formidable pathogen is the extent of its spread in the human population: 1.7 billion people, approximately one-third of the world's population, are infected with MTB. With a 50% lethality rate in untreated human tuberculosis cases, the pathogen likely exerted selective pressure in the pre-antibiotic era, explaining why a great majority of modern humans are initially resistant to tuberculosis infection. Indeed, the lifetime risk of developing clinical disease following infection is about 10%, and development of clinical disease within a year after primary infection occurs in less than 5% of cases (Fig. 1).

Among those who do develop the disease after initial exposure, the rate of the disease progression and gravity of clinical manifestations vary significantly. Pulmonary tuberculosis, the only epidemiologically significant form of the disease,

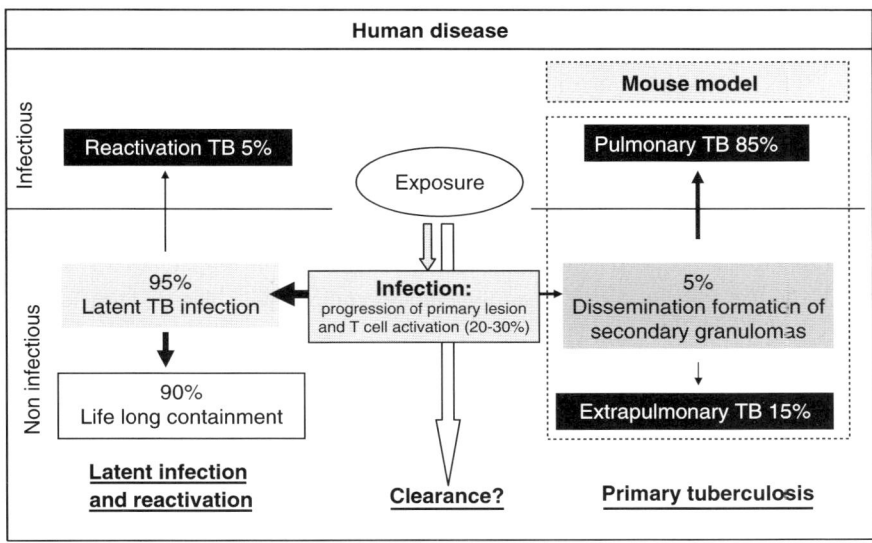

Fig. 1 Outcomes of tuberculosis infection in humans and in the mouse model. It is estimated that approximately one-third of the world's population is exposed to virulent *M. tuberculosis* during their lifetime. Of those, 20%–30% become infected and develop a T cell-mediated immune response to the bacteria, which is documented by a positive skin test (delayed-type hypersensitivity) to the purified protein derivative (PPD) of *M. tuberculosis*. More than 90% of people infected do not develop clinical manifestations of disease and are thus latently infected. They are at risk of the disease for their lifetime, however, and may develop reactivation disease as their immune system is weakened, which happens in approximately 5% of the latently infected individuals. The risk of reactivation of latent tuberculosis infection is dramatically increased by concomitant infection with human immunodeficiency virus (HIV). In contrast, in about 5% of infected individuals disease develops within the first year after exposure to the pathogen, i.e., primary tuberculosis. Of those, approximately 85% manifest pulmonary tuberculosis and become potentially infectious. The mouse model (delimited by the *dashed lines*) recapitulates primary progressive tuberculosis only

develops in 85% of all cases of clinical tuberculosis (Onyebujoh and Rook 2004). Unlike infectious agents that can be transmitted within populations by latent carriers, i.e., infected individuals that do not develop disease, MTB is an obligatory pathogen for transmission. Active pulmonary tuberculosis with extensive lung tissue damage is necessary for MTB transmission via the respiratory route.

The typical tuberculosis lesion is called a granuloma. It contains myeloid cells, mostly macrophages and their derivatives, the epithelioid and multinucleated Langhans giant cells, and varying proportions of T and B lymphocytes. A characteristic feature of those lesions is the development of a dense central necrotic area, caseous necrosis. Immunocompetent cells are organized in concentric layers surrounding the necrotic core. The bacteria in the granulomas are located extracellularly within the necrotic area as well as inside macrophages that constitute the granuloma wall. Stable granuloma formation is a hallmark of chronic persistent infection as it protects both the host from the pathogen and the pathogen from the host. This status quo, however, can be broken, which leads to an increased inflammatory reaction, bacterial multiplication, liquefaction of the necrotic masses, and erosion of the granuloma wall, giving the pathogen access to airways. Necrotic masses that contain vast numbers of the pathogen are spread via fine aerosolized particles by individuals that often remain undiagnosed for extended periods of time, during which they may expose hundreds of contacts to the pathogen. This stealth strategy enables continuous transmission even within a population in which susceptible hosts are rarely encountered, making MTB a very successful human pathogen (Flynn and Chan 2005; Hingley-Wilson et al. 2003; Rodrigo et al. 1997). Formation and subsequent decomposition of tuberculous granulomas in the lungs of immunocompetent but susceptible individuals is a key element of this strategy.

Although disseminated extrapulmonary tuberculosis is a life-threatening disease, this clinical form is a dead end from the pathogen's evolutionary perspective, because patients that develop fatal disseminated mycobacterial infections and rapidly succumb to the infection do not transmit the pathogen efficiently. Therefore, understanding host and pathogen factors that allow preferential colonization and destruction of lung tissue by the pathogen in the face of effective host immunity is necessary for the development of effective control measures.

Genetic Predisposition to Tuberculosis

Initially, Koch's discovery of MTB overturned the prevailing theory of tuberculosis pathogenesis championed by the prominent German pathologist Rudolf Virchow, that tuberculosis was a noninfectious disease or "diathesis" resulting from a heritable malfunction of host cells (Rich 1951). In the subsequent years, however, substantial heritable variation in host resistance to tuberculosis infection was demonstrated in humans as well as in animal models. In humans, the first convincing evidence was obtained in epidemiological studies of twins (Comstock 1978; Kallmann and Reisner 1943). Although the authors were able to clearly demonstrate significant heritability of susceptibility to tuberculosis by comparing concordance rates of monozygotic and dizygotic twins, they concluded that the genetic control was complex and did not follow Mendelian laws. In experimental animal models heritability of tuberculosis susceptibility or resistance was demonstrated directly by analyzing outcomes of standardized tuberculosis infection in several generations of progeny of resistant and susceptible animals. In his classical studies, Max Lurie used a rabbit model of airborne infection with virulent MTB to demonstrate using quantitative analysis that not only did individual rabbits vary in their native resistance to the infection, but their susceptibility to the infection was a heritable polygenic trait that could not be explained according to a simple Mendelian formula (Lurie et al. 1952). Early studies using inbred mouse strains and their hybrids also demonstrated complex genetic control (Lynch et al. 1965).

From the genetic perspective host resistance to tuberculosis is a complex multifactorial genetic trait in which many genetic polymorphisms contribute to the phenotype, while their individual contributions are influenced by gene–gene and gene–environment interactions (Bellamy et al. 2000; Hill 2006). It was also proposed that the genetic component of tuberculosis susceptibility in human populations is heterogeneous, representing a spectrum ranging from rare cases of monogenic control (Mendelian susceptibility to mycobacterial disease, MSMD) to truly polygenic control (Abel and Casanova 2000; Alcais et al. 2005). MSMD mutations in genes involved in the central pathway of antituberculosis immunity [interferon (IFN)-γ-mediated activation of macrophages] confer a high degree of susceptibility to mycobacteria. In MSMD patients, normally apathogenic mycobacterial species or an attenuated vaccine strain of *M. bovis* bacillus Calmette-Guerin (BCG) cause disseminated, often fatal disease due to severe disruptions in the essential pathway of antimycobacterial immunity, namely the interleukin IL-12–IFN-γ–signal transducer and activator of transcription (STAT)1 axis (Jouanguy et al. 1996; Levin et al. 1995; Newport et al. 1996; reviewed in Casanova and Abel 2002; Fortin et al. 2007)). Remarkably, the same genes were found earlier to be essential for resistance to tuberculosis infection in mice (reviewed in Flynn 2006). In fact, extreme susceptibility to MTB of IFN-γ, INF-γ receptor, and IL12p40 knockout mice provided clues for identification of the MSMD genes in humans. From an epidemiological point of view mutations causing MSMD are very rare in human populations (Casanova and Abel 2005) and arguably account for a small fraction of the tuberculosis burden (Hill 2006).

As discussed above, the most epidemiologically significant form of tuberculosis infection in humans is pulmonary tuberculosis. However, factors that predispose immunocompetent individuals to this outcome are largely unknown. Even after infection with virulent MTB, immune mechanisms in susceptible hosts in most of the cases allow for systemic control of the infection, but fail specifically in the lungs. If host genetic polymorphisms do contribute to pulmonary tuberculosis in humans, they neither confer general immunodeficiency, nor compromise host resistance to environmental and attenuated vaccine strains of mycobacteria. Identification of such virulent mycobacteria-specific genes in humans would reveal mechanisms that the pathogen has evolved to exploit in the majority of immunocompetent hosts. Genetic heterogeneity, weak effects of individual genes, and the significant impact of environmental factors, however, have made the genetic analysis in human populations especially difficult.

From this perspective, attempts to use animal models for the genetic analysis of tuberculosis susceptibility provide several important advantages: uniform environment, equal exposure to identical pathogen (no variation in virulence), limited genetic heterogeneity of the host, and the possibility of controlled breeding and repeated testing of animals that bear the same genotype at individual loci or combinations of allelic variants at several loci. Intraspecies variation in host susceptibility to tuberculosis infection appears to be a rule—it has been observed in laboratory mice (Buschman et al. 1988; Medina and North 1998), rats (Sugawara et al. 2004), guinea pigs (Cohen et al. 1987; Wright and Lewis 1921), rabbits (Dorman et al. 2004; Lurie et al. 1955), red deer (Mackintosh et al. 2004), and primates (Capuano et al. 2003; Flynn 2006). Although rabbits and guinea pigs represent a popular model for studying the pathomorphology of pulmonary tuberculosis and testing vaccines and drugs, tools for their genetic analysis have yet to be developed (Helke et al. 2005; Orme 2005).

Genetic Analysis of Tuberculosis Resistance Using Experimental Mouse Model

The mouse is by far the most popular experimental animal model in which to study tuberculosis infection because powerful immunological and genetic tools are available for this species. Genetically engineered mouse strains represent a useful tool for dissecting roles of individual genes in complex phenotypes. Studies of knockout mice greatly contributed to our knowledge of essential mechanisms of host resistance to tuberculosis (reviewed in Cooper and Flynn 1995; Flynn 2006; North and Jung 2004; Salgame 2005). This "reverse genetic" approach was extremely successful in demonstrating an essential role of T cell-mediated immunity and production of T helper (Th)1-type cytokines, e.g., IFN-γ, as well as IL-12 and TNF-α signaling and nitric oxide production (MacMicking et al. 1997) for host resistance to virulent MTB. It appears that many of the essential pathways of antituberculosis immunity are similar in man and mouse. Mutations that disrupt the IFN-γ pathway in humans were shown to be responsible for extreme susceptibility to mycobacterial infections (reviewed in Casanova and Abel 2002; Ottenhoff et al. 2005), and neutralization of TNF-α led to relapses of latent tuberculosis infection (Gardam et al. 2003; Keane 2005). To date, the utility of this "reverse genetic" approach has been mostly limited to identification of essential pathways of tuberculosis immunity, but it has not illuminated lung-specific aspects of the disease.

As comprehensively discussed by North and Jung (2004), the mouse model may faithfully recapitulate major aspects of antituberculosis immunity and pathogenesis, including the particular vulnerability of the lung. However, the utility of the mouse for dissecting the pathogenesis of human tuberculosis has been debated. Indeed, the mouse is not a natural host of MTB, the pathogen is not transmitted among the murine species, and properly organized tuberculous lung granulomas containing necrotic centers have not been previously described in the experimental mouse model. In inbred mice, infection with virulent MTB invariably leads to progressive primary disease, while this outcome of infection is usually observed in less than 5% of humans (Fig. 1). Thus, mice cannot be used to model reactivation in pulmonary disease.

To address this dilemma, one should consider the "mouse model of tuberculosis" in light of host genetic heterogeneity. In mice, as in humans, host resistance to tuberculosis is a multigenic trait in which epistatic gene interactions play a significant role in shaping the phenotype. The genetic variation among standard inbred mouse strains, however, is much narrower compared to human populations, and therefore not all aspects of the human disease are easily recapitulated using several standard inbred mouse strains. Nevertheless, as evidenced by several studies of natural variation in resistance to tuberculosis infection among inbred mouse strains, conspicuous phenotypic diversity representing various manifestations of clinical tuberculosis exists in murine species, including phenotypes relevant to the human disease (Kramnik et al. 2000; Lavebratt et al. 1999; Mitsos et al. 2003; Watson et al. 2000). Those phenotypes can be systematically dissected using a forward genetic approach, which is uniquely suited for the identification of the molecular basis of complex phenotypes in vivo, regardless of whether they are controlled by a single or multiple genes (Casanova et al. 2002; Fortier et al. 2005b). The attractiveness of this laborious and time-consuming analysis is its potential to uncover novel gene functions and molecular pathways that are particularly important for disease pathogenesis in vivo.

Three independent forward genetic studies of mouse resistance to infection with virulent MTB have been performed to date using different pairs of resistant and susceptible parental strains and different strains of virulent mycobacteria, varying the doses, routes of infection, and readouts. In a study by Apt and colleagues tuberculosis progression in progeny of A/Sn (relatively resistant) and I/St (susceptible) strains was monitored by weight loss and survival after i.v. infection with the MTB strain H37Rv (Lavebratt et al. 1999; Nikonenko et al. 2000). Both phenotypes were controlled by three major loci, which were mapped to distal mouse chromosome 3 (designated tuberculosis severity 1, *tbs1*), proximal chromosome 9 (*tbs2*) and to chromosome 17 in the vicinity of the H-2 complex (Lavebratt et al. 1999; Sanchez et al. 2003). Gros and co-workers mapped four tuberculosis-resistance loci (Mitsos et al. 2000, 2003). Survival after the i.v. challenge was controlled by loci on chromosomes 1, 3, and 7, while multiplication of MTB in the lungs after aerosol challenge was controlled by two loci on chromosomes 7 and 19. Importantly, the location of the chromosome 7 peak in both experiments was very similar, suggesting that the same locus played an important role in controlling tuberculosis infection irrespective of the route and dose of MTB infection. The third study, which utilizes the same resistant parental strain as Gros and co-workers but a different susceptible strain (C3HeB/FeJ), is discussed in detail below.

Identification of the *sst1* Locus

These studies began with the observation that the standard inbred mouse strain
C3HeB/FeJ was extremely susceptible to tuberculosis (Kramnik et al. 1998).
After systemic intravenous infection with 10^5 colony-forming units (CFU) of
MTB Erdman strain, C3HeB/FeJ mice died abruptly within 25–28 days, while
other standard inbred mouse strains, including other substrains of C3H, survived
for 10–40 weeks after infection with the same dose of MTB, the C57BL/6J (B6)
mice being among the most resistant. Although the C3HeB/FeJ substrain of the
C3H mice had no known immunodeficiency, its survival time was similar to that
of the immunodeficient severe combined immunodeficient (*scid*) mice and T cell
receptor knockout mice, and even shorter than that of the CD4 and inducible nitric
oxide synthase (iNOS) knockouts (Fig. 2). Only the immunodeficient IFN-γ,
STAT1, and tumor necrosis factor receptor (TNFR)-I knockout mice were more
susceptible to MTB. The survival time of C3HeB/FeJ mice in our studies was
much shorter than that of another susceptible strain, DBA/2, described by North,
Gros, and colleagues (Mitsos et al. 2000). After i.v. infection with a similar dose
of MTB H37Rv, the DBA/2 mice survived for about 100 days. The major distinc-
tion of tuberculosis progression in the C3HeB/FeJ mice was the development of
very unusual macroscopic lesions in their lungs starting 3 weeks after systemic
i.v. infection. Those lesions resembled abscesses rather than the typical diffuse
lung lesions observed in various other strains of immunocompetent inbred mice.

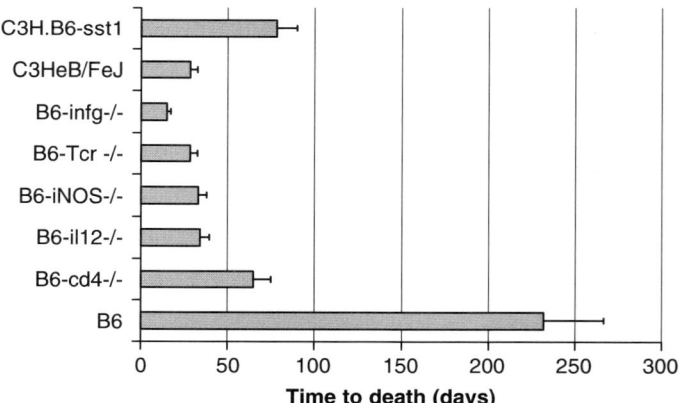

Fig. 2 Effect of the *sst1* locus on mouse survival after infection with virulent MTB. Time to death
of the *sst1* susceptible and resistant congenic mouse strains (C3HeB/FeJ and C3H.B6-*sst1*, respectively) is compared to the resistant inbred mouse strain C57BL/6J (B6) as well as to mice with
knockout of genes essential for systemic antituberculosis immunity on the B6 genetic background.
Mice were infected intravenously with 50×10^3 CFU of virulent MTB strain Erdman

Acid fast fluorescent staining, however, of the lung tissue sections with auromine O and rhodamine, a standard method of identifying mycobacteria, demonstrated that the abscess-like lesions were in fact loaded with mycobacteria localized both extracellularly within central necrotic masses and airways, as well as inside macrophages of the inflammatory lesions. Importantly, no necrotic lesions were observed in other organs. These findings were of particular interest because formation of necrotic lung lesions resembling human lesions had not been previously reported in immunocompetent mice, although it was a hallmark of experimental tuberculosis infection in guinea pigs, rabbits, and monkeys (Helke et al. 2005). In fact, the absence of necrotic centers in tuberculosis granulomas was considered a major limitation of the mouse model of tuberculosis, decreasing its utility for testing new vaccines and antituberculosis drugs. Consequently, we chose a forward genetic approach to dissect this phenotype, which held the promise of revealing yet unknown mechanism(s) underlying the exceptional vulnerability of lung tissue to tuberculosis infection.

Time to death after systemic i.v. infection with MTB was used for linkage analysis of tuberculosis susceptibility in the F_2 hybrid progeny of C57BL/6J and C3HeB/FeJ mice. The shortest survival correlated with formation of the necrotic tuberculosis lesions in the mouse lungs, which were identical to those observed in the parental C3HeB/FeJ mice. We used DNA of these extremely susceptible F_2 mice, which represented approximately 15% of the F_2 population, for a whole genome scan with microsatellite markers and found that all F_2 hybrid mice that developed necrotic lung lesions within 4 weeks post-infection were homozygous for a C3H-derived segment in the central region of mouse chromosome 1. This indicated that the recessive C3H-derived allele of the gene(s) responsible for this phenotype was encoded within that locus, which was termed *sst1* (for *s*upersusceptibility to *t*uberculosis) (Kramnik et al. 2000). We have generated the *sst1* congenic mouse strain by introgression of the C57BL/6J-derived 20-cM region of mouse chromosome 1 encompassing the *sst1* locus into the susceptible C3HeB/FeJ background and demonstrated that the presence of the *sst1*-resistant allele was sufficient to prevent formation of necrotic lung lesions after either i.v. or aerosol infection with MTB (Fig. 3), and to increase the survival of the *sst1* congenic mice under both conditions of infection (Pan et al. 2005). Analysis of the disease progression demonstrated that the *sst1*-susceptible animals (*sst1^S*) were capable of controlling multiplication of MTB in spleen and liver, and that all the bacteria were intracellular, confined to small clusters of macrophages, and no necrosis associated with the infection was observed. The specific effect of the *sst1* locus on progression of lung tuberculosis made it an especially attractive target for further analysis. Our subsequent research focused on (1) revealing functional activity of the *sst1*-encoded genes in host resistance and (2) identification of the *sst1*-encoded candidate genes using positional cloning. The functional and genetic studies were performed in parallel, which was important for subsequent prioritization and validation of the *sst1*-encoded candidate genes.

C3H   **C3H.B6-*sst1***

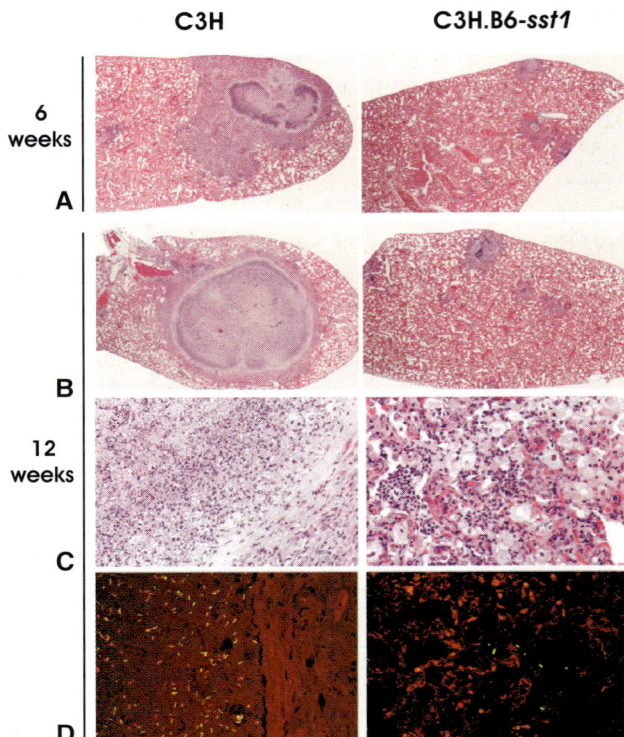

Fig. 3 A–D Progression of pulmonary tuberculosis in the *sst1* congenic inbred mice after aerosol infection with MTB. **A, B** Tuberculous lesions in the lungs of the C3HeB/FeJ (C3H) and the *sst1*-resistant congenic mouse strain C3H.B6-*sst1* at 6 weeks (**A**) and 12 weeks (**B**) after aerosol challenge with MTB. Extensive inflammation resembling caseous pneumonia develops in the lungs of the *sst1*-susceptible mice 6 weeks after infection with 15–30 CFU of *M. tuberculosis* Erdman via aerosol. Areas of necrosis are formed within the inflammatory lesions, which tend to merge and expand (**A**, *left panel*). At 12 weeks post-infection, large areas of necrosis occupy a significant portion of the lung lobe and are surrounded by a fibrotic capsule (**B**, *left panel*). Lung lesions in the *sst1*-resistant congenics were much smaller, lacked necrosis, and did not progress much between the 6th and the 12th week of infection (**A** and **B**, *right panels*). **C** Tuberculosis granuloma wall adjacent to central necrosis in the lung lesions of C3H (*sst1*^{S}) mice (*left panel*) and lung granuloma of the C3H.B6-*sst1* (*sst1*^{R}) mice (*right panel*) 12 weeks after aerosol challenge with MTB. H&E, 200×, original magnification. **D** Auromine-rhodamine staining of the acid fast bacteria (MTB), 400×, original magnification. Central necrosis with fibrous capsule is seen in lesions of the susceptible C3H mice, with numerous extracellular bacilli seen under fluorescence microscopy within necrotic masses. Lung lesions of the *sst1*-resistant congenic mice (C3H.B6-*sst1*) showed minimal necrosis, abundant lymphocytes and foamy macrophages with scant bacilli upon fluorescence microscopy

Role of the *sst1* Locus in Antituberculosis Immunity

The *sst1*-susceptible (*sst1^S*) C3HeB/FeJ and *sst1*-resistant (*sst1^R*) C3H.B6-*sst1* congenic mouse strains were compared for their ability to control multiplication of virulent MTB and *M. bovis* as well as avirulent attenuated vaccine strain *M. bovis* BCG. The effect of the *sst1* locus on survival and control of mycobacterial multiplication was significant only when the mice were infected with virulent mycobacteria. Multiplication of the attenuated mycobacteria BCG was controlled similarly in both the *sst1^R* and *sst1^S* mice, in which the bacterial load rapidly decreased. After infection with virulent TB, the survival of the *sst1^R* congenic mice was significantly longer (10–12 weeks) as compared to the parental *sst1^S* mice (3–4 weeks). The C57BL/6J parental strain, however, was much more resistant than the C3H.B6-*sst1* both in terms of survival and the ability to control multiplication of MTB in lungs, spleens, and livers. This was observed after MTB infection either via systemic or respiratory routes, indicating that the *sst1* locus was only partially responsible for the genetically controlled difference between the parental strains (Yan et al. 2006).

Comparing immune responses to tuberculosis infection of C57BL/6J and C3HeB/FeJ mouse strains, Behar and co-workers found a greater proportion of IFN-γ-producing CD4-positive T cells in the lungs (Chackerian et al. 2001) and earlier dissemination of MTB to peripheral organs after respiratory infection (Chackerian et al. 2002) in the resistant C57BL/6J mice. These findings suggested a mechanism of resistance in which earlier trafficking of the pathogen to lymphoid organs resulted in more rapid priming of adaptive immunity and better control of the infection. Defects in recruitment of the mycobacteria-specific IFN-γ-producing Th1 cells to the lungs seemed to be a plausible explanation for the dramatic differences in progression of lung tuberculosis between the parental strains. Later this group tested a set of the H-2 congenic mouse strains and found that, indeed, the C57BL/6J haplotype at the major histocompatibility complex (H-2^b) was responsible for greater CD4-positive T cell responses to mycobacterial antigens, IFN-γ production, and T cell recruitment to the lungs (Kamath et al. 2004). Survival and lung pathology, however, was controlled by non-MHC loci.

To define a specific role for the *sst1* locus in the control of tuberculosis pathology and progression in the lungs, we generated and tested reciprocal bone marrow chimeras between the *sst1^S* and *sst1^R* congenic mice. Although the *sst1*-susceptible phenotype during tuberculosis infection was expressed predominantly in the lungs, we found that the *sst1* phenotype was carried exclusively by the bone marrow-derived cells (Pan et al. 2005). However, neither the priming nor recruitment of the IFN-γ-producing CD4- and CD8-positive T cells to the lung was *sst1*-dependent. Production of IFN-γ by T cells isolated from tuberculous lung lesions of the *sst1* congenic mice was also similar (Yan et al. 2007). Adoptive transfer of naïve lymphocytes obtained from the *sst1* congenic mice into C3H.*scid* recipients did not reveal any functional differences between the *sst1*-resistant and -susceptible lymphocytes: both were equally efficient in transfer of protective immunity to tuberculosis. Considering the small contribution of humoral immunity to overall resistance to MTB infection, these experiments suggested that the *sst1*-mediated effect was most likely expressed by nonlymphoid bone marrow-derived cells.

To test this hypothesis a pair of immunodeficient *sst1* congenic mice was generated. Both the *sst1^S* and *sst1^R* mice carried a mutation in the *Prkdc* gene, which leads to severe combined immunodeficiency. In this setting, effects of the *sst1* locus could be studied in the absence of an adaptive immune response. In contrast to immunocompetent mice, after i.v. infection with a standard dose of MTB, the spread of infection in *scid* mice was fastest in the spleens and not the lungs, and the effect of the *sst1* locus on multiplication of the bacteria and survival of the mice was statistically significant but minimal—both *sst1^S* and *sst1^R* strains of *scid* mice succumbed within 1 month post-infection, although the *sst1^R* mice survived several days longer. The *Prkdc* mutation, which ablated the adaptive immune response, acted epistatically, such that the *sst1*-dependent differences were almost completely masked in immunodeficient hosts. This effect is consistent with the requirement for a T cell-mediated immune response and IFN-γ production to control MTB infection: immune defects leading to compromise of the Th1 immune response result in severe disseminated mycobacterial infections both in humans and in mice.

In a separate experiment we reconstituted adaptive immunity in the *sst1* congenic *scid* mice via adoptive transfer of mycobacteria-specific T cells shortly after the infection. The CD4-positive T cells were isolated from the BCG-immunized *sst1^R* mice and transferred into either the *sst1^S* or *sst1^R* *scid* mice. In this setting, we bypassed the initial stages of T cell activation and delivered identical mycobacteria-primed CD4-positive *sst1^R* T cells to *scid* animals that differed only at the *sst1* locus. On both *sst1^S* and *sst1^R* genetic backgrounds the mycobacteria-specific T cells significantly suppressed multiplication of MTB. This effect was especially prominent in the spleens. After an initial delay, however, necrotic lesions started to appear in the lungs of the *sst1^S* *scid* mice, and the bacterial burden in the lungs, but not other organs, rapidly increased. Thus, nonlymphoid bone marrow-derived cells appeared to be responsible for the *sst1*-mediated effect on progression of pulmonary tuberculosis. Taken together, these studies demonstrate that T cell-mediated immunity is necessary but not sufficient for protection, especially in the lungs, where the *sst1*-mediated mechanism of innate immunity appears to play a prominent role in the presence of active T cell-mediated immunity. During tuberculosis infection in vivo, *sst1*-mediated immunity is relatively organ-specific as compared to complete lack of T cell-mediated immunity, which results in systemic failure of antituberculosis host defense.

A distinctive lung-specific feature of the *sst1*-susceptible phenotype is formation of necrotic lesions. To address the effect of the *sst1* locus on cell death within the tuberculous lung lesions, we used a terminal transferase dUTP nick end labeling (TUNEL) assay to detect cells containing fragmented DNA. Within the lung lesions of the *sst1*-resistant C3H.B6-*sst1* congenic mice, cells containing TUNEL-positive nuclei (indicative of apoptosis) represented a major fraction of all TUNEL-positive cells. Meanwhile, extensive TUNEL staining in the lungs of the *sst1*-susceptible C3HeB/FeJ mice was cytoplasmic in more than 90% of TUNEL-positive cells, which is indicative of necrotic death (Yan et al. 2007). Previously, formation of necroses in the mouse lungs has been observed at terminal stages of tuberculosis progression as a result of very high bacterial loads (Flynn 2006; Mitsos et al. 2000). In contrast, in our studies the first necrotic microfoci started to appear in the tuberculous lung lesions of *sst1*-susceptible mice as early as 2 weeks post-infection. At that time the bacterial loads in the lungs of the *sst1^S* and *sst1^R* congenic mice were similar and relatively low, suggesting that the necrosis was not due to higher bacterial loads in the lungs of the *sst1^S* animals, but was a result of higher sensitivity of their lung tissue to virulent mycobacteria. The results of these experiments are consistent with the concept that apoptotic death of infected cells limits local inflammation, bacterial multiplication, and spread and is therefore beneficial for the host (Chen et al. 2006; Henson 2003; Kornfeld et al. 1999; Watson et al. 2000; Zamboni et al. 2006). Our findings suggest that the *sst1*-mediated control of progression of pulmonary tuberculosis in vivo may be directly or indirectly involved in control of cell death in the tuberculous lung lesions.

Subsequent experiments in vitro demonstrated that the *sst1* locus affects multiplication of MTB in bone marrow-derived macrophages, and death of the infected macrophages (Pan et al. 2005). In addition, innate resistance to infection with another intracellular pathogen, *Listeria monocytogenes*, was also shown to be mediated by the *sst1* locus both using infection of the *sst1* congenic *scid* mice in vivo and infection of their bone marrow-derived macrophages in vitro (Boyartchuk et al. 2004). Taken together, our experiments establish that the *sst1*-dependent susceptible phenotype is expressed by macrophages in a cell-autonomous manner.

Identification of the Candidate Gene *Ipr1*

The C57BL/6J-derived resistant allele of *sst1* is dominant. For positional cloning we therefore analyzed median survival time (MST) of backcross progeny of males that carried recombinant chromosome 1 on the C3HeB/FeJ genetic background. After three backcrosses on the susceptible background, the *sst1* effect was converted into a monogenic trait. The backcross progeny that carried the C57BL/6J-derived resistant allele displayed an MST within the range of 8–12 weeks, while the *sst1*-susceptible homozygous mice succumbed within 4 weeks after i.v. infection.

Initial mapping of the *sst1* locus to a 30-cM interval in the middle part of mouse chromosome 1 raised the possibility that the *sst1* candidate gene was identical to a previously identified host resistance gene, *Nramp1* (natural resistance-associated macrophage protein 1), the first bacterial resistance gene identified by positional cloning by Gros and co-workers (Vidal et al. 1993). This gene controls host resistance to several taxonomically unrelated intracellular macrophage parasites: avirulent vaccine strain *M. bovis* BCG (*Bcg*), *Salmonella typhimurium* (*Ity*), and *Leishmania donovani* (*Lsh*). The phenotypic expression of *sst1* locus, however, was distinct from *Bcg/Ity/Lsh*, as it was specific for virulent MTB and did not control host resistance to the *Nramp1*-dependent microorganisms avirulent *M. bovis* BCG, and *L. donovani* (A.R. Satoskar, unpublished). Using genetic recombination we reduced the *sst1* region to a 2-cM interval approximately 10–12 cM apart from the *Nramp1* gene (Kramnik et al. 2000).

Our attempts to further reduce the interval were complicated by the presence of an unusually large homogeneously stained repeat (HSR) region. This region was first described in some populations of wild mice from Western Europe (Traut et al. 2001; Weichenhan et al. 2001) and Siberia (Agulnik et al. 1993). It was estimated that this long-range repeat cluster may contain between 60 and 2,000 repeat units and extend over 6–200 Mb of *Mus musculus* chromosome 1, to make up as much as 0.1%–5% of the haploid genome. Weichenhan et al. identified component genes encoded within the HSR region and determined that it appeared only 1–2 million years ago by duplication, gene fusion, and amplification in the genus *Mus* and hypothesized that it might have become fixed in a 'selective sweep' (Traut et al. 200_; Weichenhan et al. 2001). We determined that the *sst1* critical interval encompassed the distal part of the HSR repeat region and a flanking region between the repeat region and the *NppC* gene. This region, in addition to the transcripts encoded within the repeat itself, contained a total of 22 known and predicted genes. The presence of the HSR repeat within the *sst1* candidate region discouraged further attempts to reduce the *sst1* critical region by genetic recombination, since the great majority of recombination events occurred within the repeat region. Thus, our subsequent work focused on functional evaluation of individual genes within the minimal candidate region and relied on our understanding of the specific effect of the *sst1* locus on immunity to infection described above.

All genes encoded within the candidate region were prioritized based on their expression pattern, which was established using RNA isolated from the lungs of the *sst1* congenic mouse strains during the course of tuberculosis infection in vivo, as well as from the bone marrow-derived macrophages infected with MTB in vitro. Our criteria for selecting candidate genes were based on their expression in the lung tissue and in macrophages, regulation of gene expression levels during the course of tuberculosis infection, and possible differential expression of the candidate gene(s) between the *sst1^S* and *sst1^R* mouse strains. Gene expression was analyzed using RT-PCR for known or predicted genes within the candidate region, GeneChip microarrays, and interval-specific arrays that we have constructed using clones isolated from the mouse genome bacterial artificial chromosome (BAC) libraries RPCI-23 and RPCI-24. In addition, rapid analysis of cDNA ends (RACE) analysis was performed for all *sst1*-encoded candidate genes, in which expression was detected in MTB-infected lung tissue and macrophages. The BAC arrays were included in our studies because by the time of our experiments, the HSR repeat region was represented by a gap in the mouse genome assembly due to difficulties associated with sequencing repeat regions, which suggested that our knowledge of the *sst1*-encoded genes might be incomplete. The BAC clones were isolated during our unsuccessful attempt to produce a contiguous physical map of the candidate region, which would include the HSR repeat. Nevertheless, we were able to identify BAC clones that covered the flanking regions and bridged the flanking and the HSR repeat region, as well as multiple clones containing the HSR-encoded sequences. A subset of those clones was digested with restriction enzymes and, after separation in agarose gels, transferred to membranes, which were used for comparative hybridizations with radioactively labeled probes prepared from mRNA isolated from the tuberculous lung lesions of the $sst1^S$ and $sst1^R$ congenic mice. This analysis produced the first indications that transcripts differentially expressed between the $sst1^R$ and $sst1^S$ mice were encoded within the HSR repeat.

Subsequently, the *ifi75* (interferon-inducible-75) gene encoded within the HSR repeat region emerged as a top candidate. Expression of this gene in the lungs of the $sst1^R$ congenic mice was significantly upregulated during MTB infection in vivo, but was undetectable by Northern blot analysis in the lungs of the $sst1^S$ C3HeB/FeJ mice either prior to or after the infection (Pan et al. 2005). This candidate gene was also upregulated in the $sst1^R$, but not $sst1^S$, bone marrow-derived macrophages after infection with MTB in vitro. *Ifi75* was also upregulated in $sst1^R$ macrophages primed with type I and type II interferon, most prominently by IFN-β and -γ. These data suggested that *ifi75* function may be associated with the innate mechanism of antituberculosis immunity, which is consistent with the characteristics of the *sst1* locus.

Since multiple copies of *ifi75* are encoded within the HSR repeat region (Weichenhan et al. 2001), we wanted to determine whether specific *ifi75* isoforms are expressed in tuberculous lung lesions. We performed RACE on mRNA isolated from the lungs of the MTB-infected *sst1* congenic mouse strains to reconstruct full-length *ifi75* expressed in tuberculosis lesions. One isoform of *ifi75* was predominantly expressed in the lungs of $sst1^R$ mice, and expression of this isoform was also strongly induced in $sst1^R$ macrophages by infection with MTB or *M. bovis* BCG, or by macrophage activation with type I and type II interferon. Meanwhile, the $sst1^S$ macrophages weakly expressed multiple aberrant forms of the *ifi75* transcripts under the same activation conditions. Although some of the aberrant transcripts were also present in the lung tissue of the $sst1^R$ animals, the majority of the *Ifi75*-related transcripts in the tuberculous lung lesions were represented by a single isoform, which was 92% identical to the *Mus caroli ifi75* described by Weichenhan et al. (2001). The cDNA encoding the $sst1^R$-specific isoform isolated from tuberculous lung lesions and IFN-activated macrophages was subsequently named *Ipr1* (intracellular pathogen resistance 1) to differentiate it from other *ifi75*- related sequences (*ifi75-rs*) encoded within the HSR repeat that have been or may be identified in other genetic backgrounds or cell types, or induced by different activating stimuli.

A key experiment confirming the role of *Ipr1* in host resistance to intracellular pathogens was expression of an *Ipr1* transgene in *Ipr1*-negative macrophages. Transgenic mice were generated directly on the C3HeB/FeJ background. A modified human scavenger receptor A (hSR-A) promoter was used to drive expression of the *Ipr1* transgene specifically in mature macrophages of the $sst1^S$ (and *Ipr1*-negative) genetic background. We observed that expression of *Ipr1* improved macrophage ability to control multiplication of two species of pathogenic intracellular bacteria, MTB and *L. monocytogenes*. Although both *Ipr1*-positive and *Ipr1*-negative bone marrow-derived macrophages eventually died after infection with either pathogen, we noticed that monolayers of C3HeB/FeJ macrophages were destroyed more rapidly than transgenic macrophages. Membrane damage in C3HeB/FeJ cells could be detected by flow cytometry even in the absence of signs of apoptosis. *Ipr1*-expressing bone marrow-derived macrophages controlled bacterial multiplication better and displayed signs of apoptotic cell death, such as annexin V staining of plasma membranes and mitochondrial membrane permeability transition (Pan et al. 2005).

Genetic Basis of the *Ipr1* Variation

The fact that the candidate gene was encoded within the repeat region posed several questions: How many copies of this gene are present within the repeat region? Are all copies similar in terms of their sequence, tissue-specific regulation, and function? What specific genetic lesion differentiates the *sst1*-resistant and -susceptible alleles?

Previously, the genome of another murine species, *M. caroli*, was shown to contain single copies of genes that constitute the HSR repeat in *M. musculus* (Traut et al. 2001; Weichenhan et al. 2001). Weichenhan and co-workers determined the genomic structure of *M. caroli ifi75* and found that it contained 12 exons. To compare the number of individual exons in *ifi75* in *sst1^R* versus *sst1^S* mice, we used quantitative PCR to amplify genomic DNA from the *sst1* congenic strains using primer pairs specific for individual exons. *M. caroli* genomic DNA was used as a standard for quantitation. We determined that in both strains the number of copies of each of the 12 individual exons of *ifi75* ranged from 5 to 40. Thus, approximately 40 copies of *ifi75* were present in both genetic backgrounds. Most of the HSR repeat units, however, encoded incomplete *ifi75* copies; we subsequently referred to them as *ifi75*-related sequences (*ifi75-rs*). In addition, the *sst1*-susceptible genome contained fewer copies of exons 1, 2, and 4 of the *ifi75* gene. This was confirmed using single strand conformation polymorphism (SSCP) analysis (see supplemental Figs. 3c and d in Pan et al. 2005). Taken together, our data demonstrated that individual copies of *ifi75-rs* are nonidentical within the same genetic background as well as between strains.

We also found that the lack of *Ipr1* expression in C3HeB/FeJ mice was due to a recent mutation, because other substrains of C3H tested in our experiments still expressed the *Ipr1* gene. The ability of several C3H substrains to resist experimental tuberculosis infection was quantitatively compared to that of the C3HeB/FeJ and the C3H.B6-*sst1* congenic mice. With the exception of the C3HeB/FeJ, all other C3H mice were similar to the *sst1*-resistant congenic C3H.B6-*sst1* mice in terms of their survival and control of MTB multiplication in the lungs. The C3HeB/FeJ was the only substrain that developed necrotic lung lesions within the first month of tuberculosis infection. Given the high degree of genetic similarity between the C3H substrains, correlation between *Ipr1* expression and the *sst1*-resistant phenotype provided independent evidence for the candidacy of the *Ipr1* gene.

The C3HeB/FeJ substrain of C3H was derived by Fekete (Fe) in the 1950s using transfer of C3H embryos into C57BL/6J females (designated as eB). The C3H inbred mice are highly susceptible to mouse mammary tumor virus (MMTV), which is transmitted with milk from mothers to their progeny. The C57BL/6J mice are resistant to MMTV and do not transmit the virus. The litters were raised by the C57BL/6J mothers, which prevented transmission of the milk-borne MMTV and rendered the C3HeB/FeJ mice MMTV-free. The genetic defect that resulted in reduction of *Ipr1* expression might have been a random event that occurred after separation of C3HeB/FeJ from other stocks of C3H in the 1950s, or it might have been triggered by the embryo transfer. Another intriguing possibility is that the presence of MMTV might have exerted selective pressure to preserve functional copy(s) of the *Ipr1* gene in C3H inbred mice, which was lost after eliminating the virus. This speculation is consistent with reports demonstrating interactions between the human homolog of the Ipr1 protein, SP110, with viral proteins in yeast two-hybrid screens (discussed in the following section). Unusual expansion of the HSR repeat to up to 2,000 copies per genome in some populations of wild mice may also suggest that the high number of repeat elements within the HSR is maintained due to selective pressure exerted by natural infectious agents. Perhaps the interferon-inducible *Ipr1*-mediated mechanism plays a broader role in host immunity and possibly in adaptation to other environmental stressors. This hypothesis may also provide a tentative explanation for decreased numbers of functional HSR-encoded sequences in laboratory mouse strains, which are not exposed to the everyday dangers of free living.

Recent studies revealed that structural variation within normal genomes is much greater than previously estimated. While initial analysis of genetic variation in mammals focused primarily on single nucleotide polymorphisms (SNPs), regions of structural variation (deletions, insertions, and segmental genome duplications) were less studied, primarily due to difficulties associated with their sequence assembly. Application of novel high-resolution methods to genomic analysis demonstrated appreciable amounts of variation in copy numbers between normal genomes (Sebat et al. 2004). Redon et al. identified 1,447 copy number variation (CNV) regions in humans, estimated that in total those regions covered approximately 12% of the human genome, and revealed marked variation in CNVs in human populations (Redon et al. 2006). Copy number variation was also detected among inbred mouse strains (Adams et al. 2005; Lakshmi et al. 2006). It has been recently demonstrated that CNVs had significant impact on gene expression variation, suggesting their important contribution to phenotypic diversity, evolution, and disease (Stranger et al. 2007). The CNV regions contain hundreds of genes, including disease loci (Redon et al. 2006).

It has been noted that regions of segmental genome duplications are enriched for genes involved in immunity. For example, macrophage-mediated resistance to *Legionella pneumophila* in mice is controlled by the *Naip5/Birc1* gene (Fortier et al. 2005a; Ren et al. 2006), a putative cytosolic microbe sensor, which is encoded within a complex region containing a cluster of closely linked paralogs generated by duplications from a single progenitor gene (Endrizzi et al. 2000). Interestingly, an independently evolved orthologous genomic segment exists in humans, where it is involved in a noninfectious disease phenotype, spinal muscular atrophy (Growney et al. 2000). In another example, segmental duplications containing the *CCL3L1* gene (CCR5 ligand) were linked to HIV-1 infection in humans. Possession of *CCL3L1* in lower copy number than the population average was associated with markedly enhanced susceptibility to acquired immunodeficiency syndrome (AIDS) (Gonzalez et al. 2005). In this case, the benefit of increased copy number may simply be due to a higher level of CCL3L1 protein production, which reduces viral cell entry via binding to the HIV-1 co-receptor CCR5. It is possible, however, that closely related genes that evolve within duplicated regions of the genome may generate functional diversity and thus facilitate recognition or elimination of pathogens. Further analysis of functional and structural variants of proteins encoded by the *Ipr1* gene and its human homolog SP110 in genetically diverse individuals may provide insight into mechanisms associated with CNVs that mediate host resistance to pathogenic microorganisms and, possibly, other immune-related phenotypes.

Structure and Function of the Mouse Ipr1 Protein and Its Human Homolog SP110

In humans, the most structurally related homolog of the predicted mouse Ipr1 protein is SP110 (41% identity), a member of the Speckled protein 100-kDa (Sp100) protein family. Three related nuclear proteins, SP100, SP110, and SP140 are encoded within a single cluster on human chromosome 2q37. This region is highly conserved between mice, rats, and humans, although no long-range repeat similar to the mouse HSR repeat was reported in humans and rats. In humans, *SP110* is a single gene represented by three isoforms, a, b and c, that are products of alternative splicing. Expression of both *Ipr1* and *SP110* is regulated by interferons, suggesting their possible role in immunity in both species (Grotzinger et al. 1996; Kadereit et al. 1993). Using a yeast two-hybrid screen, the SP110b protein has been found to interact physically with two viral proteins, Epstein–Barr virus SM protein (Nicewonger et al. 2004) and hepatitis C virus core protein (Watashi et al. 2003), suggesting that SP110b may also play a role in host response to viral infections.

The SP110b isoform is the closest human homolog of mouse Ipr1. Both proteins contain a putative Sp100-like protein–protein interaction domain, chromatin-associated SAND domain, a bipartite nuclear localization signal (NLS) and a single LXXLL nuclear receptor co-activator motif. All other members of the Sp100 family also contain the Sp100 and SAND domains, and may contain known chromatin association domains, such as plant homeobox domain (PHD), high mobility group (HMG), and Bromo domains, which indicate their involvement in transcriptional control and chromatin remodeling. In humans, SP100, SP110, and SP140 produce multiple isoforms as a result of differential mRNA splicing. They are called Speckled proteins (SP) because in the nucleus they are not distributed uniformly, but form aggregates, which are reported to colocalize with structures called nuclear bodies (NBs) (Bloch et al. 2000). NBs contain two permanent components, the PML (promyelocytic leukemia) and SP100 proteins. Many proteins that play an important regulatory role in cell activation, division, and apoptosis (Hofmann and Will 2003) dynamically localize to NBs (Hofmann and Will 2003; Maul et al. 2000; Regad and Chelbi-Alix 2001; Zhong et al. 2000).

The SAND domain (named after Sp100, AIRE-1, NucP41/75, DEAF-1) is a conserved approx. 80-residue region found in a number of nuclear proteins, many of which function in chromatin-mediated transcriptional regulation. These include Sp100, NUDR (nuclear DEAF-1 related), GMEB (glucocorticoid modulatory element binding) (Bottomley et al. 2001; Surdo et al. 2003), and AIRE-1 (autoimmune regulator 1) proteins (Purohit et al. 2005). The DNA binding surface of the SAND domain has been mapped to a conserved KDWK motif (Bottomley et al. 2001), which is also present in the Ipr1 and SP110b proteins. Proteins containing the SAND domain have a modular structure, and the SAND domain can be associated with a number of other modules, which have been implicated in interactions with chromatin or transcription factors. Most frequently the SAND domain is associated with the N-terminal Sp100 domain.

The Sp100-like domain is approximately 100 amino acid residues in length and rich in hydrophobic residues. The Sp100-like domain was found to be required for dimerization of Sp100 and its localization to the NBs (Sternsdorf et al. 1999). We found that deletion of the Sp100-like domain of Ipr1 prevents its association with nuclear speckles and produces a diffuse nuclear localization pattern. Perhaps this domain is required for the interactions of Ipr1 with the nuclear matrix or other structural elements in the nucleus. Indeed, AIRE-1 also contains the Sp100 domain and was found to be tightly associated with nuclear matrix (Tao et al. 2005).

The LXXLL nuclear receptor binding motif was originally identified in nuclear receptor co-activators (reviewed in Savkur and Burris 2004). This motif, however, was also found in nuclear receptor co-repressors (e.g., NcoR) (Horlein et al. 1995), other transcription regulators (e.g., PIAS3, protein inhibitor of activated STAT3) (Jang et al. 2004), and chromatin proteins (e.g., SCC3, Sister chromatid cohesion protein-3) (Lara-Pezzi et al. 2004). Interestingly, PIAS3 suppressed nuclear factor (NF)-κB-mediated transcription by interacting with the p65/RelA subunit via its LXXLL motif (Jang et al. 2004), while SCC3 had NF-κB coactivator activity that also depended on one of its LXXLL motifs (Lara-Pezzi et al. 2004). Watashi et al. showed that Sp110b is a transcriptional cofactor negatively regulating retinoic acid receptor α-mediated transcription (Watashi et al. 2003). Perhaps this interaction also involves the LXXLL motif. The vitamin D receptor is an attractive candidate to interact directly with Ipr1/SP110b via LXXLL motifs and control macrophage interactions with MTB. Indeed, vitamin D receptor activity was recently found to mediate antimycobacterial activity of human macrophages stimulated via a Toll-like receptor (Liu et al. 2006), and its transcriptional activity was shown to be dependent on interaction with coactivators via an LXXLL motif (Pike et al. 2003).

An exciting picture of the Ipr1/Sp110b function begins to emerge from these studies. Ipr1/Sp110b might connect structural components of the nucleus with chromatin, participate in its reorganization, and help recruit transcription factors and other proteins to specific nuclear domains. This may affect transcriptional activity via facilitation or interruption of communication between promoters, enhancers and distant *cis* regulatory elements, and other components of chromatin. Regulation of this protein by interferons and infection suggests that its specific functional activity is important for adjustment of nuclear processes to challenges imposed by infectious agents and, possibly, other stressors.

A recent publication by Roscioli et al. demonstrated that in humans rare inactivating mutations in the *SP110* gene were associated with a specific autosomal recessive primary immunodeficiency, hepatic veno-occlusive disease with immunodeficiency (VODI) (Roscioli et al. 2006). Patients homozygous for the mutant allele of Sp110 presented between 3–7 months of age with a combined T and B cell immunodeficiency, and were very susceptible to a number of bacterial, viral, and fungal infections, although no mycobacterial infections were observed in that study. Macrophage function has not been studied in these patients.

To date, four studies investigated the impact of common *SP110* polymorphisms on tuberculosis susceptibility. In family-based association studies in three West African countries, two SNPs were found to associate with tuberculosis (Tosh et al. 2006). However, population-based association studies in Ghana, Russia, and South Africa failed to detect significant association between common sequence variations of the *SP110* gene with tuberculosis (Babb et al. 2007; Szeszko et al. 2007; Thye et al. 2006). In the mouse, the *sst1* locus controls not susceptibility to MTB per se, but the type of progression of pulmonary tuberculosis. Lack of *Ipr1* expression is associated with formation of extensive necroses within tuberculous lung lesions. This phenotype, however, has not been incorporated into the design of human association studies. Obviously, the role of the *SP110*-mediated pathway in progression of pulmonary tuberculosis, as well as other infectious diseases, deserves further experimental, biochemical, and genetic analysis.

Multigenic Control of Tuberculosis Resistance and Susceptibility

Our studies indicate that the *sst1*/Ipr1-mediated pathway of immunity is necessary but not sufficient to protect host from virulent MTB. Indeed, the C3H.B6-*sst1* mice that carry the *sst1*-resistant allele on the C3H genetic background are significantly more susceptible than the resistant parental C57BL/6J strain. In addition, the reciprocal congenic strain B6.C3H-*sst1* that carries the *sst1*-susceptible allele on the resistant genetic background is also more resistant than the C3H.B6-*sst1*, indicating that the *sst1* locus is not a sole determinant of susceptibility to MTB in our genetic model (Kramnik et al. 1998; Kramnik et al. 2000). To identify non-*sst1* loci involved in susceptibility, we crossed the *sst1*-resistant congenic strain C3H.B6-*sst1* with the parental C57BL/6J strain to eliminate the strong effect of the *sst1*-susceptible allele. This allowed easier mapping of four additional tuberculosis-resistance loci on chromosomes 7, 12, 15, and 17 (Yan et al. 2006). The C57BL/6J-derived allele of the chromosome 7 locus had the highest linkage scores in these experiments. To study this locus further, we have generated a chromosome 7 consomic strain, which carries a C57BL/6J-derived chromosome 7, while the rest of the genome, including the *sst1*-susceptible allele, is from C3H. In these mice, the isolated effect of the C57BL/6J-derived chromosome 7 on survival after tuberculosis infection was very small—the median survival time increased by less than a week as compared to the susceptible parental C3HeB/FeJ mice. However, interactions of the *sst1* and chromosome 7 loci produced a remarkable synergistic effect on survival, control of bacterial replication, and lung pathology. The survival time of the C3HeB/FeJ mice that carried the C57BL/6J-derived resistant alleles at both the *sst1* and the chromosome 7 loci increased from 4 weeks to approximately 20 weeks. Thus, the synergistic interactions of the two C57BL/6J-derived resistance loci identified in our crosses accounted for more than a half of the dramatic difference in tuberculosis susceptibility between the C3HeB/FeJ and C57BL/6J inbred mouse strains.

We observed that mice carrying the $sst1^S$ allele developed necrotic lesions in their lungs, albeit at different rates. The most resistant B6.C3H-*sst1* mice carrying the $sst1^S$ allele on a C57BL/6J genetic background developed lung necrosis about 10–12 weeks post-infection. Progression of the necrotic lung lesions in these mice was limited by thick granuloma wall and resulted in chronic disease similar to pulmonary tuberculosis in adult humans. Thus, in our model, formation of lung necroses was controlled by the *sst1* locus irrespective of other genes, while the rate of pulmonary disease progression, the extent of necrotic inflammation, and the survival of animals were controlled by *sst1* interactions with other genes. Further dissection of the genetic architecture of tuberculosis susceptibility using the mouse model will include: (1) identification of specific functional effects of individual non-*sst1* loci; (2) discovery of causal genetic variants encoded within each locus; (3) identification of molecular pathways of immunity that these polymorphisms affect; and (4) understanding how individual host resistance loci interact to produce tuberculosis-resistant or susceptible phenotypes.

Conclusions

Tuberculosis susceptibility, even in a simple genetic model produced by breeding of two immunocompetent mouse strains, is a multigenic trait in which epistatic gene interactions play a prominent role in shaping the resistant phenotype. This genetic architecture reflects complex interactions that develop during the course of tuberculosis infection in immunocompetent individuals, and no single mutation accounts for a failure of host immunity. Identification of genes and polymorphisms that contribute to the outcome of tuberculosis infection in vivo, using forward genetics in an experimental mouse model of infection, will help reconstruct the biochemical and cellular pathways that those genes control and determine how they fit into a complex hierarchy of regulatory networks at the whole organism level.

Although genetic and phenotypic variation in human hosts is much greater than in laboratory mice, genetically defined mouse models allow in-depth analysis of a key element of the MTB virulence strategy—lung colonization and destruction in genetically susceptible, but immunocompetent, individuals. This is useful not only to reach deeper understanding of tuberculosis pathogenesis, but also for testing novel antituberculosis vaccine candidates and drugs to identify those that protect or cure the lung most efficiently.

References

Abel L, Casanova JL (2000) Genetic predisposition to clinical tuberculosis: bridging the gap between simple and complex inheritance. Am J Hum Genet 67:274–277

Adams DJ, Dermitzakis ET, Cox T, Smith J, Davies R, Banerjee R, et al (2005) Complex haplotypes, copy number polymorphisms and coding variation in two recently divergent mouse strains. Nat Genet 37:532–536

Agulnk S, Plass C, Traut W, Winking H (1993) Evolution of a long-range repeat family in chromosome 1 of the genus Mus. Mamm Genome 4:704–710

Alcais A, Fieschi C, Abel L, Casanova JL (2005) Tuberculosis in children and adults: two distinct genetic diseases. J Exp Med 202:1617–1621

Babb C, Keet EH, van Helden PD, Hoal EG (2007) SP110 polymorphisms are not associated with pulmonary tuberculosis in a South African population. Hum Genet 121:521–522

Bellamy R, Beyers N, McAdam KP, Ruwende C, Gie R, Samaai P, et al (2000) Genetic susceptibility to tuberculosis in Africans: a genome-wide scan. Proc Natl Acad Sci U S A 97: 8005–8009

Bleed D, Dye C, Raviglione MC (2000) Dynamics and control of the global tuberculosis epidemic. Curr Opin Pulm Med 6:174–179

Bloch DB, Nakajima A, Gulick T, Chiche JD, Orth D, de La Monte SM, et al (2000) Sp110 localizes to the PML-Sp100 nuclear body and may function as a nuclear hormone receptor transcriptional coactivator. Mol Cell Biol 20:6138–6146

Bottomley MJ, Collard MW, Huggenvik JI, Liu Z, Gibson TJ, Sattler M (2001) The SAND domain structure defines a novel DNA-binding fold in transcriptional regulation. Nat Struct Biol 8:626–633

Boyartchuk V, Rojas M, Yan BS, Jobe O, Hurt N, Dorfman DM, et al (2004) The host resistance locus sst1 controls innate immunity to Listeria monocytogenes infection in immunodeficient mice. J Immunol 173:5112–5120

Buschman E, Apt AS, Nickonenko BV, Moroz AM, Averbakh MH, Skamene E (1988) Genetic aspects of innate resistance and acquired immunity to mycobacteria in inbred mice. Springer Semin Immunopathol 10:319–336

Capuano SV 3rd, Croix DA, Pawar S, Zinovik A, Myers A, Lin PL, et al (2003) Experimental Mycobacterium tuberculosis infection of cynomolgus macaques closely resembles the various manifestations of human M. tuberculosis infection. Infect Immun 71:5831–5844

Casanova JL, Abel L (2002) Genetic dissection of immunity to mycobacteria: the human model. Annu Rev Immunol 20:581–620

Casanova JL, Abel L (2005) Inborn errors of immunity to infection: the rule rather than the exception. J Exp Med 202:197–201

Casanova JL, Schurr E, Abel L, Skamene E (2002) Forward genetics of infectious diseases: immunological impact. Trends Immunol 23:469–472

Chackerian AA, Perera TV, Behar SM (2001) Gamma interferon-producing CD4+ T lymphocytes in the lung correlate with resistance to infection with Mycobacterium tuberculosis. Infect Immun 69:2666–2674

Chackerian AA, Alt JM, Perera TV, Dascher CC, Behar SM (2002) Dissemination of Mycobacterium tuberculosis is influenced by host factors and precedes the initiation of T-cell immunity. Infect Immun 70:4501–4509

Chen M, Gan H, Remold HG (2006) A mechanism of virulence: virulent Mycobacterium tuberculosis strain H37Rv, but not attenuated H37Ra, causes significant mitochondrial inner
membrane disruption in macrophages leading to necrosis. J Immunol 176:3707–3716

Cohen MK, Bartow RA, Mintzer CL, McMurray DN (1987) Effects of diet and genetics on
Mycobacterium bovis BCG vaccine efficacy in inbred guinea pigs. Infect Immun 55:314–319

Comstock GW (1978) Tuberculosis in twins: a re-analysis of the Prophit survey. Am Rev Respir
Dis 117:621–624

Cooper AM, Flynn JL (1995) The protective immune response to Mycobacterium tuberculosis.
Curr Opin Immunol 7:512–516

Dorman SE, Hatem CL, Tyagi S, Aird K, Lopez-Molina J, Pitt ML, et al (2004) Susceptibility to
tuberculosis: clues from studies with inbred and outbred New Zealand White rabbits. Infect
Immun 72:1700–1705

Endrizzi MG, Hadinoto V, Growney JD, Miller W, Dietrich WF (2000) Genomic sequence analysis of the mouse Naip gene array. Genome Res 10:1095–1102

Flynn JL (2006) Lessons from experimental Mycobacterium tuberculosis infections. Microbes
Infect 8:1179–1188

Flynn JL, Chan J (2005) What's good for the host is good for the bug. Trends Microbiol
13:98–102

Fortier A, Diez E, Gros P (2005a) Naip5/Birc1e and susceptibility to Legionella pneumophila.
Trends Microbiol 13:328–335

Fortier A, Min-Oo G, Forbes J, Lam-Yuk-Tseung S, Gros P (2005b) Single gene effects in mouse
models of host: pathogen interactions. J Leukoc Biol 77:868–877

Fortin A, Abel L, Casanova JL, Gros P (2007) Host genetics of mycobacterial diseases in mice
and men: forward genetic studies of BCG-osis and tuberculosis. Annu Rev Genomics Hum
Genet 8:163–192

Gagneux S, Deriemer K, Van T, Kato-Maeda M, de Jong BC, Narayanan S, et al (2005) Variable
host-pathogen compatibility in Mycobacterium tuberculosis. Proc Natl Acad Sci USA
103:2869–2873

Gardam MA, Keystone EC, Menzies R, Manners S, Skamene E, Long R, et al (2003) Anti-tumour
necrosis factor agents and tuberculosis risk: mechanisms of action and clinical management.
Lancet Infect Dis 3:148–155

Gonzalez E, Kulkarni H, Bolivar H, Mangano A, Sanchez R, Catano G, et al (2005) The influence
of CCL3L1 gene-containing segmental duplications on HIV-1/AIDS susceptibility. Science
307:1434–1440

Gradmann C (2006) Robert Koch and the white death: from tuberculosis to tuberculin. Microbes
Infect 8:294–301

Grotzinger T, Jensen K, Will H (1996) The interferon (IFN)-stimulated gene Sp100 promoter
contains an IFN-gamma activation site and an imperfect IFN-stimulated response element
which mediate type I IFN inducibility. J Biol Chem 271:25253–25260

Growney JD, Scharf JM, Kunkel LM, Dietrich WF (2000) Evolutionary divergence of the mouse
and human Lgn1/SMA repeat structures. Genomics 64:62–81

Helke KL, Mankowski JL, Manabe YC (2005) Animal models of cavitation in pulmonary tuberculosis. Tuberculosis (Edinb) 86:337–348

Henson PM (2003) Possible roles for apoptosis and apoptotic cell recognition in inflammation and
fibrosis. Am J Respir Cell Mol Biol 29:S70–S76

Hill AV (2006) Aspects of genetic susceptibility to human infectious diseases. Annu Rev Genet
40:469–486

Hingley-Wilson SM, Sambandamurthy VK, Jacobs WR Jr (2003) Survival perspectives from the
world's most successful pathogen, Mycobacterium tuberculosis. Nat Immunol 4:949–955

Hofmann TG, Will H (2003) Body language: the function of PML nuclear bodies in apoptosis
regulation. Cell Death Differ 10:1290–1299

Horlein AJ, Naar AM, Heinzel T, Torchia J, Gloss B, Kurokawa R, et al (1995) Ligand-independent
repression by the thyroid hormone receptor mediated by a nuclear receptor co-repressor.
Nature 377:397–404

Jang I-D, Yoon K, Shin YJ, Kim J, Lee SY (2004) PIAS3 suppresses NF-kappaB-mediated transcription by interacting with the p65/RelA subunit. J Biol Chem 279:24873–24880

Jouanguy E, Altare F, Lamhamedi S, Revy P, Emile JF, Newport M, et al (1996) Interferon-gamma-receptor deficiency in an infant with fatal bacille Calmette-Guerin infection. N Engl J Med 335:1956–1961

Kadereit S, Gewert DR, Galabru J, Hovanessian AG, Meurs EF (1993) Molecular cloning of two new interferon-induced, highly related nuclear phosphoproteins. J Biol Chem 268:24432–24441

Kallmann FJ, Reisner D (1943) Twin studies on the significance of genetic factors in tuberculosis. Am Rev Tuberc 47:549–574

Kamath AB, Alt J, Debbabi H, Taylor C, Behar SM (2004) The major histocompatibility complex haplotype affects T-cell recognition of mycobacterial antigens but not resistance to Mycobacterium tuberculosis in C3H mice. Infect Immun 72:6790–6798

Kaufmann SH, Schaible UE (2005) 100th anniversary of Robert Koch's Nobel Prize for the discovery of the tubercle bacillus. Trends Microbiol 13:469–475

Kaufmann SH, Cole ST, Mizrahi V, Rubin E, Nathan C (2005) Mycobacterium tuberculosis and the host response. J Exp Med 201:1693–1697

Keane J (2005) TNF-blocking agents and tuberculosis: new drugs illuminate an old topic. Rheumatology 44:714–720

Kornfeld H, Mancino G, Colizzi V (1999) The role of macrophage cell death in tuberculosis. Cell Death Differ 6:71–78

Kramnik I, Demant P, Bloom BB (1998) Susceptibility to tuberculosis as a complex genetic trait: analysis using recombinant congenic strains of mice. Novartis Found Symp 217:120–131; discussion 132–137

Kramnik I, Dietrich WF, Demant P, Bloom BR (2000) Genetic control of resistance to experimental infection with virulent Mycobacterium tuberculosis. Proc Natl Acad Sci USA 97:8560–8565

Lakshmi B, Hall IM, Egan C, Alexander J, Leotta A, Healy J, et al (2006) Mouse genomic representational oligonucleotide microarray analysis: detection of copy number variations in normal and tumor specimens. Proc Natl Acad Sci U S A 103:11234–11239

Lara-Fezzi E, Pezzi N, Prieto I, Barthelemy I, Carreiro C, Martinez A, et al (2004) Evidence of a transcriptional co-activator function of cohesin STAG/SA/Scc3. J Biol Chem 279:6553–6559

Lavebratt C, Apt AS, Nikonenko BV, Schalling M, Schurr E (1999) Severity of tuberculosis in mice is linked to distal chromosome 3 and proximal chromosome 9. J Infect Dis 180:150–155

Levin M, Newport MJ, D'Souza S, Kalabalikis P, Brown IN, Lenicker HM, et al (1995) Familial disseminated atypical mycobacterial infection in childhood: a human mycobacterial susceptibility gene? Lancet 345:79–83

Liu PT, Stenger S, Li H, Wenzel L, Tan BH, Krutzik SR, et al (2006) Toll-like receptor triggering of a vitamin D-mediated human antimicrobial response. Science 311:1770–1773

Lurie MB, Zappasodi P, Dannenberg AM Jr, Weiss GH (1952) On the mechanism of genetic resistance to tuberculosis and its mode of inheritance. Am J Hum Genet 4:302–314

Lurie MB, Zappasodi P, Tickner C (1955) On the nature of genetic resistance to tuberculosis in the light of the host-parasite relationships in natively resistant and susceptible rabbits. Am Rev Tuberc 72:297–329

Lynch CJ, Pierce-Chase CH, Dubos R (1965) A genetic study of susceptibility to experimental tuberculosis in mice infected with mammalian tubercle bacilli. J Exp Med 121:1051–1070

Mackintosh CG, de Lisle GW, Collins DM, Griffin JF (2004) Mycobacterial diseases of deer. N Z Vet J 52:163–174

MacMicking J, Xie QW, Nathan C (1997) Nitric oxide and macrophage function. Annu Rev Immunol 15:323–350

Maul GG, Negorev D, Bell P, Ishov AM (2000) Review: properties and assembly mechanisms of ND10, PML bodies, or PODs. J Struct Biol 129:278–287

Medina E, North RJ (1998) Resistance ranking of some common inbred mouse strains to Mycobacterium tuberculosis and relationship to major histocompatibility complex haplotype and Nramp1 genotype. Immunology 93:270–274

Mitsos LM, Cardon LR, Fortin A, Ryan L, LaCourse R, North RJ, et al (2000) Genetic control of susceptibility to infection with Mycobacterium tuberculosis in mice. Genes Immun 1:467–477

Mitsos LM, Cardon LR, Ryan L, LaCourse R, North RJ, Gros P (2003) Susceptibility to tuberculosis: a locus on mouse chromosome 19 (Trl-4) regulates Mycobacterium tuberculosis replication in the lungs. Proc Natl Acad Sci U S A 100:6610–6615

Newport MJ, Huxley CM, Huston S, Hawrylowicz CM, Oostra BA, Williamson R, et al (1996) A mutation in the interferon-gamma-receptor gene and susceptibility to mycobacterial infection. N Engl J Med 335:1941–1949

Nicewonger J, Suck G, Bloch D, Swaminathan S (2004) Epstein-Barr virus (EBV) SM protein induces and recruits cellular Sp110b to stabilize mRNAs and enhance EBV lytic gene expression. J Virol 78:9412–9422

Nikonenko BV, Averbakh MM Jr, Lavebratt C, Schurr E, Apt AS (2000) Comparative analysis of mycobacterial infections in susceptible I/St and resistant A/Sn inbred mice. Tuber Lung Dis 80:15–25

North RJ, Jung YJ (2004) Immunity to tuberculosis. Annu Rev Immunol 22:599–623

Onyebujoh P, Rook GA (2004) Tuberculosis. Nat Rev Microbiol 2:930–932

Orme IM (2005) Mouse and guinea pig models for testing new tuberculosis vaccines. Tuberculosis (Edinb) 85:13–17

Orme IM (2006) Safety issues regarding new vaccines for tuberculosis with an emphasis on post-exposure vaccination. Tuberculosis (Edinb) 86:68–73

Ottenhoff TH, Verreck FA, Hoeve MA, van de Vosse E (2005) Control of human host immunity to mycobacteria. Tuberculosis (Edinb) 85:53–64

Pan H, Yan BS, Rojas M, Shebzukhov YV, Zhou H, Kobzik L, Higgins DE, Daly MJ, Bloom BR, Kramnik I (2005) Ipr1 gene mediates innate immunity to tuberculosis. Nature 434:767–772

Pike JW, Pathrose P, Barmina O, Chang CY, McDonnell DP, Yamamoto H, Shevde NK (2003) LXXLL peptide antagonize 1 Synthetic 25-dihydroxyvitamin D3-dependent transcription. J Cell Biochem 88:252–258

Purohit S, Kumar PG, Laloraya M, She JX (2005) Mapping DNA-binding domains of the autoimmune regulator protein. Biochem Biophys Res Commun 327:939–944

Redon R, Ishikawa S, Fitch KR, Feuk L, Perry GH, Andrews TD, et al (2006) Global variation in copy number in the human genome. Nature 444:444–454

Regad T, Chelbi-Alix MK (2001) Role and fate of PML nuclear bodies in response to interferon and viral infections. Oncogene 20:7274–7286

Ren T, Zamboni DS, Roy CR, Dietrich WF, Vance RE (2006) Flagellin-deficient Legionella mutants evade caspase-1- and Naip5-mediated macrophage immunity. PLoS Pathog 2:e18

Rich AR (1951) The pathogenesis of tuberculosis, 2nd edn. Charles C Thomas, Springfield, p 1028

Rodrigo T, Cayla JA, Garcia de Olalla P, Galdos-Tanguis H, Jansa JM, Miranda P, et al (1997) Characteristics of tuberculosis patients who generate secondary cases. Int J Tuberc Lung Dis 1:352–357

Roscioli T, Cliffe ST, Bloch DB, Bell CG, Mullan G, Taylor PJ, et al (2006) Mutations in the gene encoding the PML nuclear body protein Sp110 are associated with immunodeficiency and hepatic veno-occlusive disease. Nat Genet 38:620–622

Salgame P (2005) Host innate and Th1 responses and the bacterial factors that control Mycobacterium tuberculosis infection. Curr Opin Immunol 17:374–380

Sanchez F, Radaeva TV, Nikonenko BV, Persson AS, Sengul S, Schalling M, et al (2003) Multigenic control of disease severity after virulent Mycobacterium tuberculosis infection in mice. Infect Immun 71:126–131

Savkur RS, Burris TP (2004) The coactivator LXXLL nuclear receptor recognition motif. J Pept Res 63:207–212

Sebat J, Lakshmi B, Troge J, Alexander J, Young J, Lundin P, et al (2004) Large-scale copy number polymorphism in the human genome. Science 305:525–528

Sternsdorf T, Jensen K, Reich B, Will H (1999) The nuclear dot protein sp100, characterization of domains necessary for dimerization, subcellular localization, and modification by small ubiquitin-like modifiers. J Biol Chem 274:12555–12566

Stranger BE, Forrest MS, Dunning M, Ingle CE, Beazley C, Thorne N, et al (2007) Relative impact of nucleotide and copy number variation on gene expression phenotypes. Science 315:848–853

Sugawara I, Yamada H, Mizuno S (2004) Pulmonary tuberculosis in spontaneously diabetic goto kakizaki rats. Tohoku J Exp Med 204:135–145

Surdo PL, Bottomley MJ, Sattler M, Scheffzek K (2003) Crystal structure and nuclear magnetic resonance analyses of the SAND domain from glucocorticoid modulatory element binding protein-1 reveals deoxyribonucleic acid and zinc binding regions. Mol Endocrinol 17:1283–1295

Szeszko JS, Healy B, Stevens H, Balabanova Y, Drobniewski F, Todd JA, et al (2007) Resequencing and association analysis of the SP110 gene in adult pulmonary tuberculosis. Hum Genet 121:155–160

Tao Y, Kupfer R, Stewart BJ, Williams-Skipp C, Crowell CK, Patel DD, et al (2006) AIRE recruits multiple transcriptional components to specific genomic regions through tethering to nuclear matrix. Mol Immunol 43:335–345

Thye T, Browne EN, Chinbuah MA, Gyapong J, Osei I, Owusu-Dabo E, et al (2006) No associations of human pulmonary tuberculosis with Sp110 variants. J Med Genet 43:e32

Tosh K, Campbell SJ, Fielding K, Sillah J, Bah B, Gustafson P, Manneh K, Lisse I, Sirugo G, Bennett S, Aaby P, McAdam KP, Bah-Sow O, Lienhardt C, Kramnik I, Hill AV (2006) Variants In the SP110 gene are associated with genetic susceptibility to tuberculosis In West Africa. Proc Natl Acad Sci U S A 103:10364–10368

Traut W, Rahn IM, Winking H, Kunze B, Weichehan D (2001) Evolution of a 6–200 Mb long-range repeat cluster in the genus Mus. Chromosoma 110:247–252

Vidal SM, Malo D, Vogan K, Skamene E, Gros P (1993) Natural resistance to infection with intracellular parasites: isolation of a candidate for Bcg. Cell 73:469–485

Watashi K, Hijikata M, Tagawa A, Doi T, Marusawa H, Shimotohno K (2003) Modulation of retinoid signaling by a cytoplasmic viral protein via sequestration of Sp110b, a potent transcriptional corepressor of retinoic acid receptor, from the nucleus. Mol Cell Biol 23:7498–7509

Watson VE, Hill LL, Owen-Schaub LB, Davis DW, McConkey DJ, Jagannath C, et al (2000) Apoptosis in mycobacterium tuberculosis infection in mice exhibiting varied immunopathology. J Pathol 190:211–220

Weichenhan D, Kunze B, Winking H, van Geel M, Osoegawa K, de Jong PJ, et al (2001) Source and component genes of a 6–200 Mb gene cluster in the house mouse. Mamm Genome 12:590–594

WHO (2006) Global tuberculosis control—surveillance, planning. financing. In: WHO Report 2006. WHO, Geneva

Wright S, Lewis PA (1921) Factors in the resistance of guinea pigs to tuberculosis, with especial regard to inbreeding and heredity. Am Nat 55:20–50

Yan BS, Kirby A, Shebzukhov YV, Daly MJ, Kramnik I (2006) Genetic architecture of tuberculosis resistance in a mouse model of infection. Genes Immun 7:201–210

Yan ES, Pichugin AV, Jobe O, Helming L, Eruslanov EB, Gutierrez-Pabello JA, Rojas M, Shebzukhov YV, Kobzik L, Kramnik I (2007) Progression of pulmonary tuberculosis and efficiency of bacillus Calmette-Guerin vaccination are genetically controlled via a common sst1-mediated mechanism of innate immunity. J Immunol 179:6919–6932

Zamboni DS, Kobayashi KS, Kohlsdorf T, Ogura Y, Long EM, Vance RE, et al (2006) The Birc1e cytosolic pattern-recognition receptor contributes to the detection and control of Legionella pneumophila infection. Nat Immunol 7:318–325

Zhong S, Salomoni P, Pandolfi PP (2000) The transcriptional role of PML and the nuclear body. Nat Cell Biol 2:E85–90

Part II
Self-Reactivity

Scurfy, the *Foxp3* Locus, and the Molecular Basis of Peripheral Tolerance

M.W. Appleby, F. Ramsdell(✉)

Contents

Abstract The ability to rapidly and efficiently recognize and eliminate pathogens while sparing normal self tissue is a hallmark of the mammalian immune system. When it fails, however, autoimmune disease results. The genetic and environmental factors that control the process of making such distinctions, not to mention the specific targeted tissues, are extraordinarily complex in the human population; only now are we characterizing the candidate genes responsible for these responses to pathogens. The examination of specific traits in murine models of disease has led to the identification of many of the candidate genes for human disease. The study of mouse mutations (both induced and spontaneous) has also greatly advanced our understanding of the immune responses and autoimmune disease. Here, we describe the use of classical mouse genetics to identify one gene centrally involved in the control of immune responses. Furthermore, although mutations in the orthologous human gene result in a virtually identical phenotype to that seen in the mouse, it is unlikely that studying the human disease populations alone would have successfully identified this gene. Thus, despite the complete sequencing of the human and mouse genomes, the examination of murine mutations remains a powerful and unbiased tool to connect genotype and phenotype.

F. Ramsdell
ZymoGenetics Inc., 1201 Eastlake Ave EastSeattle, WA 98102, USA
ramsdell@zgi.com

B. Beutler (ed.), *Immunology, Phenotype First: How Mutations Have Established New Principles and Pathways in Immunology.* Current Topics in Microbiology and Immunology 321. © Springer-Verlag Berlin Heidelberg 2008

Introduction

The process of scientific discovery is often thought of as a continuum in which our understanding of a system is advanced through the integration of knowledge acquired over a series of incremental steps. Under appropriate circumstances, however, it is possible for scientific understanding to take a more substantial leap forward and in recent years the exploitation of phenotype-driven gene discovery programs has afforded us one such route to rapid discovery. Thus by working with disease populations it has been possible to shed new light on fundamentals of biology by uncovering the molecular basis of normal processes that have gone awry. The murine immune system represents particularly fertile ground for the exploitation of these phenotype-driven approaches: phenotypic abnormalities that compromise immune development are seldom sufficiently devastating to result in embryonic lethality, and genetic abnormalities compromising immune function are generally well tolerated in the typical pathogen-free environment that the laboratory mouse calls home. But such phenotypic abnormalities can often be revealed at the developmental level by flow cytometric analysis of the immune system and at the functional level by experimental challenge. As a result, inherited mutations affecting the murine immune system have proved to be a valuable source for the identification of novel genes that have shaped our thinking of immune function, including Fas and Fas ligand revealed by *lpr* and *gld* mouse strains and the Tlr signaling pathway uncovered by the *Lps* locus.

A number of years ago we became interested in a novel mutant mouse strain, the *scurfy* mouse, that had originated at Oak Ridge National Laboratory (ORNL) in the 1940s. The mouse exhibited a profound phenotype characterized by massive lymphoproliferation, extensive multiorgan immune infiltration, and the overproduction of multiple cytokines, which resulted in early juvenile lethality (Russell et al. 1959; Godfrey et al. 1991a). We reasoned that the phenotype present in these animals was reflective of massive T cell dysregulation and that the identification of the gene mutated in these animals might help uncover a key regulator of immune function. We also reasoned that mutations in this gene product would likely affect the human population, but that the rapid and aggressively fatal nature of the *scurfy* mutation might make their identification using traditional familial human genetics difficult. With this in mind we set about identifying the molecular basis of the *scurfy* mouse mutation.

Scurfy: The Early Years

The *scurfy (sf)* mouse mutation arose spontaneously in 1949 at the ORNL in Oak Ridge, Tennessee. The Laboratory itself had something of a spontaneous origin, being built in secret in 1943 as part of the Manhattan project, on farmland in the mountains of east Tennessee. The wartime race to develop the atomic bomb opened a number of scientific avenues for subsequent exploration in the post World War II arena. Included in these was the pressing need to understand the human consequences of exposure to ionizing radiation encountered either as fallout from nuclear weapons tests or from the domestic use of nuclear power. In order to do this a mouse genetics program devoted to the investigation of the effects of radiation was initiated at ORNL under the guidance of Dr. Bill Russell. In 1951 Dr. Russell published the first results of these experiments, involving the analysis of more than 85,000 animals generated either from irradiated or control parents (Russell 1951). Dr. Russell also developed an elegant mechanism for facilitating the study of germ cell mutations, which allowed the detection of recessive mutations in first generation offspring. This method, known as the specific locus test, took advantage of an established tester strain of mice that had been bred to be homozygous at a number of autosomal recessive visible loci. Mutagen-treated animals were then mated to these tester strain mice: under normal circumstances the progeny from these crosses would receive one functional allele at each of the autosomal recessive visible loci from the mutagenized parent and one mutant allele from the tester strain. But a germ cell mutation in one of these visible marker loci would be uncovered when mutagenized animals were crossed onto the tester strain, allowing the detection of mutations in this first generation (Russell et al. 1958; Silver 1995). The construction of this tester strain represented a substantial breeding exercise, requiring the breeding to homozygosity of all seven recessive alleles, and ironically the *scurfy* mutation arose spontaneously from this program.

As the name suggests the original *scurfy* animals were characterized by an early scaling of the skin that was particularly apparent on the ears, tail, and feet and which was followed by a generalized wasting, with most animals dying around the time of weaning (Russell et al. 1959). Early studies at ORNL focused on the mechanism of inheritance of this mutant phenotype. Studies conducted by Russell and colleagues showed that female animals occasionally exhibited the *scurfy* phenotype and that these animals had an X^{sf}/O genotype. This led Lee Russell and colleagues to propose in 1959 that the Y chromosome was the male determining factor in mice, and that, by inference, the Y chromosome might confer maleness in other mammals including man (Welshons and Russell 1959).

Despite the seminal nature of these initial observations and their implications for our understanding of sex determination, the *scurfy* mutant mouse drifted into PubMed obscurity. Any additional early characterization of the *scurfy* mutation was limited to observations of the animal's external appearance and comments on the animal's early mortality. Analogies were drawn between the characteristic scaling and other skin abnormalities observed in *scurfy* and those present in X-linked ichthyosis of humans (Lyon et al. 1990; Godfrey et al. 1991b).

Scurfy: A Novel Immunoregulatory Gene

A more systematic evaluation of the *scurfy* phenotype and a dismissal of this ichthyosis association had to wait until the early 1990s, when studies by Lyon and colleagues (1990) and Godfrey and colleagues (1991a) demonstrated substantial differences at the pathophysiological and clinical level between *scurfy* and ichthyosis. *Scurfy* mutant mice developed bloody diarrhea, and hematological studies indicated that platelet and erythrocyte counts were reduced in *scurfy* animals and that these mice were severely anemic. By histopathology, *scurfy* animals exhibited splenomegaly and enlarged lymph nodes, with lympho-histiocytic proliferation and infiltration of peripheral lymph nodes, spleen, liver, and skin. It thus appeared as if the *scurfy* phenotype had an underlying immune basis that distinguished it from X-linked ichthyosis. The unique nature of the *scurfy* mutation was further confirmed by mapping studies, which placed the *scurfy* locus near the centromere of the X chromosome, separate from the steroid sulfatase gene that had been implicated in ichthyosis (Lyon et al. 1990).

A handful of publications then followed that further emphasized the immunologic nature of the *scurfy* phenotype. It became apparent that this was not a classic X-linked immunodeficiency but rather was a disease characterized by immune dysregulation with an absolute requirement for T cells. Studies from Oak Ridge demonstrated that *scurfy* mice that had been subjected to neonatal thymectomy had a prolonged life and less severe disease when compared to euthymic *scurfy* controls, while the transfer of the *scurfy* mutant allele onto either a nude or severe combined immunodeficiency (SCID) background resulted in abolition of disease (Godfrey et al. 1991b, 1994). Disease progression also exhibited a requirement for the exposure of developing T cells to endogenous antigen. When the *scurfy* mutation was bred onto a T cell receptor (TCR) transgenic line, the resultant *scurfy*/TCR transgenic animals (in which 75%–95% of the T cells expressed TCR for an exogenous antigen) had ameliorated disease. This disease could be blocked entirely in a *scurfy*/TCR-transgenic/Rag1 knockout background in which only T cells reactive to the exogenous antigen develop (Zahorsky-Reeves and Wilkinson 2001). Disease progression appeared to exhibit an absolute requirement for CD4[+] T cells: monoclonal antibody depletion of CD4[+] T cells but not CD8[+] T cells resulted in a retardation of *scurfy* disease, and life expectancy was also extended when *scurfy* animals were crossed onto a CD4-null but not CD8-null background (Blair et al. 1994a). CD4[+] T cells from *scurfy* animals were also able to transfer disease when transplanted into H-2 compatible nude mice, unlike CD8[+] T cells. In addition the CD4[+] T cells present in the *scurfy* animal appeared to have a dysregulated phenotype, expressing activation markers and demonstrating a hyper-responsiveness to stimulation through the TCR and a decreased requirement for costimulation (Blair et al. 1994a; Clark et al. 1999). Thus the *scurfy* gene product appeared to play a key role in the generation of a functional and appropriately regulated population of CD4[+] T cells.

The *Scurfy* Phenotype Is Caused by a Mutation in *Foxp3*

The *scurfy* locus was initially mapped to a 1.7-cM interval in the proximal region of the mouse X chromosome (Lyon et al. 1990; Blair et al. 1994b). Today, the completion of the mouse and human genome initiatives would make the identification of genes within this region [real as well as predicted open reading frames (ORFs)] a simple computational exercise using publicly available resources. In the late 1990s, however, such resources were at a primitive stage, making this a considerable logistical challenge. Nevertheless, the compelling nature of the phenotype persuaded us that further mapping and gene identification efforts were warranted.

Through an intersubspecific backcross, our group, led by Mary Brunkow, was able to further localize the *scurfy* locus to a 0.3-cM region (Brunkow et al. 2001). By using a combination of high resolution genetic and physical mapping and large scale sequence analysis, Brunkow and colleagues identified 20 candidate genes within this genomic region, including several genes predicted based on sequence analysis only. Initial prioritization of these candidate genes based on T cell-specific mRNA expression was not informative: no mutations were detected in those genes restricted to lymphocyte expression. Further prioritization based on drugability characteristics (wishful thinking) was similarly unsuccessful. Ultimately, DNA sequencing of all genes from both normal and *scurfy* mice identified a single gene (the last gene on our prioritization scale) with a mutation in the coding sequence. This ORF had strong similarity with the DNA-binding domain of the forkhead family of proteins and contained a 2-bp insertion in the predicted coding region. This insertion was contained in affected *scurfy* animals but absent from non-*scurfy* siblings, absent from seven other mouse strains, and absent from the analogous human cDNA. This insertion resulted in a frameshift and the subsequent generation of a truncated gene product lacking the carboxy terminal forkhead domain. Confirmation that this insertion was causal of the *scurfy* mutant phenotype came from transgenesis, when a 30.8-kb genomic fragment was used to rescue the mutant phenotype (Brunkow et al. 2001). In compliance with accepted nomenclature standards for the forkhead family, the gene mutated in *scurfy* mice was given the mundane designation *Foxp3*. Since there is no required/accepted nomenclature for the protein, we adopted a more descriptive name for the protein: scurfin (Brunkow et al. 2001).

Mutations in *Foxp3* Cause Disease in Humans

Given the severe nature of the *scurfy* mutant phenotype one might expect that mutations in the human gene would be equally catastrophic. A number of X-linked human immunodeficiencies and immunodysregulatory disorders have been described, and studies in the late 1980s mapped one of these, Wiskott-Aldrich syndrome (WAS), to a *scurfy* syntenic region (Lyon et al. 1990). The gene responsible for WAS was cloned by Derry and colleagues and shown to be a 502 amino acid-containing protein containing putative SH3 binding domains and a nuclear localization signal (Derry et al. 1994). However, the subsequent identification of the mouse homolog of the WAS gene followed by sequence analysis and transcript analysis failed to reveal any disease-specific alterations between normal and *scurfy* mice (Derry et al. 1995).

Several investigators have reported isolated cases of infant males with a variety of immune-related symptoms culminating in early lethality, including enteropathy, type I diabetes, eczema, and hyperthyroidism. That these individuals might be suffering from a common disorder with an underlying genetic component was first proposed by Powell et al., working with a family in which multiple males across three generations (connected through females) had various combinations of intractable diarrhea, eczema, hemolytic anemia, diabetes mellitus, or thyroid autoimmunity (Powell et al. 1982). Linkage analysis of this and other families suggested that this disease locus lay close to the centromere of the X chromosome, close to (but not allelic with) the WAS locus and thus close to the *Foxp3* locus (reviewed in Wildin and Freitas 2005). The multiplicity of symptoms associated with this disorder was summarized in the name conferred upon it: IPEX, for immune dysfunction/polyendocrinopathy/enteropathy/X-linked. Over time, a small number of familial clusters of IPEX were reported (e.g., Peake et al. 1996; Levy-Lahad and Wildin 2001).

While this familial disease had been recognized for years, little progress beyond the association with WAS had been made in the identification of the gene responsible. We were intrigued by the complex immune dysfunction seen in IPEX patients and by its map location, which placed it close to *Foxp3*, and the cloning of the gene responsible for *scurfy* enabled us to establish collaborations to test for the presence of mutations in this gene. In a multinational effort led by Dr. Bob Wildin and working with collaborators in Italy, Australia, France, and Israel we were able to identify five unrelated and ethnically diverse families, each of which contained at least two males affected with IPEX. Sequence analysis of DNA from one male from each of these families indicated that four of these five males carried mutations in exons 10 or 11, within the winged-helix domain of *Foxp3*. Where material was available we were able to show that carriers were heterozygous for these mutations and that an unaffected male sibling lacked the mutation. To determine the normal spectrum of variation in exons 10 and 11 these two exons were sequenced in 240 unaffected ethnically diverse individuals. No sequence variation was found in any of these individuals (Wildin et al. 2001). At the same time Bennett et al. were able to take advantage of an extended family with a history of IPEX disease over four generations: a G to A transition, resulting in an Ala to Thr substitution at residue 384 of the winged-helix domain, segregated with disease in all members of the family tested, with two affected males being hemizygous for the mutation. The significance of this substitution was confirmed by sequence analysis of 500 control X chromosomes, none of which showed the same polymorphism. Analysis of a second family of Japanese origin also revealed a *Foxp3* mutation, in this case a 2-bp deletion within the *Foxp3* termination codon, resulting in a predicted addition of 25 amino acids (Bennett et al. 2001). Thus the cloning of a genetic mutation responsible for a lethal mouse disorder led directly to the identification of the gene responsible for a lethal human disorder, reaffirming the utility of using the mouse as a genetic tool to support human genetic studies. In addition to *Foxp3*, mutations in several other forkhead family proteins have been shown to result in autoimmune disease in mice. Mutations in Foxn1 in mice and humans result in a relatively diminished T cell response, whereas mutations in Foxo3a and Foxj1 can lead to a progressive autoimmune disease that progresses with age. It remains to be definitively determined whether these family members have a role in human disease.

Tolerance

The original rationale for choosing to work on the *scurfy* mutation was based on the autoimmune nature of the phenotype of the mouse (Godfrey et al. 1991a). It seemed apparent that defining the mutation would provide a significant insight into the mechanism(s) by which the immune system developed or was controlled. There were several examples of mutations in genes that led to disorders of immunological development (most notably several mutations that led to a SCID-like phenotype), but no specific mutations in which a defect in tolerance had been established, and the *scurfy* mouse seemed like it might represent such an example. It has been known for some time that there are multiple processes to maintain tolerance within the immune system. Pioneering studies by Kappler and Marrack (Kappler et al. 1987; MacDonald et al. 1988), among others, indicated T cells that recognized "self" antigens could be eliminated during their development. A similar phenomenon occurs for B cells during their development (Goodnow et al. 1990; Basten et al. 1991). This process of clonal deletion was postulated to be a major mechanism by which the immune system removed those cells that could react to self tissues, but maintain a diverse repertoire to respond to pathogens. Ultimately, the use of TCR [and B cell receptor (BCR)] transgenic mice, in which the antigen-specific receptor was predetermined on all T (or B) cells, allowed for a dramatic visualization of this process (Kisielow et al. 1988; Sha et al. 1988; Nemazee and Burki 1989). In these types of studies it was possible to control the dose of antigen, the timing of antigen presence, and even the nature of the cell that presented the antigen, to understand more fully the process of clonal deletion.

A major issue for the clonal deletion model, however, was how tolerance to antigens not expressed within the thymus during T cell development was induced. It seemed apparent that there were tissue-specific antigens (TSA) that would not be present within the thymic microenvironment, and that there must be a mechanism to prevent or control reactivity to these tissues. While many models have been proposed, experimental evidence has supported two major mechanisms to maintain tolerance to TSA, the first being the "promiscuous" expression of TSA within the thymus and the second model being the presence of "suppressor" cells within the peripheral milieu that prevent autoreactivity. As is commonly the case in immunology, both theories have ultimately proved to be correct.

The expression of TSA within the thymus could derive either from the transport of such antigens to the thymus or from specific gene expression within the thymus. Several studies demonstrated that the genes for at least some TSA are in fact expressed in thymic stromal cells during thymic development (Klein and Kyewski 2000; Derbinski et al. 2001). Further studies showed that the transcription factor

AIRE (autoimmune regulator) is in part responsible for this expression, resulting in the deletion of T cells reactive to antigens that are normally expressed only in specific tissues of the body (Anderson et al. 2002, 2005). The process of thymic clonal deletion could thus ensure that as T cells developed they were exposed to normal self antigens. Those cells that reacted strongly with these antigens were then programmed to undergo apoptosis and thus be eliminated from the pool of potentially reactive cells that entered the peripheral immune system. Importantly, in the absence of AIRE, an organ-specific autoimmunity called APECED (autoimmune polyendocrinopathy-candidiasis-ectodermal dystrophy) develops (Aaltonen et al. 1997; Nagamine et al. 1997). While this disease is not as severe as IPEX, this nonetheless reflects the importance of antigen-specific clonal deletion in maintaining tolerance.

This system of clonal deletion is not perfect at eliminating self-reactive cells. It is clear that normal mice and humans, as well as autoimmune individuals, possess T cells capable of reacting with self antigens. There have been a number of alternative models described for controlling these self-reactive cells. Two predominant theories are the functional inactivation of T cells (loosely termed anergy for the current discussion) and the generation of a population of T cells capable of suppressing self-reactive cells. These suppressor cells are today more commonly referred to as regulatory T cells (T_R). Although there are numerous in vitro and in vivo model systems in which anergy can be demonstrated, the data suggesting that this is a significant component of normal tolerance in vivo is not strong at present. In part, this may be because the anergic state is difficult to measure (due to the relative lack of a response) and because it may be transient in nature. Thus, while anergy may be important for maintaining tolerance to self in vivo, this has been difficult to prove experimentally.

T_R cells to a great extent represent the reincarnation of the suppressor T cell populations described in the 1970s and 1980s. Although this population of cells has a somewhat "checkered" history and fell out of research favor for many years (Shevach 2000), seminal studies from Sakaguchi and colleagues established that a minor population of CD4$^+$ T cells (those co-expressing CD25) was capable of inhibiting the response of autoantigen-specific cells (Sakaguchi et al. 1995). The CD4$^+$25$^+$ subset of T_R cells is most often referred to as nT_R cells or natural regulatory T cells. These comprise approximately 10% of all CD4$^+$ T cells in the mouse. Thymectomy of mice within the first 3 days of life dramatically reduces the number of these cells and also results in the development of a broad-spectrum, tissue-specific autoimmunity (largely directed at endocrine tissues) (Sakaguchi et al. 1985). Similarly, antibody-mediated elimination of CD4$^+$25$^+$ cells causes a pathology that resembles that observed following thymectomy (Sakaguchi et al. 1995). In vitro studies have demonstrated that when purified, the addition of CD4$^+$25$^+$ cells could inhibit proliferation and interleukin (IL)-2 production by the CD4$^+$25$^-$ subset of cells (Thornton and Shevach 1998). Finally, in vivo studies demonstrated that the co-transfer of CD4$^+$25$^+$ cells could inhibit an autoimmune-induced inflammatory bowel disease in SCID animals (Mottet et al. 2003). It has been historically far more challenging to demonstrate a corresponding subset of cells in humans, although in vitro data for such activities does exist (Baecher-Allan and Hafler 2006). In addition, there are also descriptions of subtypes of T_R cells with somewhat different properties in terms of their phenotypes and mechanisms of action (for a review see Shevach 2002). Thus, the data indicate that both in vitro and in vivo, such CD4$^+$25$^+$ T_R cells could act to suppress the activities of CD4$^+$25$^-$ cells, and one possible explanation for the break in tolerance observed in the *scurfy* mice could be the loss of nT_R cells.

Foxp3 and Tolerance

The nature of the pathology observed in *scurfy* mice suggested that the etiology of the disease might be due to a defect in tolerance. The nature of the mutation suggested that this defect would lie within the T cell compartment since this was the major population of cells that appeared to express the gene. We thus began to analyze the various forms of tolerance that had been described for T cells to determine what process(es) might have been affected by the mutation. Our earlier studies had suggested, in fact, that clonal deletion was operative within *scurfy* mice. This was based on examination of the repertoire of TCRs in mice carrying the *scurfy* mutation and indicated that those specific TCR families expected to be deleted were, in fact, deleted normally. More conclusive studies by Zahorsky-Reeves and Wilkinson demonstrated that *scurfy* mice carrying only an ovalbumin (OVA)-specific TCR (due to a RAG-1^{null} mutation) did not succumb to disease and that thymic deletion of these cells appeared normal in the presence of antigen (Zahorsky-Reeves and Wilkinson 2001). This suggested that, at least for the TCR–antigen combinations tested, deletion appeared normal. Because mice in which T cells could only recognize OVA failed to develop disease, the data further indicated that the T cells within the *scurfy* mice must recognize endogenous antigens in order to initiate pathology.

Since CD4$^+$25$^+$ T_R cells appeared to be critical for maintaining tolerance, Roli Khattri in our group examined the expression of *Foxp3* in CD4$^+$ T cell subsets. It was immediately apparent that the CD4$^+$25$^+$ subset was highly enriched for *Foxp3* mRNA expression compared to virtually all other cell types (Khattri et al. 2003). This suggested that the disease seen in *scurfy* mice was due to an inability to generate nT_R cells. Two other pieces of data supported this theory. First, we were unable to identify any suppressor activity in CD4$^+$25$^+$ cells from *scurfy* mice. Because CD25 is expressed on all activated cells, and many CD4$^+$ cells in *scurfy* mice are activated, we further attempted to isolate subsets of CD25$^+$ cells in an effort to identify suppressor activity, without success. The second, and more important, piece of data to suggest that *Foxp3* was involved in the generation of nT_R cells derived from a more detailed analysis of the *Foxp3* transgenic mice generated previously. These animals were developed to prove that the mutation in *Foxp3* was in fact the causal mutation in the *scurfy* strain as discussed. In five independent lines, each expressing a distinct amount of *Foxp3* message, crossing of the transgenic animal to *scurfy* mice resulted in the prevention of disease in genotypically *sf*/Y animals. However, when all of these lines were bred onto an otherwise wildtype background, the resulting animals displayed a reduction in the number of peripheral T cells. Interestingly, the reduction in T cells was directly proportional to the amount of transgene expression. A variety of in vitro and in vivo analyses indicated that there was also a functional defect in the T cells from these transgenic mice. The more transgene expressed, the less responsive these cells were to stimulation. This was particularly obvious when IL-2 production was examined. Thus, the cells were virtually unresponsive in vitro, very much like nT_R cells. When tested in suppressor assays, however, it was discovered that the transgenic cells (even those that failed to express CD25) could mediate suppression toward normal T cells. This result was confirmed by others using retroviral transduction of *Foxp3* into CD4$^+$25$^-$ cells and demonstrating suppressor activity (Hori et al. 2003; Fontenot et al. 2003) in the transduced cells. Further studies using both the transgenic animals and the retrovirally transduced cells demonstrated that *Foxp3*-expressing cells could act as suppressor cells in vivo.

Thus, the cloning of the mutation in *scurfy* mice had identified a transcription factor involved in the generation of nT_R cells. The presence of *Foxp3* within most tissues (as assessed by Northern blot and PCR techniques) suggested that nT_R cells were also present within these tissues. Analyses of *Foxp3*–green fluorescent protein (GFP) knockin mice confirmed the presence of *Foxp3*-positive cells in a variety of nonlymphoid tissues. Initially it was this presence of *Foxp3* message in most tissues that led us to think that *Foxp3* was unlikely to be the gene responsible for disease in *scurfy* mice, as we had reasoned (incorrectly) that the mutated gene would be most highly expressed in lymphoid tissues. The data, however, support a model in which nT_R cells reside within peripheral tissues and are critical for preventing autoimmune responses. The data also demonstrate that this is a dominant form of tolerance in which autoreactive T cells are maintained in a quiescent state due to the inhibitory effects of nT_R cells. Unlike clonal deletion, suppression by nT_R cells can act to inhibit autoimmune responses that arise as a consequence of pathogen-specific T cells inadvertently recognizing normal self tissues due to similarities between pathogen and tissue antigens.

One of the most controversial and highly studied areas of research involves the induction of *Foxp3* expression. In the thymus there are a number of interactions that are required for selection of nT_R cells, including TCR-MHC II, CD28, and IL-2. The specific regions of the *Foxp3* promoter are just now being characterized, and the integration of factors that regulate expression is not yet fully determined (Mantel et al. 2006). While continued *Foxp3* expression in peripheral cells is critical to maintain tolerance, it remains unclear whether transient induction of *Foxp3* in responding T cells is necessary for tolerance, particularly in humans. The autoimmune pathology observed in day 3 thymectomized mice or in mice depleted of CD25$^+$ T_R cells is substantially less severe than that observed in *scurfy* mice. This could reflect the fact that these manipulations result in only partial depletion of nT_R cells, or the need to generate *Foxp3*$^+$ T_R cells subsequent to thymic development. The absolute requirement for *Foxp3* expression in peripheral T cells could support either model. Nonetheless, the induced expression of *Foxp3*, its stabilization in peripheral T cells, or controlling both together presents a unique opportunity for therapeutic intervention in autoimmune disease. Regardless of whether this leads directly to the generation of T_R cells or simply a reduced responsiveness to stimulation, it could result in a diminished T cell response and thus diminished disease.

A final point emphasizes the utility of such mouse mutational analyses for biological annotation: when first identified, *Foxp3* was not found within the public EST database and was not present on any of the commercial microarray chips. Genes whose function is restricted to a particular cellular subset, especially a rare or not easily accessible subset, may be very difficult to functionally annotate if starting from expression data alone. Even when the relevant cellular distribution is unknown in advance, such as with *scurfy*, the existence of a demonstrable phenotypic effect of the mutation enables such annotation.

Mechanism of Action

How *Foxp3* acts to generate or maintain nT_R cells is still unclear. The original model suggested that *Foxp3* might act in much the same way that T-bet and GATA-3 are involved in the commitment of cells to specific differentiation pathways (Th1 and Th2, respectively). Recent data from two groups, however, suggest that *Foxp3* is not required to initiate the process of nT_R cell development (Lin et al. 2007; Gavin et al. 2007). In these studies, cells that express a nonfunctional *Foxp3* can still develop a number of nT_R characteristics. These cells, however, do not mediate suppressive activity. The data also support previous conclusions that *Foxp3* expression must be maintained in nT_R cells in the periphery in order to maintain tolerance. This followed from the observation that mice that expressed *Foxp3* only in the thymus (via a transgene) remain susceptible to disease in a manner very similar to *scurfy* mice. The overall conclusions to date suggest that during T cell development, some factor drives a subpopulation of T cells toward a regulatory lineage. One consequence of this process is the induction of *Foxp3*, the expression of which is absolutely required for the maintenance and suppressive activity of nT_R cells, which are in turn absolutely necessary for the normal control of the immune system. The factors responsible for the initial commitment to the nT_R lineage may involve TCR affinity (Picca et al. 2006), the nature of the antigen-presenting cell, the type and magnitude of costimulatory molecule engagement, and the cytokines present within the thymic microenvironment during development (Watanabe et al. 2005). Data from Aschenbrenner et al. (2007) suggest that medullary thymic epithelial cells have the ability to determine this fate. Since the ability to control and induce *Foxp3* (and more importantly, the suppressive state) is of great potential therapeutic value, characterizing the factors that induce and maintain *Foxp3* expression will remain a very active area of interest for some time to come.

From a more mechanistic perspective, whether *Foxp3* is involved in epigenetic or acute transcriptional events is yet to be determined. For T-bet and GATA-3, a key component of their function appears to be the ability to remodel chromatin structure, although their overall mechanism of action is still not completely understood (Murphy and Reiner 2002). Most studies on *Foxp3* have focused on direct transcriptional activity, although one report suggests that chromatin remodeling via histone deacetylase binding and activation may be involved (Chen et al. 2006). As noted earlier, there is no apparent transcriptional activation domain for *Foxp3*, and preliminary data suggested that the protein is capable of inhibiting IL-2 transcription directly (Schubert et al. 2001). Recent data suggest that the *Foxp3* protein can dimerize with other transcription factors, notably NFATc (nuclear factor of activated T cells, cytoplasmic), and can thus alter the interactions of NFATc with AP-1 to inhibit IL-2 production (Wu et al. 2006). This is similar to the manner in which both GATA-3 and T-bet can interact with NFAT. Studies also indicate that *Foxp3* interacts with other transcriptional elements, including AML1, and can affect transcription of IL-2 through this pathway in an apparently independent manner (Ono et al. 2007). In addition to IL-2, chromatin immunoprecipitation (ChIP) assays have recently been performed and suggest that *Foxp3* binds to a number of relevant promoter sequences, including Ctla-4, CD25, and glucocorticoid-induced TNFR-related gene (GITR), among many others (Marson et al. 2007; Zheng et al. 2007). Combined with mRNA analyses, the data suggest that *Foxp3* binding (likely in a multimeric form with other factors) can both augment and inhibit transcription. This has been observed with other Fox-family members, and can depend upon the homo- or heterodimerization of these proteins.

The structure of the *Foxp3* protein predicts a number of functional domains, including zinc finger, leucine zipper, and forkhead binding domains. It would be predicted that the leucine zipper and zinc finger domains are involved in dimerization. Indeed, both *Foxp3* homodimerization and heterodimerization with NFAT and nuclear factor (NF)-κB have been described (Bettelli et al. 2005; Lopes et al. 2006). The proline-rich N-terminal portion of *Foxp3* is important for modulating gene expression as well, apparently independent of *Foxp3* dimerization with NFAT and possibly by recruitment of transcriptional corepressors, coactivators, or both (Ono et al. 2007; Lopes et al. 2006). In humans, an additional splice variant lacking exon 2 is also expressed at the protein level. At this point, no significant functional distinctions between the full-length protein and the variant lacking exon 2 have been identified, although this exon codes for sequences within the N-terminal domain of *Foxp3*. Emerging data clearly suggest that *Foxp3* binds to and forms a stable complex with NFATc that results in a pattern of gene expression distinct from AP-1:NFATc complexes. Determining which other factors are involved in the control of gene expression awaits further experimentation.

While the mutation discovered in the *scurfy* mouse results in a truncation and complete loss of function, there has been a variety of mutations identified throughout the *Foxp3* gene from human patients. These mutations include insertions, deletions, and missense mutations in the forkhead domain as well as other regions of the protein. There are also several examples of noncoding mutations that significantly affect mRNA levels. Changes within the forkhead domain have been shown to alter DNA binding (or intracellular localization) whereas mutations within other domains, such as the leucine zipper, can alter dimerization. The individual mutations are now being examined for their specific effect on functional activity to better understand the mechanism(s) by which *Foxp3* controls immune responses. To date there have been approximately 20 distinct IPEX families with identified *Foxp3* mutations. It is interesting to note that all coding polymorphisms identified within the human *Foxp3* gene have resulted in IPEX disease. At present, no studies have demonstrated a convincing association between *Foxp3* and any autoimmune disease (other than IPEX), suggesting that this pathway is tightly regulated and that even minor alterations in expression or function lead to catastrophic disease.

Scurfy: Prospects

A number of aspects of *Foxp3* identification merit comment. The mutation arose spontaneously at ORNL from among a large-scale mouse genetics program. The fact that it was identified and subsequently established for future generations is a testament to the enthusiasm of the ORNL staff. We ourselves were fortunate, both in learning of this fascinating but little-studied animal and in being able to make the leap between the murine disease phenotype and human disease syndrome. The identification of the *scurfy* gene in the mouse led to a new understanding of the basic principles of immune regulation and tolerance. At the same time it brought resolution to a long-running series of family disease studies that had been initiated in the early 1980s and importantly offered a diagnostic tool for the identification of IPEX carriers. In the absence of the mouse mutation this identification of the human gene would have been a logistical challenge.

The study of the *Foxp3* mutant mouse provides a clear illustration of the power of using monogenic diseases in a phenotype-first approach. The compelling biology of the *scurfy* mutation and the phenotypic similarity to knockouts of two key immunoregulatory molecules, CTLA-4 and TGF-β, convinced us that the underlying mutation might reveal an equally important immunoregulatory gene. The resultant identification of the gene responsible for this disorder provided a transformative insight into a fundamental mechanism for controlling immune function. As evidenced by the number of PubMed citations (nine in 2001, greater than 1,000 by 2007), this result represents the type of substantial leap in understanding possible through a phenotype-driven discovery program.

Monogenic diseases in both the mouse and in humans have played an important historical role in revealing the mechanistic basis of normal and disease processes. Yet despite considerable successes in disease mapping and cloning, a sizeable proportion of the genome remains to be annotated. Furthermore, the existing collection of spontaneous mouse mutations is limited and there remains a gulf between the spectrum of phenotypes afflicting these animals and those which one might expect to find based on the spectrum of genetic diseases in humans: classical mouse mutations are representative of only a subset of those diseases afflicting the human population. This disparity (the "phenotype gap") likely reflects a historical bias

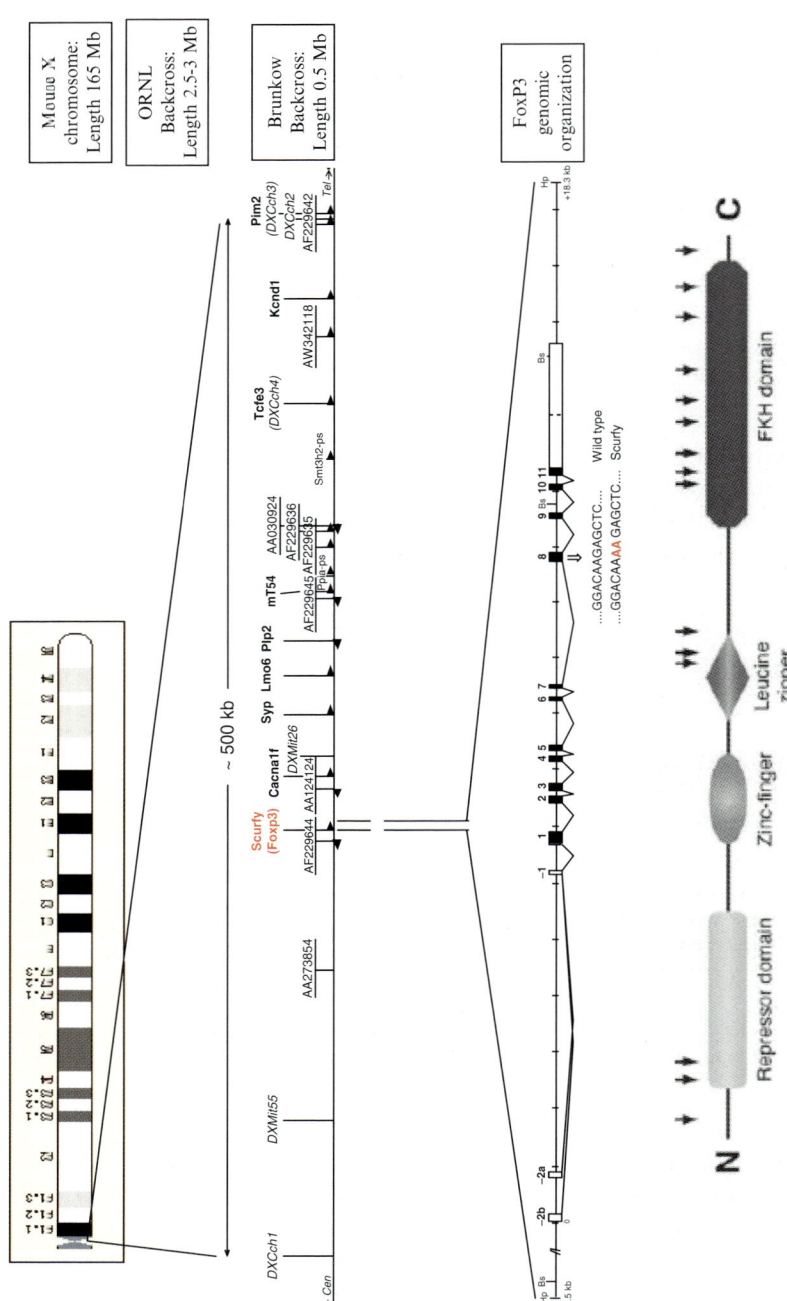

Fig. 7.1 Positional cloning of the Foxp3 gene. An interspecific backcross established a 0.5 Mb region containing 20 candidate genes responsible for the scurfy phenotype. cDNA sequencing identified a mutation in the Foxp3 gene as the only change between affected and unaffected animals. The domain structure for the Foxp3 protein is shown, with arrows representing mutations found in human IPEX patients

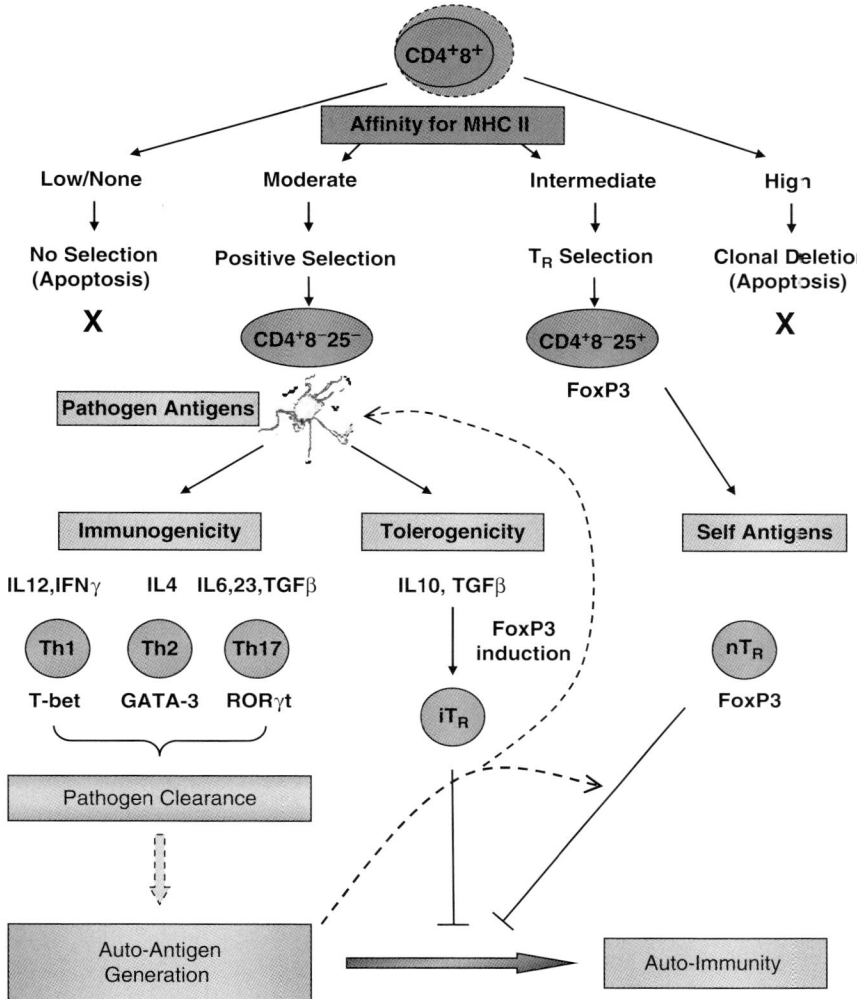

Fig. 7.2 A model for the continuum of development of Regulatory T Cell development in the thymus (top section) and periphery (lower section). Multiple factors control the expression of Foxp3, as well as other genes required for regulatory T cell development and activity (see text)

toward the identification of easily discernible visible mutant phenotypes (Brown and Peters 1996). A number of groups have set out to close this phenotype gap by combining traditional mouse mutagenesis, based on that pioneered by ORNL, with high throuput phenotyping (Beutler et al. 2006; Cook et al. 2006). Just as the *scurfy* mutation arose spontaneously from the directed mutagenesis activities at ORNL, we can only hope that these latest genome-wide efforts will spawn equally elucidative phenotypes.

References

Aaltonen J, Björses P, Perheentupa J, Horelli-Kuitunen N, Palotie A, Peltonen L, Su Lee Y, Francis F, Henning S, Thiel C, Leharach H, Yaspo ML (1997) An autoimmune disease, APECED, caused by mutations in a novel gene featuring two PHD-type zinc-finger domains. The Finnish-German APECED Consortium. Autoimmune Polyendocrinopathy-Candidiasis-Ectodermal Dystrophy. Nat Genet 17:399–403

Anderson MS, Venanzi ES, Klein L, Chen Z, Berzins SP, Turley SJ, von Boehmer H, Bronson R, Dierich A, Benoist C, Mathis D (2002) Projection of an immunological self shadow within the thymus by the aire protein. Science 298:1395–1401

Anderson MS, Venanzi ES, Chen Z, Berzins SP, Benoist C, Mathis D (2005) The cellular mechanism of Aire control of T cell tolerance. Immunity 23:227–239

Aschenbrenner K, D'Cruz LM, Vollmann EH, Hinterberger M, Emmerich J, Swee LK, Rolink A, Klein L (2007) Selection of Foxp3+ regulatory T cells specific for self antigen expressed and presented by Aire+ medullary thymic epithelial cells. Nat Immunol 8:351–358

Baecher-Allan C, Hafler DA (2006) Human regulatory T cells and their role in autoimmune disease. Immunol Rev 212:203–216

Basten A, Brink R, Peake P, Adams E, Crosbie J, Hartley S, Goodnow CC (1991) Self tolerance in the B-cell repertoire. Immunol Rev 122:5–19

Bennett CL, Christie J, Ramsdell F, Brunkow ME, Ferguson PJ, Whitesell L, Kelly TE, Saulsbury FT, Chance PF, Ochs HD (2001) The immune dysregulation, polyendocrinopathy, enteropathy, X-linked syndrome (IPEX) is caused by mutations of FOXP3. Nat Genet 27:20–21

Bettelli E, Dastrange M, Oukka M (2005) Foxp3 interacts with nuclear factor of activated T cells and NF-kappa B to repress cytokine gene expression and effector functions of T helper cells. Proc Natl Acad Sci U S A 102:5138–5143

Beutler B, Jiang Z, Georgel P, Crozat K, Croker B, Rutschmann S, Du X, Hoebe K (2006) Genetic analysis of host resistance: Toll-like receptor signaling and immunity at large. Annu Rev Immunol 24:353–389

Blair PJ, Bultman SJ, Haas JC, Rouse BT, Wilkinson JE, Godfrey VL (1994a) CD4+CD8- T cells are the effector cells in disease pathogenesis in the scurfy (sf) mouse. J Immunol 153:3764–3774

Brown SD, Peters J (1996) Combining mutagenesis and genomics in the mouse—closing the phenotype gap. Trends Genet 12:433–435

Blair PJ, Carpenter DA, Godfrey VL, Russell LB, Wilkinson JE, Rinchik EM (1994b) The mouse scurfy (sf) mutation is tightly linked to Gata1 and Tfe3 on the proximal X chromosome. Mamm Genome 5:652–654

Brunkow ME, Jeffery EW, Hjerrild KA, Paeper B, Clark LB, Yasayko SA, Wilkinson JE, Galas D, Ziegler SF, Ramsdell F (2001) Disruption of a new forkhead/winged-helix protein, scurfin, results in the fatal lymphoproliferative disorder of the scurfy mouse. Nat Genet 27:68–73

Chen C, Rowell EA, Thomas RM, Hancock WW, Wells AD (2006) Transcriptional regulation by Foxp3 is associated with direct promoter occupancy and modulation of histone acetylation. J Biol Chem 281:36828–36834

Clark LB, Appleby MW, Brunkow ME, Wilkinson JE, Ziegler SF, Ramsdell F (1999) Cellular and molecular characterization of the scurfy mouse mutant. J Immunol 162:2546–2554

Cook MC, Vinuesa CG, Goodnow CC (2006) ENU-mutagenesis: insight into immune function and pathology. Curr Opin Immunol 18:627–633

Derbinski J, Schulte A, Kyewski B, Klein L (2001) Promiscuous gene expression in medullary thymic epithelial cells mirrors the peripheral self. Nat Immunol 2:1032–1039

Derry JM, Ochs HD, Francke U (1994) Isolation of a novel gene mutated in Wiskott-Aldrich syndrome. Cell 79:922

Derry JM, Wiedemann P, Blair P, Wang Y, Kerns JA, Lemahieu V, Godfrey VL, Wilkinson JE, Francke U (1995) The mouse homolog of the Wiskott-Aldrich syndrome protein (WASP) gene is highly conserved and maps near the scurfy (sf) mutation on the X chromosome. Genomics 29:471–477

Fontenot JD, Gavin MA, Rudensky AY (2003) Foxp3 programs the development and function of CD4+CD25+ regulatory T cells. Nat Immunol 4:330–336

Gavin MA, Rasmussen JP, Fontenot JD, Vasta V, Manganiello VC, Beavo JA, Rudensky AY (2007) Foxp3-dependent programme of regulatory T-cell differentiation. Nature 445:771–775

Godfrey VL, Wilkinson JE, Russell LB (1991a) X-linked lymphoreticular disease in the scurfy (sf) mutant mouse. Am J Pathol 138:1379–1387

Godfrey VL, Wilkinson JE, Rinchik EM, Russell LB (1991b) Fatal lymphoreticular disease in the scurfy (sf) mouse requires T cells that mature in a sf thymic environment: potential model for thymic education. Proc Natl Acad Sci U S A 88:5528–5532

Godfrey VL, Rouse BT, Wilkinson JE (1994) Transplantation of T cell-mediated, lymphoreticular disease from the scurfy (sf) mouse. Am J Pathol 145:281–286

Goodnow CC, Adelstein S, Basten A (1990) The need for central and peripheral tolerance in the B cell repertoire. Science 248:1373–1379

Hori S, Nomura T, Sakaguchi S (2003) Control of regulatory T cell development by the transcription factor Foxp3. Science 299:1057–1061

Kappler JW, Roehm N, Marrack P (1987) T cell tolerance by clonal elimination in the thymus. Cell 49:273–280

Khattri R, Cox T, Yasayko SA, Ramsdell F (2003) An essential role for Scurfin in CD4+CD25+ T regulatory cells. Nat Immunol 4:337–342

Kisielow P, Bluthmann H, Staerz UD, Steinmetz M, von Boehmer H (1988) Tolerance in T-cell-receptor transgenic mice involves deletion of nonmature CD4+8+ thymocytes. Nature 333:742–746

Klein L, Kyewski B (2000) "Promiscuous" expression of tissue antigens in the thymus: a key to T-cell tolerance and autoimmunity? J Mol Med 78:483–494

Levy-Lahad E, Wildin RS (2001) Neonatal diabetes mellitus, enteropathy, thrombocytopenia, and endocrinopathy: further evidence for an X-linked lethal syndrome. J Pediatr 138:577–580

Lin W, Haribhai D, Relland LM, Truong N, Carlson MR, Williams CB, Chatila TA (2007) Regulatory T cell development in the absence of functional Foxp3. Nat Immunol 8:359–638

Lopes JE, Torgerson TR, Schubert LA, Anover SD, Ocheltree EL, Ochs HD, Ziegler SF (2006) Analysis of FOXP3 reveals multiple domains required for its function as a transcriptional repressor. J Immunol 177:3133–3142

Lyon MF, Peters J, Glenister PH, Ball S, Wright E (1990) The scurfy mouse mutant has previously unrecognized hematological abnormalities and resembles Wiskott-Aldrich syndrome. Proc Natl Acad Sci U S A 87:2433–2437

MacDonald HR, Pedrazzini T, Schneider R, Louis JA, Zinkernagel RM, Hengartner H (1988) Intrathymic elimination of Mlsa-reactive (V beta 6+) cells during neonatal tolerance induction to Mlsa-encoded antigens. J Exp Med 167:2005–2010

Mantel PY, Ouaked N, Ruckert B, Karagiannidis C, Welz R, Blaser K, Schmidt-Weber CB (2006) Molecular mechanisms underlying FOXP3 induction in human T cells. J Immunol 176:3593–3602

Marson A, Kretschmer K, Frampton GM, Jacobsen ES, Polansky JK, MacIsaac D, Levine SS, Fraenkel E, von Boehmer H, Young RA (2007) Foxp3 occupancy and regulation of key target genes during T-cell stimulation. Nature 445:931–935

Mottet C, Uhlig HH, Powrie F (2003) Cutting edge: cure of colitis by CD4+CD25+ regulatory T cells. J Immunol 170:3939–3943

Murphy KM, Reiner SL (2002) The lineage decisions of helper T cells. Nat Rev Immunol 2:933–944

Nagamine K, Peterson P, Scott HS, Kudoh J, Minoshima S, Heino M, Krohn KJ, Lalioti MD, Mullis PE, Antonarakis SE, Kawasaki K, Asakawa S, Ito F, Shimizu N (1997) Positional cloning of the APECED gene. Nat Genet 17:393–398

Nemazee DA, Burki K (1989) Clonal deletion of B lymphocytes in a transgenic mouse bearing anti-MHC class I antibody genes. Nature 337:562–566

Ono M, Yaguchi H, Ohkura N, Kitabayashi I, Nagamura Y, Nomura T, Miyachi Y, Tsukada T, Sakaguchi S (2007) Foxp3 controls regulatory T-cell function by interacting with AML1/Runx1. Nature 446:685–689

Peake JE, McCrossin RB, Byrne G, Shepherd R (1996) X-linked immune dysregulation, neonatal insulin dependent diabetes, and intractable diarrhoea. Arch Dis Child Fetal Neonatal Ed 74: F195–199

Picca CC, Larkin J 3rd, Boesteanu A, Lerman MA, Rankin AL, Caton AJ (2006) Role of TCR specificity in CD4+ CD25+ regulatory T-cell selection. Immunol Rev 212:74–85

Powell BR, Buist NR, Stenzel P (1982) An X-linked syndrome of diarrhea, polyendocrinopathy, and fatal infection in infancy. J Pediatr 100:731–737

Russell WL (1951) X-ray-induced mutations in mice. Cold Spring Harb Symp Quant Biol 16:327–336

Russell WL, Russell LB, Kelly EM (1958) Radiation dose rate and mutation frequency. Science 128:1546–1550

Russell WL, Russell LB, Gower JS (1959) Exceptional Inheritance of a sex-linked gene in the mouse explained on the basis that the X/O sex-chromosome constitution is female. Proc Natl Acad Sci USA 45:554–560

Sakaguchi S, Fukuma K, Kuribayashi K, Masuda T (1985) Organ-specific autoimmune diseases induced in mice by elimination of T cell subset. I Evidence for the active participation of T cells in natural self-tolerance; deficit of a T cell subset as a possible cause of autoimmune disease. J Exp Med 61:72–87

Sakaguchi S, Sakaguchi N, Asano M, Itoh M, Toda M (1995) Immunologic self-tolerance maintained by activated T cells expressing IL-2 receptor alpha-chains (CD25). Breakdown of a single mechanism of self-tolerance causes various autoimmune diseases. J Immunol 155:1151–1164

Schubert LA, Jeffery E, Zhang Y, Ramsdell F, Ziegler SF (2001) Scurfin (FOXP3) acts as a repressor of transcription and regulates T cell activation. J Biol Chem 276:37672–37679

Sha WC, Nelson CA, Newberry RD, Kranz DM, Russell JH, Loh DY (1988) Positive and negative selection of an antigen receptor on T cells in transgenic mice. Nature 336:73–76

Shevach EM (2000) Regulatory T cells in autoimmmunity*. Annu Rev Immunol 18:423–449

Shevach EM (2002) CD4+ CD25+ suppressor T cells: more questions than answers. Nat Rev Immunol 2:389–400

Silver LM (1995) Mouse genetics: concepts and applications. Oxford University Press, New York, pp 114–132

Thornton AM, Shevach EM (1998) CD4+CD25+ immunoregulatory T cells suppress polyclonal T cell activation in vitro by inhibiting interleukin 2 production. J Exp Med 188:287–296

Watanabe N, Wang YH, Lee HK, Ito T, Wang YH, Cao W, Liu YJ (2005) Hassall's corpuscles instruct dendritic cells to induce CD4+CD25+ regulatory T cells in human thymus. Nature 436:1181–1185

Welshons WJ, Russell LB (1959) The Y-chromosome as the bearer of the male determining factors in the mouse. Proc Natl Acad Sci USA 45:560–566

Wildin RS, Freitas A (2005) IPEX and FOXP3: clinical and research perspectives. J Autoimmun 25 Suppl:56–62

Wildin RS, Ramsdell F, Peake J, Faravelli F, Casanova JL, Buist N, Levy-Lahad E, Mazzella M, Goulet O, Perroni L, Bricarelli FD, Byrne G, McEuen M, Proll S, Appleby M, Brunkow ME (2001) X-linked neonatal diabetes mellitus, enteropathy and endocrinopathy syndrome is the human equivalent of mouse scurfy. Nat Genet 27:18–20

Wu Y, Borde M, Heissmeyer V, Feuerer M, Lapan AD, Stroud JC, Bates DL, Guo L, Han A, Ziegler SF, Mathis D, Benoist C, Chen L, Rao A (2006) FOXP3 controls regulatory T cell function through cooperation with NFAT. Cell 126:375–387

Zahorsky-Reeves JL, Wilkinson JE (2001) The murine mutation scurfy (sf) results in an antigen-dependent lymphoproliferative disease with altered T cell sensitivity. Eur J Immunol 31:196–204

Zheng Y, Josefowicz SZ, Kas A, Chu TT, Gavin MA, Rudensky AY (2007) Genome-wide analysis of Foxp3 target genes in developing and mature regulatory T cells. Nature 445:936–940

Fevers, Genes, and Innate Immunity

J.G. Ryan, D.L. Kastner(✉)

Contents

Abstract The characterization of patients with recurrent inflammatory syndromes into distinct clinical phenotypes provided early clues to the mode of inheritance of these conditions and facilitated the subsequent identification of causative gene mutations. The prototype autoinflammatory syndrome, familial Mediterranean fever, is characterized by self-limiting episodes of localized inflammation. Hallmarks of the classical autoimmune response are largely absent. The use of positional cloning techniques led to the identification of the causative gene, *MEFV*, and its product pyrin. This previously unrecognized protein plays an important role in modulating the innate immune response. Cryopyrin, the protein encoded by *CIAS1*, is mutated in a spectrum of autoinflammatory conditions, the cryopyrinopathies. In response to a wide range of potential pathogens, it forms a macromolecular complex termed the "inflammasome," resulting in caspase-1 activation and subsequent release of the active proinflammatory cytokine interleukin-1β (IL-1β). The role of an established biochemical pathway in regulating inflammation was uncovered by the discovery that the hyperimmunoglobulin D with periodic fever syndrome (HIDS) results from mutations in *MVK*, which encodes an enzyme in the isoprenoid pathway. The discovery that mutations in the gene encoding tumor necrosis factor (TNF) receptor 1

D.L. Kastner
Genetics and Genomics Branch, National Institute of Arthritis and Musculoskeletal
and Skin Diseases, Bethesda, MD 20892, USA
kastnerd@mail.nih.gov

B. Beutler (ed.), *Immunology, Phenotype First: How Mutations Have Established New Principles and Pathways in Immunology*. Current Topics in Microbiology and Immunology 321. © Springer-Verlag Berlin Heidelberg 2008

(TNFR1) cause a proinflammatory phenotype was unanticipated, as it seemed more likely that such mutations would instead have resulted in an immunodeficiency pattern. This review describes the clinical phenotypes of autoinflammatory syndromes, the underlying gene mutations, and current concepts regarding their pathophysiology.

Introduction

The study of Mendelian recurrent inflammatory syndromes, through the identification of new proteins and the recognition of novel roles for established biochemical pathways, has led to a deeper understanding of the innate immune response. Each of these syndromes is characterized by episodic inflammation without a clear antigenic stimulus. In addition, features typical of the autoimmune diseases are notable by their absence, namely autoreactive antibodies and T cells. The term "autoinflammatory diseases" was proposed to encompass this new group of disorders (McDermott et al. 1999). These conditions result from the aberrant activation of the innate, rather than the adaptive, immune system. In the case of familial Mediterranean fever, the discovery of the causative gene resulted in the identification of a novel protein called pyrin. The discovery that hyperimmunoglobulin D with periodic syndrome resulted from a mutation in an enzyme in the isoprenoid biosynthesis pathway has suggested a novel role for this established biochemical pathway. In this chapter we will discuss the Mendelian autoinflammatory diseases, the discovery of causative genes, and current concepts regarding their pathophysiology. In addition, we will describe how knowledge of the basic science underlying these disorders has led to targeted therapies that have proven life altering for many patients with these diseases.

Familial Mediterranean Fever

Familial Mediterranean fever (FMF) [OMIM 249100 (Online Mendelian Inheritance in Man 2008)] is the prototype autoinflammatory disease. Early reports highlighted a preponderance of individuals of Mediterranean ancestry with this condition, leading to the adoption of the term FMF. It is the most common of the autoinflammatory diseases, with a modest male preponderance, and is most frequently observed in Jewish, Armenian, Arab, Turkish, and southern Italian populations (Aksentijevich et al. 1999). Carrier rates in certain high-risk populations can reach 1 in 3.

FMF is characterized by acute attacks of fever, and localized inflammation of the peritoneum, pleura, joints, or skin, sometimes in combination. Typically, episodes last 12–72 hours. Episodes may vary in nature; childhood episodes may be manifested by fever alone, while other features may develop progressively with time. Abdominal symptoms range from mild discomfort to severe pain and abdominal rigidity. The most serious complication of FMF is the development of AA amyloidosis. Prior to the advent of effective therapy for FMF, in many patients the development of amyloidosis led to chronic renal failure by age 40 (Samuels et al. 1998).

In the 1960s, segregation analysis in Israeli families manifesting typical FMF symptoms established FMF as a single-gene recessive disorder with incomplete penetrance. Attempts to identify the FMF gene by functional hypothesis-driven approaches were not productive and positional cloning was ultimately employed. Linkage studies in 1992 placed the FMF susceptibility locus on the short arm of chromosome 16, and this area of interest was narrowed by analyses of genetic recombinations in families and conserved haplotypes in populations. All genes within a refined 200-kb interval were screened for disease-associated mutations; and two independent consortia identified *MEFV* (The International FMF Consortium 1997; The French FMF Consortium 1997). An online database (Infevers 2008) has been established and provides an updated list of mutations and polymorphisms in *MEFV* and other autoinflammatory diseases. Over 50 disease-associated *MEFV* mutations have been described, with many clustered on exon 10 (Infevers 2008).

MEFV (*ME*diterranean *FE*ver) consists of 10 exons, and covers approximately 15 kb of DNA. It encodes a 781-amino acid protein named pyrin (to denote fever) or marenostrin (from the Latin for the Mediterranean sea). Pyrin is expressed in skin, peritoneal fibroblasts (Matzner et al. 2000), synovial fibroblasts, granulocytes, dendritic cells, and monocytes (Diaz et al. 2004). Pyrin is a member of the tripartite motif (TRIM) family of proteins, and is composed of four domains. At the N-terminal end of pyrin is the pyrin domain (PYD), a 92-amino acid motif, encoded by exon 1 of *MEFV*. This domain bears structural homologies to caspase-recruitment (CARD) domains, death domains, and death effector domains, and together these four motifs constitute the death fold family (Fairbrother et al. 2001). Variants of the pyrin domain are present in approximately 20 proteins, each of which plays a role in modulating the innate immune response. The PYD of pyrin engages in homotypic interactions with an adaptor protein called ASC (apoptosis-associated speck-like protein with a CARD) influencing the activation of interleukin (IL)-1β. Deletion of the PYD of pyrin abolishes its interaction with ASC (Richards et al. 2001; Yu et al. 2006).

The C-terminal end of pyrin contains a B-box zinc-finger domain (B-box), an α-helical coiled-coil domain (CC), and a B30.2 (PRYSRPY) domain. The B-box domain is both necessary and sufficient for pyrin's interactions with proline serine threonine phosphatase interacting protein (PSTPIP1) (Shoham et al. 2003). The B-box has recently been shown to interact with the PYD and thereby to block its interaction with ASC, thus serving as an intramolecular inhibitor (Yu et al. 2007).

The CC domain of pyrin mediates the formation of a homotrimer, a process required for pyrin's recently demonstrated induction of ASC oligomerization and subsequent caspase-1 activation (Yu et al. 2007) . The CC domain is also necessary, but not by itself sufficient, for pyrin's interaction with PSTPIP1 (Shoham et al. 2003).

The B30.2 domain of pyrin is responsible for interactions with the NACHT (Koonin and Aravind 2000) domain of NALP3, a component of the inflammasome (Papin et al. 2007). The B30.2 domain interacts, albeit weakly, with pro-caspase-1, and more avidly with active cleaved caspase-1 (Chae et al. 2006; Papin et al. 2007). There is also speculation that the B30.2 domain of pyrin acts as an intracellular pathogen-associated molecular pattern (PAMP) sensor, and that mutations in pyrin may bind PAMPs more avidly and thereby confer a heightened immune response to potential pathogens with possible survival benefit (Yepiskoposyan and Harutyunyan 2007). In support of this theory is the recognition of the role for members of the TRIM family proteins in control of retroviral infections (Yap et al. 2004). Interestingly, the amino acid changes that cause FMF are often present as wildtype in other species. For several human mutations, the mutant represents the reappearance of an ancestral amino acid state. Studies in primates suggest that these mutations are indeed counter-evolutionary changes selected to cope with a sporadically encountered pathogen (Schaner et al. 2001).

There is a general consensus that pyrin plays a role in modulating caspase-1 activity and subsequent IL-1β release; there is disagreement, however, as to its net effect on levels of IL-1β. Findings in keeping with a net negative effect include the demonstration that pyrin competitively binds with ASC, via PYD, preventing ASC binding to caspase-1 (Chae et al. 2003). Pyrin also binds caspase-1, via its B30.2 domain, thus reducing caspase-1 activation (Chae et al. 2006; Papin et al. 2007). In addition, pyrin's competitive interaction with ASC may prevent the formation of the NALP3 inflammasome. The "sequestration hypothesis" has been proposed to encompass pyrin's net negative effect on IL-1β release. Further support for an inhibitory role for wildtype pyrin comes from mouse constructs. Mice expressing truncated pyrin produce increased amounts of activated caspase-1 and IL-1β in response to stimuli (Chae et al. 2003). Most mutations in patients with FMF affect the B30.2 domain, which is responsible for protein–protein interactions. Recent data that common mutations in pyrin result in impaired binding of pyrin to caspase-1 imply that these mutations may lead to clinical disease by impairing pyrin's antiinflammatory interactions with caspase-1 (Chae et al. 2006). However, the impact of mutations in the B30.2 domain has been variable (Papin et al. 2007).

A net positive effect of pyrin on IL-1β levels is suggested by data that fresh human monocytes have elevated pyrin protein and mRNA compared to monocyte-derived macrophages, a finding that parallels their ability to release active IL-1β in response to lipopolysaccharide (LPS) stimulation (Seshadri et al. 2007). In contrast to the competitive binding described previously, it has been suggested that pyrin's interaction with ASC modulates the formation of the "pyroptosome," a protein complex involved in "pyroptosis," a recently described caspase-1-dependent form of inflammatory cell death. The adaptor protein ASC contains an N-terminal PYD and C-terminal CARD. In response to various stimuli, including LPS and potassium flux, ASC self associates via its PYD domain, and forms a supramolecular assembly, termed the pyroptosome (Fernandes-Alnemri et al. 2007). This ASC supramolecular assembly activates caspase-1, thus leading to elevated IL-1β. This process is independent of the recently described inflammasomes formed by members of the NALP family. Moreover, data using THP-1 human monocytic cell lines suggest that PSTPIP1 binding to pyrin may lead to PYD interaction with ASC, pyroptosome assembly, and procaspase-1 activation (Yu et al. 2006, 2007).

Colchicine has been the mainstay in the therapy of FMF since the 1970s (Goldfinger 1972). Clinical trials support the role of colchicine in the treatment of acute episodes, in the prevention of FMF attacks (Zemer et al. 1974), and in reducing the risk of AA amyloidosis. The induction of *MEFV* mRNA by the addition of a combination of colchicine and interferon (IFN)-α suggests a role for *MEFV* in the antiinflammatory actions of these agents (Centola et al. 2000). Pyrin's close association with actin filaments and microtubules suggests a role for pyrin in directed migration that can be modulated by colchicine (Mansfield et al 2001). Colchicine displays a dose responsive effect on microtubule function and structure. At high concentrations colchicine disrupts microtubules by inhibiting polymerization at the "plus" or growing terminus. Low concentrations inhibit tubulin exchange at microtubule ends without affecting polymerization. High doses of colchicine inhibit the processing of caspase-1, a finding replicated with nocodazole, a compound with microtubule-inhibiting properties (Yu et al. 2007). The low concentrations resulting from the usual doses given to patients with FMF, however, are insufficient to disrupt microtubule arrangement patterns, but may instead affect microtubule dynamics, resulting in defective trafficking of cell adhesion molecules. As not all patients benefit from colchicine, in some, adjunctive therapy with anakinra, an IL-1 receptor antagonist, has proved beneficial, supporting the role of IL-1β in the pathogenesis of FMF (Calligaris et al. 2007; Chae et al. 2006).

Cryopyrin-Associated Periodic Syndromes

The cryopyrinopathies or cryopyrin-associated periodic syndromes (CAPS) correspond to a spectrum of dominantly inherited disorders. They include familial cold autoinflammatory syndrome (FCAS)/familial cold urticaria, Muckle–Wells syndrome (MWS) and neonatal onset multisystem inflammatory disease (NOMID)/ chronic infantile neurologic cutaneous and articular syndrome (CINCA). All three may present with fever and urticaria-like skin rash and varying degrees of joint and neurologic involvement. FCAS (OMIM 120100) is generally considered the mildest, with distinct cold-induced episodic attributes. NOMID (OMIM 607115) is typically the most severe, with nearly continuous symptoms that may fluctuate in severity. Persistent central nervous system inflammation may result in intellectual impairment and loss of vision. NOMID is associated with a deforming arthropathy (Prieur 2001). MWS (OMIM 191900) is intermediate, with urticarial rash that is not cold-induced, and some patients develop sensorineural hearing loss. The clinical boundaries of these conditions have become blurred and a greater degree of overlap is now recognized. Patients with CAPS may develop AA amyloidosis and subsequent renal failure.

Independent linkage studies placed the susceptibility locus for both MWS and FCAS on chromosome 1q (Cuisset et al. 1999; Hoffman et al. 2000). In 2001, mutations in a 9-exon gene were identified in both FCAS and MWS families (Hoffman et al. 2001); the next year mutations in the same gene were identified in patients with NOMID (Aksentijevich et al. 2002; Feldmann et al. 2002). The gene named *CIAS1* (for cold-induced autoinflammatory syndrome-1) (NALP3/PYPAF1/NLRP3, OMIM

606416) encodes the protein cryopyrin. Cryopyrin is composed of an N-terminal pyrin (PYD) domain, a NACHT/nucleotide-binding oligomerization domain (NOD) and a leucine-rich repeat (LRR) domain. Cryopyrin is expressed in the cytoplasm of non-keratinized epithelial cells, uroepithelial cells, granulocytes, dendritic cells, and both T and B cells. It is also weakly expressed in monocytes (Kummer et al. 2007). Cryopyrin is a member of the CATERPILLER family (Ting et al. 2006) and is also called NALP3 (for NACHT domain-, Leucine-rich-repeat-, and Pyrin domain-containing protein 3) (Tschopp et al. 2003). Cryopyrin bears homologies with the extended NALP family of proteins, the plant cytosolic resistance (R) proteins, which mediate resistance to a variety of fungi, viruses, and bacteria, and the NOD family, a member of which, NOD2/CARD15, is mutated in patients with Crohn's disease and Blau syndrome (Miceli-Richard et al. 2001; Rosé et al. 2006).

The PYD of cryopyrin is involved in cognate interactions with other proteins containing a PYD. The NACHT domain is thought to regulate oligomerization. The LRR domain, which is found in a number of proteins including the Toll-like receptors (TLRs), may mediate interactions with numerous intracellular and extracellular potential pathogens.

Stimulation of cryopyrin leads to the formation of a macromolecular complex called the "NALP3 inflammasome." This inflammasome is formed by homotypic interactions between the PYD domain of cryopyrin and ASC, which in turn interacts via its CARD domain with caspase-1. Cryopyrin also interacts with another adaptor protein CARDINAL, which recruits additional caspase-1. The resultant homo-oligomerization of procaspase-1 is thought to facilitate autocatalytic activation to caspase-1. Active caspase-1 cleaves pro-IL-1β into mature proinflammatory IL-13 (Tschopp et al. 2003).

The demonstration that the NALP3 inflammasome activates IL-1β release in response to gram-negative bacteria in the absence of cell surface TLR4 (Kanneganti et al. 2007) strongly suggests a role for cryopyrin in the intracellular control of infectious agents. Cryopyrin's role as an intracellular sensor of so-called PAMPs has expanded greatly recently. Other activators of the inflammasome include bacterial RNA, imidazoquinoline compounds and the gram-positive bacterial toxins nigericin and maitotoxin (Kanneganti et al. 2006; Mariathasan et al. 2006). Knockout models suggest that cryopyrin plays a central role in the robust inflammatory response to both uric acid and calcium pyrophosphate (CPPD) crystals (Martinon et al. 2006). These findings suggest that both gout (uric acid) and pseudogout (CPPD) are, at least in part, autoinflammatory diseases. The means by which cryopyrin senses PAMPs remains unclear; homologies to the LRR domain present in both TLRs and NOD2/CARD15, however, may suggest a role for this domain in pathogen sensing.

The inflammasome complex alone does not appear to be sufficient for the IL-1β-mediated inflammatory response since knockout experiments implicate SGT1 and HSP90 as being essential for inflammasome activity (Mayor et al. 2007). The precise role of these proteins in modulating the inflammatory response remains uncertain. Cryopyrin may also induce cell death upon stimulation with bacteria or other pathogens independent of ASC and IL-1β (Willingham et al. 2007).

Mutations in cryopyrin lead to constitutive activation, although the molecular mechanism is not clear. Modeling of the cryopyrin structure suggests that the LRR domain self-associates with the NACHT domain, thus preventing activation and interaction with the adaptor protein CARDINAL. Mutations in either the NACHT or LRR domains may prevent self-association, resulting in direct assembly of the inflammasome complex. Most of the described mutations are found in exon 3 of *CIAS1*, which encodes the NACHT domain. Current models of cryopyrin mutants inadequately explain the spectrum of disease seen in CAPS (Aksentijevich et al. 2007; Hentgen et al. 2005), reflecting the limitations of in silico techniques.

Early insights into the role of the inflammasome, supported by the findings that monocytes from patients with CAPS showed increased caspase-1 activation and increased IL-1β release, prompted clinical trials of IL-1 inhibition in patients with CAPS. The use of anakinra, an IL-1 receptor inhibitor, in the treatment of all three syndromes has been met with considerable success, consistent with the key role of IL-1β in CAPS (Hawkins et al. 2003). The use of anakinra in patients with NOMID, the most severe of these conditions, resulted in complete remission in both peripheral and central nervous system (CNS) inflammation in a majority of subjects. Discontinuation of therapy led to a rapid relapse in symptoms, supporting the need for continuous IL-1 blockade in this condition (Goldbach-Mansky et al. 2006). The use of IL-1 blockade represents a significant advance in the treatment of CAPS.

Syndrome of Pyogenic Arthritis, Pyoderma Gangrenosum and Acne

The syndrome of pyogenic arthritis, pyoderma gangrenosum and acne (PAPA) was first described in a large family who attended the Mayo Clinic (Lindor et al. 1997); another family in Texas was later noted to have similar clinical features (Wise et al. 2000). From childhood, patients have episodic destructive arthritis that is sometimes triggered by minor trauma. Arthritis may lead to periosteal proliferation and ankylosis. Skin manifestations usually occur after puberty and range from severe cystic acne on the face, chest, or back to pyoderma gangrenosum, an ulcerating skin lesion that may be triggered by minor trauma.

Studies of both of the originally described families established linkage to chromosome 15q (Wise et al. 2000). Two different missense mutations were identified in the gene encoding PSTPIP1. This protein interacts with pyrin, the protein mutated in FMF, and is largely restricted to the hematopoietic tissues, being prominent in spleen and peripheral blood leukocytes (Li et al. 1998; Shoham et al. 2003).

PSTPIP1 protein contains an N-terminal CIP4 domain, a coiled-coil (CC) domain, and an SH3 domain. The coiled-coil and SH3 domains are important for protein interactions and both are necessary for PSTPIP1's interaction with pyrin's B-box domain (Shoham et al. 2003). PSTPIP1 also interacts via its CC domain with the C-terminal proline-rich homology domain of PTP-PEST (protein tyrosine phosphatase with a proline, glutamate, serine, threonine domain). The mutations identified in PAPA patients affect the coiled-coil domain of PSTPIP1 and lead to decreased binding of PSTPIP1 to PTP-PEST, which in turn leads to hyperphosphorylation of PSTPIP1. The hyperphosphorylation of PSTPIP1 increases its avidity for pyrin (Shoham et al. 2003; Yu et al. 2007). Cell lines co-transfected with PAPA-associated PSTPIP1 mutants and with pyrin demonstrate elevated production of interleukin-1β (Shoham et al. 2003). While it is agreed that mutant PSTPIP1 binds pyrin with greater avidity, the precise mechanism by which increased IL-1β production results is unclear. It has been proposed that when mutant PSTPIP1 binds more avidly to pyrin, it results in the sequestration of an antiinflammatory pyrin resulting in a net increase in IL-1β production (Shoham et al. 2003). Alternatively, when mutant PSTPIP1 avidly binds pyrin it may permit the unfolding of pyrin to its proinflammatory state, permitting the interaction of PYD with ASC and subsequent pyroptosome-mediated caspase-1 activation (Yu et al. 2007).

As denoted by its alternative name CD2-binding protein 1 (CD2BP1), PSTPIP1 interacts not only with CD2 but also Wiskott–Aldrich syndrome protein (WASp). WASp co-localizes with actin to form the immunologic synapse in natural killer (NK) cells (Orange et al. 2002). Thus, PSTPIP1 may play a role in the adaptive immune system through both CD2 binding and WASp-induced polymerization with actin, with potential effects on the formation of immunologic synapses in antigen recognition (Badour et al. 2003).

Therapeutic strategies have been informed by evidence that LPS-induced IL-1β secretion is markedly increased in cells from PAPA patients compared to controls (Shoham et al. 2003). In contrast, cytokines such as IL-2, IL-5, and IFN-γ were undetectable. Anecdotal reports suggest that anakinra, an IL-1 receptor antagonist, is beneficial (Dierselhuis et al. 2005); however, both the variable natural history and rarity of this condition suggest that definitive clinical trials of targeted therapies will prove difficult.

TNF Receptor-Associated Periodic Syndrome

Clinical descriptions of families of individuals with prolonged fever and localized inflammation were the first hints of an autosomal-dominant recurrent fever syndrome. Early clinical reports highlighted the Celtic ethnicity of affected individuals, resulting in the term "familial Hibernian fever" (McDermott et al. 1997), while smaller family series described a broader North European ancestry and used the term "autosomal-dominant recurrent fever syndrome." Now known as tumor necrosis factor (TNF) receptor-associated periodic syndrome (TRAPS), patients typically have episodes lasting at least 1 week and sometimes as long as 6–8 weeks. Characteristic manifestations include migratory erythema which may occur on the torso or limbs and spreads distally, with myalgia in the underlying muscle group. Ocular involvement with conjunctivitis or periorbital edema is common. TRAPS is associated with an increased risk of AA amyloidosis in up to 15% of affected individuals.

In 1998, linkage studies placed the susceptibility locus of a subset of these individuals to a region of chromosome 12p13 (McDermott et al. 1998; Mulley et al. 1998). Within a year *TNFRSF1A* (OMIM entry 191190) was identified as the causative gene (McDermott et al. 1999). Dominantly inherited mutations were identified in families of diverse ancestry, and the term TRAPS (OMIM entry 142680) is used to describe all patients with mutations in *TNFRSF1A* irrespective of ancestry.

TNFRSF1A encodes a 55-kDa receptor (TNFR1/p55) for the cytokine TNF. This receptor has four extracellular cysteine-rich domains, a transmembrane domain, and an intracellular death domain. TNFR1 is expressed on a wide range of cell types and can mediate apoptosis and function as a regulator of inflammation. Of the initial six mutations that were described, five were single-nucleotide substitutions resulting in amino acid substitutions in highly conserved extracellular cysteine domains (McDermott et al. 1999). These cysteine residues are required to maintain the stability of the extracellular domain by forming disulfide bonds. A further mutation disrupted a highly conserved intrachain hydrogen bond in the extracellular domain. Mutations in the intracellular or transmembrane domains have not been identified.

Initial studies of affected families suggested that disease-associated mutations are highly penetrant. Not all mutations, however, are associated with such high penetrance or typical disease. Two substitutions occur in over 1% of the Caucasian (R92Q) and African-American (P46L) populations, and one substitution occurs in up to 9% of selected African (P46L) populations. While these substitutions may lead to a proinflammatory phenotype, patients typically do not appear to have typical TRAPS (Tchernitchko et al. 2005).

The pathophysiology of TRAPS remains unclear. In healthy subjects, TNF stimulates TNFR1, which recruits several proteins to form a complex resulting in the activation of nuclear factor-κB (NF-κB), while an alternate pathway leads to apoptosis (Chen and Goeddel 2002). TNFR1 stimulation results in cleavage of the extracellular domains of the receptor following activation. Cleaved soluble TNFR1 (sTNFR1) acts as a decoy receptor for TNF. In patients with TRAPS, low levels of cleaved soluble TNFR1 led to the hypothesis that mutations lead to impaired cleavage of the extracellular domain of TNFR1 by matrix metalloproteinases following stimulation. Thus, the usual regulatory processes in terminating TNF signaling were impaired, with insufficient sTNFR1 to act as a TNF blocker in serum and excess activated TNFR1 remaining on the cell surface. This was supported by early laboratory studies (McDermott et al. 1999); subsequent reports, however, demonstrated variable rates of cleavage across disease-associated mutations, and thus did not fully explain the pathophysiology of this disease. Defective intracellular processing of mutant TNFR1 has also been identified. Following synthesis, mutant TNFR1 is unable to traffic appropriately from the endoplasmic reticulum to the cell surface (Lobito et al. 2006; Todd et al. 2007). It has been postulated that mutant TNFR1 is retained in the endoplasmic reticulum resulting in the proinflammatory unfolded protein response. Thus, inflammation may occur without direct ligand interactions with TNFR1. Alternatively, mutant receptors may be retained within the cell, autoaggregate, and inappropriately activate proinflammatory cascades

(Rebelo et al. 2006). Collectively this is termed the "ligand-independent" hypothesis. Mutant TNFR1 may also result in prolonged survival of inflammatory cells, since neutrophils from patients with TRAPS demonstrate impaired TNF-mediated apoptosis (D'Osualdo et al. 2006).

The initial "defective shedding" hypothesis, whereby the decoy receptor for TNF cleaved soluble TNFR1, is decreased in patients with TRAPS, led to efforts to restore the balance in favor of inhibition of TNF using etanercept. Etanercept is a p75 TNF receptor fusion protein that binds serum TNF and prevents its engagement with cell surface TNFR1. Use of this agent has been beneficial in terms of clinical and laboratory parameters (Hull et al. 2002). In keeping with the alternative "ligand-independent" hypothesis, in which inflammation results from non-TNF-mediated pathways, the use of anakinra, an IL-1 receptor antagonist, has also been reported to be of benefit (Simon et al. 2004).

Hyperimmunoglobulinemia D with Periodic Fever Syndrome

In 1984 a Dutch group described six patients with periodic fever and elevations in immunoglobulin D (van der Meer et al. 1984). In 1999 two independent Dutch groups identified the gene responsible for Hyperimmunoglobulinemia D with periodic fever syndrome (HIDS), an autosomal-recessive condition. Traditional linkage analysis enabled one group to localize the causative gene (Drenth et al. 1999), while the other group identified elevated mevalonate in the urine of patients with HIDS and decreased enzyme activity in skin fibroblasts (Houten et al. 1999). The causative gene, *MVK*, encodes an enzyme involved in the isoprenoid biosynthesis pathway, and this unanticipated finding suggested a new role for this pathway in regulating inflammatory responses. The isoprenoid metabolism pathway generates a wide variety of important compounds for cell function. Branches of the pathway synthesize over 20,000 compounds including sterols, which includes cholesterol, and the nonsterol isoprene compounds. Two isoprenoid moieties, farnesyl or geranylgeranyl, are added to proteins during posttranslational modification, thus promoting membrane association.

HIDS episodes usually start in infancy, and may be triggered by immunizations. Episodes may occur once or twice per month and typically last 3–7 days. Typical episodes are characterized by initial chills and headache with subsequent fevers and diffuse tender lymphadenopathy. Diarrhea frequently occurs and a number of cutaneous manifestations have been described including painful erythematous macules. Joint symptoms include arthralgia and polyarticular large joint arthritis. Episodes typically occur less frequently in adulthood and are usually less severe (Drenth et al. 1994).

Mutations in *MVK* that result in complete loss of mevalonate kinase (MK) enzymatic activity cause the related condition mevalonic aciduria, a rare metabolic disease with mental retardation, failure to thrive, and early death, in addition to the features seen in HIDS. In contrast, HIDS-associated *MVK* mutations result in residual MK enzymatic activity, in the range of 1%–8% of normal (Mandey et al. 2006a). Interestingly, in vitro experiments demonstrate that MK enzymatic activity is temperature-sensitive, with decreased activity at higher temperatures (Houten et al. 2002).

Mutations in *MVK* are found throughout the gene, and most HIDS patients are compound heterozygotes for missense mutations. A number of mutations are more strongly associated with either HIDS or MA. Mutations resulting in a base pair change at position 377 (V377I) are most commonly associated with HIDS, and result in modest decreases in enzymatic activity, in contrast to predictions that this mutation would not affect enzymatic activity based on modeling studies (Mandey et al. 2006b). This mutation exhibits a founder effect in the Dutch population, and likely explains the higher prevalence of HIDS in this population. Population-based studies indicate that 0.6% of Dutch people carry the V377I mutation. Given the marked underrepresentation of homozygote V377I patients in HIDS cohorts, it has been suggested that the homozygous state results in either a milder phenotype or none at all (Houten et al. 2003).

The activity of the isoprenoid pathway is tightly controlled. An early rate-limiting step, undertaken by HMG-CoA (3-hydroxy-3-methyl-glutaryl-CoA) reductase, has been extensively studied. The identification of this enzyme, and use of the "statin" group of HMG-CoA reductase inhibitors, has been a major advance in the treatment of hypercholesterolemia. The next step in isoprenoid synthesis is MK, resulting in the phosphorylation of mevalonate to 5-phosphomevalonate. MK deficiency results in an increase in HMG-CoA reductase activity, which may increase mevalonate concentrations.

In HIDS there is no general deficiency in isoprenoid end products, and serum cholesterol levels are only slightly decreased. Mevalonate levels are increased to detectable levels in urine during attacks.

Manipulation of the isoprenoid pathway with statins, in an effort to reduce mevalonate levels, has been considered to have antiinflammatory effects, although contradictory reports have emerged. The use of statins in patients with MA resulted in acute flares in two patients within weeks of commencement of a statin; in contrast, six HIDS patients treated for 6 months did show a decrease in symptoms (Simon et al. 2004).

Peripheral blood mononuclear cells (PBMCs) from patients with HIDS show excess IL-1β production in response to LPS stimulation, a finding that can be reversed by the addition of geranylgeranyl, an isoprenoid deficient in HIDS (Mandey et al. 2006a). In contrast, the addition of mevalonate, which is elevated in HIDS, also reduced IL-1β production, suggesting that it is not central to the proinflammatory phenotype. Apoptosis of activated cells is a key mechanism in the termination of the inflammatory response and, in keeping with the protracted inflammatory response seen in HIDS, defective apoptosis has been observed in PBMCs from patients with HIDS (Bodar et al. 2007).

Therapeutic options in HIDS are limited. As stated earlier, there are conflicting results regarding the usefulness of statins. Manipulation of the isoprenoid biosynthesis pathways to augment the production of nonsterol isoprenoids has been suggested as a potential therapeutic option based on in vitro studies (Schneiders et al. 2006). Elevations in urinary leukotrienes during HIDS episodes led to the trial of oral leukotriene receptor antagonism, using montelukast, with anecdotal reports suggesting clinical benefit. The demonstration of elevated serum TNF led to a pilot study involving the use of etanercept, the p75 TNF receptor fusion protein, which demonstrated clinical benefit (Takada et al. 2003).

Future Directions

The study of rare autoinflammatory syndromes has informed us of novel proteins involved in the innate immune response. These proteins provide further evidence for the complexity of this ancient host defense system. Many of these recently described proteins are involved in intracellular pathogen sensing, a previously under-recognized role for the innate immune system. Despite the progress made in recent years, there remain a significant number of patients with recurrent fevers in whom the previously described gene defects cannot be found. Efforts are ongoing to identify new genes. Regarding the known genes and their products, the accumulating evidence highlights the difficulties encountered in unraveling their interactions. Further information regarding the roles of these proteins should in time allow clear elucidation of their complex interplay with the cell and host environment.

References

Aksentijevich I, Torosyan Y, Samuels J, Centola M, Pras E, Chae JJ, Oddoux C, Wood G, Azzaro MP, Palumbo G, Giustolisi R, Pras M, Ostrer H, Kastner DL (1999) Mutation and haplotype studies of familial Mediterranean fever reveal new ancestral relationships and evidence for a high carrier frequency with reduced penetrance in the Ashkenazi Jewish population. Am J Hum Genet 4:949–962

Aksentijevich I, Nowak M, Mallah M, Chae JJ, Watford WT, Hofmann SR, Stein L, Russo R, Goldsmith D, Dent P, Rosenberg HF, Austin F, Remmers EF, Balow JE Jr, Rosenzweig S, Komarow H, Shoham NG, Wood G, Jones J, Mangra N, Carrero H, Adams BS, Moore TL, Schnikler K, Hoffman H, Lovell DJ, Lipnick R, Barron K, O'Shea JJ, Kastner DL, Goldbach-Mansky R (2002) De novo CIAS1 mutations, cytokine activation, and evidence for genetic heterogeneity in patients with neonatal-onset multisystem inflammatory disease (NOMID): a new member of the expanding family of pyrin-associated autoinflammatory diseases. Arthritis Rheum 12:3340–3348

Aksentijevich I, Putnam C, Remmers EF, Mueller JL, Le J, Kolodner RD, Moak Z, Chuang M, Austin F, Goldbach-Mansky R, Hoffman HM, Kastner DL (2007) The clinical continuum of cryopyrinopathies: novel CIAS1 mutations in North American patients and a new cryopyrin model. Arthritis Rheum 4:1273–1285

Badour K, Zhang J, Shi F, McGavin MK, Rampersad V, Hardy LA, Field D, Siminovitch KA (2003) The Wiskott-Aldrich syndrome protein acts downstream of CD2 and the CD2AP and PSTPIP1 adaptors to promote formation of the immunological synapse. Immunity 1:141–154

Bodar EJ, van der Hilst JC, van Heerde W, van der Meer JW, Drenth JP, Simon A (2007) Defective apoptosis of peripheral-blood lymphocytes in hyper-IgD and periodic fever syndrome. Blood 6:2416–2418

Calligaris L, Marchetti F, Tommasini A, Ventura A (2007) The efficacy of anakinra in an adolescent with colchicine-resistant familial Mediterranean fever. Eur J Pediatr Jun 23 [Epub ahead of print]

Centola M, Wood G, Frucht DM, Galon J, Aringer M, Farrell C, Kingma DW, Horwitz ME, Mansfield E, Holland SM, O'Shea JJ, Rosenberg HF, Malech HL, Kastner DL (2000) The gene for familial Mediterranean fever, MEFV, is expressed in early leukocyte development and is regulated in response to inflammatory mediators. Blood 10:3223–3231

Chae JJ, Komarow HD, Cheng J, Wood G, Raben N, Liu PP, Kastner DL (2003) Targeted disruption of pyrin, the FMF protein, causes heightened sensitivity to endotoxin and a defect in macrophage apoptosis. Mol Cell 3:591–604

Chae JJ, Wood G, Masters SL, Richard K, Park G, Smith BJ, Kastner DL (2006) The B30.2 domain of pyrin, the familial Mediterranean fever protein, interacts directly with caspase-1 to modulate IL-1beta production. Proc Natl Acad Sci U S A 26:9982–9987

Chen G, Goeddel D (2002) TNF-R1 signaling: a beautiful pathway. Science 5573:1634–1635

Cuisset L, Drenth JP, Berthelot JM, Meyrier A, Vaudour G, Watts RA, Scott DG, Nicholls A, Pavek S, Vasseur C, Beckmann JS, Delpech M, Grateau G (1999) Genetic linkage of the Muckle-Wells syndrome to chromosome 1q44. Am J Hum Genet 4:1054–1059

D'Osualdo A, Ferlito F, Prigione I, Obici L, Meini A, Zulian F, Pontillo A, Corona F, Barcellona R, Di Duca M, Santamaria G, Traverso F, Picco P, Baldi M, Plebani A, Ravazzolo R, Ceccherini I, Martini A, Gattorno M (2006) Neutrophils from patients with TNFRSF1A mutations display resistance to tumor necrosis factor-induced apoptosis: pathogenetic and clinical implications. Arthritis Rheum 3:998–1008

Diaz A, Hu C, Kastner DL, Schaner P, Reginato AM, Richards N, Gumucio DL (2004) Lipopolysaccharide-induced expression of multiple alternatively spliced MEFV transcripts in human synovial fibroblasts: a prominent splice isoform lacks the C-terminal domain that is highly mutated in familial Mediterranean fever. Arthritis Rheum 11:3679–3689

Dierselhuis MP, Frenkel J, Wulffraat NM, Boelens JJ (2005) Anakinra for flares of pyogenic arthritis in PAPA syndrome. Rheumatology (Oxford) 3:406–408

Drenth JP, Haagsma CJ, van der Meer JW (1994) Hyperimmunoglobulinemia D and periodic fever syndrome. The clinical spectrum in a series of 50 patients. International Hyper-IgD Study Group. Medicine (Baltimore) 3:133–144

Drenth JP, Cuisset L, Grateau G, Vasseur C, van de Velde-Visser SD, de Jong JG, Beckmann JS, van der Meer JW, Delpech M (1999) Mutations in the gene encoding mevalonate kinase cause hyper-IgD and periodic fever syndrome. International Hyper-IgD Study Group. Nat Genet 2:178–181

Fairbrother W, Gordon N, Humke E, O'Rourke K, Starovasnik M, Yin J, Dixit V (2001) The PYRIN domain: a member of the death domain-fold superfamily. Protein Sci 9:1911–1918

Feldmann J, Prieur AM, Quartier P, Berquin P, Certain S, Cortis E, Teillac-Hamel D, Fischer A, de Saint Basile G (2002) Chronic infantile neurological cutaneous and articular syndrome is caused by mutations in CIAS1, a gene highly expressed in polymorphonuclear cells and chondrocytes. Am J Hum Genet 1:198–203

Fernandes-Alnemri T, Wu J, Yu J, Datta P, Miller B, Jankowski W, Rosenberg S, Zhang J, Alnemri E (2007) The pyroptosome: a supramolecular assembly of ASC dimers mediating inflammatory cell death via caspase-1 activation. Cell Death Differ 9:1590–1604

French FMF Consortium (1997) A candidate gene for familial Mediterranean fever. Nat Genet 1:25–31

Goldbach-Mansky R, Dailey NJ, Canna SW, Gelabert A, Jones J, Rubin BI, Kim HJ, Brewer C, Zalewski C, Wiggs E, Hill S, Turner ML, Karp BI, Aksentijevich I, Pucino F, Penzak SR, Haverkamp MH, Stein L, Adams BS, Moore TL, Fuhlbrigge RC, Shaham B, Jarvis JN, O'Neil K, Vehe RK, Beitz LO, Gardner G, Hannan WP, Warren RW, Horn W, Cole JL, Paul SM, Hawkins PN, Pham TH, Snyder C, Wesley RA, Hoffmann SC, Holland SM, Butman JA,

Kastner DL (2006) Neonatal-onset multisystem inflammatory disease responsive to interleukin-1beta inhibition. N Engl J Med 6:581–592

Goldfinger S (1972) Colchicine for familial Mediterranean fever. N Engl J Med 25:1302

Hawkins P, Lachmann H, McDermott M (2003) Interleukin-1-receptor antagonist in the Muckle-Wells syndrome. N Engl J Med 25:2583–2584

Hentgen V, Despert V, Lepretre AC, Cuisset L, Chevrant-Breton J, Jego P, Chales G, Gall EL, Delpech M, Grateau G (2005) Intrafamilial variable phenotypic expression of a CIAS1 mutation: from Muckle-Wells to chronic infantile neurological cutaneous and articular syndrome. J Rheumatol 4:747–751

Hoffman HM, Wright FA, Broide DH, Wanderer AA, Kolodner RD (2000) Identification of a locus on chromosome 1q44 for familial cold urticaria. Am J Hum Genet 5:1693–1698

Hoffman HM, Mueller JL, Broide DH, Wanderer AA, Kolodner RD (2001) Mutation of a new gene encoding a putative pyrin-like protein causes familial cold autoinflammatory syndrome and Muckle-Wells syndrome. Nat Genet 3:301–305

Houten SM, Kuis W, Duran M, de Koning TJ, van Royen-Kerkhof A, Romeijn GJ, Frenkel J, Dorland L, de Barse MM, Huijbers WA, Rijkers GT, Waterham HR, Wanders RJ, Poll-The BT (1999) Mutations in MVK, encoding mevalonate kinase, cause hyperimmunoglobulinaemia D and periodic fever syndrome. Nat Genet 2:175–177

Houten SM, Frenkel J, Rijkers GT, Wanders RJ, Kuis W, Waterham HR (2002) Temperature dependence of mutant mevalonate kinase activity as a pathogenic factor in hyper-IgD and periodic fever syndrome. Hum Mol Genet 25:3115–3124

Houten SM, van Woerden CS, Wijburg FA, Wanders RJ, Waterham HR (2003) Carrier frequency of the V377I (1129G>A) MVK mutation, associated with Hyper-IgD and periodic fever syndrome, in the Netherlands. Eur J Hum Genet 2:196–200

Hull KM, Drewe E, Aksentijevich I, Singh HK, Wong K, McDermott EM, Dean J, Powell RJ, Kastner DL (2002) The TNF receptor-associated periodic syndrome (TRAPS): emerging concepts of an autoinflammatory disorder. Medicine (Baltimore) 5:349–368

Infevers (2008) http://fmf.igh.cnrs.fr/infevers/. Cited 18 January 2008

International FMF Consortium (1997) Ancient missense mutations in a new member of the RoRet gene family are likely to cause familial Mediterranean fever. Cell 4:797–807

Kanneganti T, Lamkanfi M, Kim Y, Chen G, Park J, Franchi L, Vandenabeele P, Núñez G (2007) Pannexin-1-mediated recognition of bacterial molecules activates the cryopyrin inflammasome independent of Toll-like receptor signaling. Immunity 4:433–443

Kanneganti TD, Ozoren N, Body-Malapel M, Amer A, Park JH, Franchi L, Whitfield J, Barchet W, Colonna M, Vandenabeele P, Bertin J, Coyle A, Grant EP, Akira S, Nunez G (2006) Bacterial RNA and small antiviral compounds activate caspase-1 through cryopyrin/Nalp3. Nature 7081:233–236

Koorin EV, Aravind L (2000) The NACHT family—a new group of predicted NTPases implicated in apoptosis and MHC transcription activation. Trends Biochem Sci 25:223–224

Kummer JA, Broekhuizen R, Everett H, Agostini L, Kuijk L, Martinon F, van Bruggen R, Tschopp J (2007) Inflammasome components NALP 1 and 3 show distinct but separate expression profiles in human tissues suggesting a site-specific role in the inflammatory response. J Histochem Cytochem 5:443–452

Li J, Nishizawa K, An W, Hussey RE, Lialios FE, Salgia R, Sunder-Plassmann R, Reinherz EL (1998) A cdc15-like adaptor protein (CD2BP1) interacts with the CD2 cytoplasmic domain and regulates CD2-triggered adhesion. EMBO J 24:7320–7336

Lindor N, Arsenault T, Solomon H, Seidman C, McEvoy M (1997) A new autosomal dominant disorder of pyogenic sterile arthritis, pyoderma gangrenosum, and acne: PAPA syndrome. Mayo Clin Proc 7:611–615

Lobito AA, Kimberley FC, Muppidi JR, Komarow H, Jackson AJ, Hull KM, Kastner DL, Screaton GR, Siegel RM (2006) Abnormal disulfide-linked oligomerization results in ER retention and altered signaling by TNFR1 mutants in TNFR1-associated periodic fever syndrome (TRAPS). Blood 4:1320–1327

Mandey SH, Kuijk LM, Frenkel J, Waterham HR (2006a) A role for geranylgeranylation in interleukin-1beta secretion. Arthritis Rheum 11:3690–3695

Mandey SH, Schneiders MS, Koster J, Waterham HR (2006b) Mutational spectrum and genotype-phenotype correlations in mevalonate kinase deficiency. Hum Mutat 8:796–802

Mansfield E, Chae JJ, Komarow HD, Brotz TM, Frucht DM, Aksentijevich I, Kastner DL (2001) The familial Mediterranean fever protein, pyrin, associates with microtubules and colocalizes with actin filaments. Blood 3:851–859

Mariathasan S, Weiss DS, Newton K, McBride J, O'Rourke K, Roose-Girma M, Lee WP, Weinrauch Y, Monack DM, Dixit VM (2006) Cryopyrin activates the inflammasome in response to toxins and ATP. Nature 7081:228–232

Martinon F, Petrilli V, Mayor A, Tardivel A, Tschopp J (2006) Gout-associated uric acid crystals activate the NALP3 inflammasome. Nature 7081:237–241

Matzner Y, Abedat S, Shapiro E, Eisenberg S, Bar-Gil-Shitrit A, Stepensky P, Calco S, Azar Y, Urieli-Shoval S (2000) Expression of the familial Mediterranean fever gene and activity of the C5a inhibitor in human primary fibroblast cultures. Blood 2:727–731

Mayor A, Martinon F, De Smedt T, Petrilli V, Tschopp J (2007) A crucial function of SGT1 and HSP90 in inflammasome activity links mammalian and plant innate immune responses. Nat Immunol 5:497–503

McDermott EM, Smillie DM, Powell RJ (1997) Clinical spectrum of familial Hibernian fever: a 14-year follow-up study of the index case and extended family. Mayo Clin Proc 9:806–817

McDermott MF, Ogunkolade BW, McDermott EM, Jones LC, Wan Y, Quane KA, McCarthy J, Phelan M, Molloy MG, Powell RJ, Amos CI, Hitman GA (1998) Linkage of familial Hibernian fever to chromosome 12p13. Am J Hum Genet 6:1446–1451

McDermott MF, Aksentijevich I, Galon J, McDermott EM, Ogunkolade BW, Centola M, Mansfield E, Gadina M, Karenko L, Pettersson T, McCarthy J, Frucht DM, Aringer M, Torosyan Y, Teppo AM, Wilson M, Karaarslan HM, Wan Y, Todd I, Wood G, Schlimgen R, Kumarajeewa TR, Cooper SM, Vella JP, Amos CI, Mulley J, Quane KA, Molloy MG, Ranki A, Powell RJ, Hitman GA, O'Shea JJ, Kastner DL (1999) Germline mutations in the extracellular domains of the 55 kDa TNF receptor, TNFR1, define a family of dominantly inherited autoinflammatory syndromes. Cell 1:133–144

Miceli-Richard C, Lesage S, Rybojad M, Prieur AM, Manouvrier-Hanu S, Hafner R, Chamaillard M, Zouali H, Thomas G, Hugot JP (2001) CARD15 mutations in Blau syndrome. Nat Genet 1:19–20

Mulley J, Saar K, Hewitt G, Ruschendorf F, Phillips H, Colley A, Sillence D, Reis A, Wilson M (1998) Gene localization for an autosomal dominant familial periodic fever to 12p13. Am J Hum Genet 4:884–889

Online Mendelian Inheritance in Man (2008) http:/www.ncbi.nlm.nih.gov/entrez/query.fcgi?db=OMIM. Cited 18 January 2008

Orange JS, Ramesh N, Remold-O'Donnell E, Sasahara Y, Koopman L, Byrne M, Bonilla FA, Rosen FS, Geha RS, Strominger JL (2002) Wiskott-Aldrich syndrome protein is required for NK cell cytotoxicity and colocalizes with actin in NK cell-activating immunologic synapses. Proc Natl Acad Sci U S A 17:11351–11356

Papin S, Cuenin S, Agostini L, Martinon F, Werner S, Grätter C, Grätter M, Tschopp J (2007) The SPRY domain of Pyrin, mutated in familial Mediterranean fever patients, interacts with inflammasome components and inhibits proIL-1beta processing. Cell Death Differ 14:1457–1466

Prieur AM (2001) A recently recognised chronic inflammatory disease of early onset character-ised by the triad of rash, central nervous system involvement and arthropathy. Clin Exp Rheumatol 1:103–106

Rebelo S, Bainbridge S, Amel-Kashipaz M, Radford P, Powell R, Todd I, Tighe P (2006) Modeling of tumor necrosis factor receptor superfamily 1A mutants associated with tumor necrosis factor receptor-associated periodic syndrome indicates misfolding consistent with abnormal function. Arthritis Rheum 8:2674–2687

Richards N, Schaner P, Diaz A, Stuckey J, Shelden E, Wadhwa A, Gumucio DL (2001) Interaction between pyrin and the apoptotic speck protein (ASC) modulates ASC-induced apoptosis. J Biol Chem 42:39320–39329

Rosé CD, Wouters CH, Meiorin S, Doyle TM, Davey MP, Rosenbaum JT, Martin TM (2006) Pediatric granulomatous arthritis: an international registry. Arthritis Rheum 10:3337–3344

Samuels J, Aksentijevich I, Torosyan Y, Centola M, Deng Z, Sood R, Kastner DL (1998) Familial Mediterranean fever at the millennium. Clinical spectrum, ancient mutations, and a survey of 100 American referrals to the National Institutes of Health. Medicine (Baltimore) 4:268–297

Scharer P, Richards N, Wadhwa A, Aksentijevich I, Kastner D, Tucker P, Gumucio D (2001) Episodic evolution of pyrin in primates: human mutations recapitulate ancestral amino acid states. Nat Genet 3:318–321

Schneiders M, Houten S, Turkenburg M, Waterham H (2006) Manipulation of isoprenoid biosynthesis as a possible therapeutic option in mevalonate kinase deficiency. Arthritis Rheum 7:2306–2313

Seshadri S, Duncan MD, Hart JM, Gavrilin MA, Wewers MD (2007) Pyrin levels in human monocytes and monocyte-derived macrophages regulate IL-1beta processing and release. J Immunol 2:1274–1281

Shoham NG, Centola M, Mansfield E, Hull KM, Wood G, Wise CA, Kastner DL (2003) Pyrin binds the PSTPIP1/CD2BP1 protein, defining familial Mediterranean fever and PAPA syndrome as disorders in the same pathway. Proc Natl Acad Sci U S A 23:13501–13506

Simon A, Drewe E, van der Meer JW, Powell RJ, Kelley RI, Stalenhoef AF, Drenth JP (2004) Simvastatin treatment for inflammatory attacks of the hyperimmunoglobulinemia D and periodic fever syndrome. Clin Pharmacol Ther 5:476–483

Takada K, Aksentijevich I, Mahadevan V, Dean J, Kelley R, Kastner D (2003) Favorable preliminary experience with etanercept in two patients with the hyperimmunoglobulinemia D and periodic fever syndrome. Arthritis Rheum 9:2645–2651

Tchernitchko D, Chiminqgi M, Galacteros F, Prehu C, Segbena Y, Coulibaly H, Rebaya N, Loric S (2005) Unexpected high frequency of P46L TNFRSF1A allele in sub-Saharan West African populations. Eur J Hum Genet 4:513–515

Ting JP, Kastner DL, Hoffman HM (2006) CATERPILLERs, pyrin and hereditary immunological disorders. Nat Rev Immunol 3:183–195

Todd I, Radford PM, Daffa N, Bainbridge SE, Powell RJ, Tighe PJ (2007) Mutant tumor necrosis factor receptor associated with tumor necrosis factor receptor-associated periodic syndrome is altered antigenically and is retained within patients' leukocytes. Arthritis Rheum 8:2765–2773

Tschopp J, Martinon F, Burns K (2003) NALPs: a novel protein family involved in inflammation. Nat Rev Mol Cell Biol 2:95–104

van der Meer J, Vossen J, Radl J, van Nieuwkoop J, Meyer C, Lobatto S, van Furth R (1984) Hyperimmunoglobulinaemia D and periodic fever: a new syndrome. Lancet 8386:1087–1090

Willingham S, Bergstralh D, O'Connor W, Morrison A, Taxman D, Duncan J, Barnoy S, Venkatesan M, Flavell R, Deshmukh M, Hoffman H, Ting J (2007) Microbial pathogen-induced necrotic cell death mediated by the inflammasome components CIAS1/cryopyrin/NLRP3 and ASC. Cell Host Microbe 3:147–159

Wise C, Bennett L, Pascual V, Gillum J, Bowcock A (2000) Localization of a gene for familial recurrent arthritis. Arthritis Rheum 9:2041–2045

Yap MW, Nisole S, Lynch C, Stoye JP (2004) Trim5alpha protein restricts both HIV-1 and murine leukemia virus. Proc Natl Acad Sci U S A 29:10786–10791

Yepiskoposyan L, Harutyunyan A (2007) Population genetics of familial Mediterranean fever: a review. Eur J Hum Genet 15:911–916

Yu J, Fernandes-Alnemri T, Datta P, Wu J, Juliana C, Solorzano L, McCormick M, Zhang Z, Alnemri E (2007) Pyrin activates the ASC pyroptosome in response to engagement by autoinflammatory PSTPIP1 mutants. Mol Cell 2:214–227

Yu JW, Wu J, Zhang Z, Datta P, Ibrahimi I, Taniguchi S, Sagara J, Fernandes-Alnemri T, Alnemri ES (2006) Cryopyrin and pyrin activate caspase-1, but not NF-kappa B, via ASC oligomerization. Cell Death Differ 2:236–249

Zemer D, Revach M, Pras M, Modan B, Schor S, Sohar E, Gafni J (1974) A controlled trial of colchicine in preventing attacks of familial Mediterranean fever. N Engl J Med 18:932–934

Itchy Mice: The Identification of a New Pathway for the Development of Autoimmunity

L.E. Matesic(✉), N.G. Copeland, N.A. Jenkins

Contents

Abstract *Itchy* mice possess a loss-of-function mutation in a HECT-domain-containing ubiquitin ligase (E3), Itch. Homozygous *itchy* mice develop a systemic and progressive autoimmune disease that proves lethal beginning at 6 months of age. Numerous targets of Itch-mediated ubiquitination have been identified, and some of these have defined physiological roles for Itch signaling in T cell anergy and T cell differentiation. Studies of *itchy* mice have also allowed for the identification of a novel pathway involved in autoimmunity: noncanonical Notch signaling. In *itchy* mice carrying an activated *Notch1* transgene, there are increased amounts

L.E. Matesic
Department of Biological Sciences, University of South Carolina, Columbia, SC 29208 USA
lmatesic@biol.sc.edu

B. Beutler (ed.), *Immunology, Phenotype First: How Mutations Have Established
New Principles and Pathways in Immunology.* Current Topics in Microbiology
and Immunology 321. © Springer-Verlag Berlin Heidelberg 2008

of full-length Notch1, which can complex with p56^{lck} and PI3K to activate a cell survival signal that is mediated by phospho-AKT. This, in turn, leads to a reduction in apoptosis in the thymus and may have consequences in T cell tolerance. A role for noncanonical Notch signaling in autoimmune disease is also supported by numerous mouse knockout studies, and suggests possible new therapeutic approaches for the treatment of autoimmune disease.

Abbreviations HECT: Homologous to E6-AP carboxy terminus; Ub: UbiquitinE1 Ubiquitin-activating enzyme; E2: Ubiquitin-conjugating enzyme; E3: Ubiquitin ligase; RING Really interesting new gene; Ndfip1: Nedd4 family interacting protein 1; ICN Intracellular fragment of Notch; *Su(dx):* Suppressor of *deltex*; FL: Full length

Introduction

Autoimmune disease is a collection of more than 80 discrete clinical entities including systemic lupus erythematosus, type I diabetes, and multiple sclerosis. This group of diseases is estimated to affect upwards of 3% of the United States population and therefore significantly contributes to healthcare costs, morbidity, and mortality (Jacobson et al. 1997). Common to all autoimmune disease is the loss of self vs nonself discrimination in the adaptive immune system. This loss of tolerance ultimately results in the destruction of the body's own tissues by immune effector cells. Most often, autoimmune disease is initiated by the malfunction of a T cell. Normally, T cells play a prominent role in the elimination of invading pathogens. They develop in the thymus through a well-defined program (Fig. 1) that assures a diverse T cell repertoire with a number of safeguards in place to protect against autoreactivity. One such defense is central tolerance, an instructive process occurring in the thymus that identifies and eliminates potentially self-reactive thymocytes through negative selection. Central tolerance requires the presentation of self-antigens by thymic epithelial cells. Since not all self-antigens are expressed and thus displayed by these cells, it is possible for a self-reactive cell to escape into the circulation. Any such escapees are controlled through measures collectively known as peripheral tolerance. Specific mechanisms of peripheral tolerance include the induction of T cell anergy (Schwartz 2003), T cell apoptosis through activation-induced cell death (Zhang et al. 2004), and the generation of suppressive regulatory T cells (Sakaguchi 2004). In autoimmune disease, loss of self-tolerance can result from defects in central tolerance, peripheral tolerance, or both.

Despite the plethora of human patients and mouse models, progress toward the identification of key molecules involved in autoimmunity has been slow. This is likely due to the complex nature of these diseases, in which environmental factors

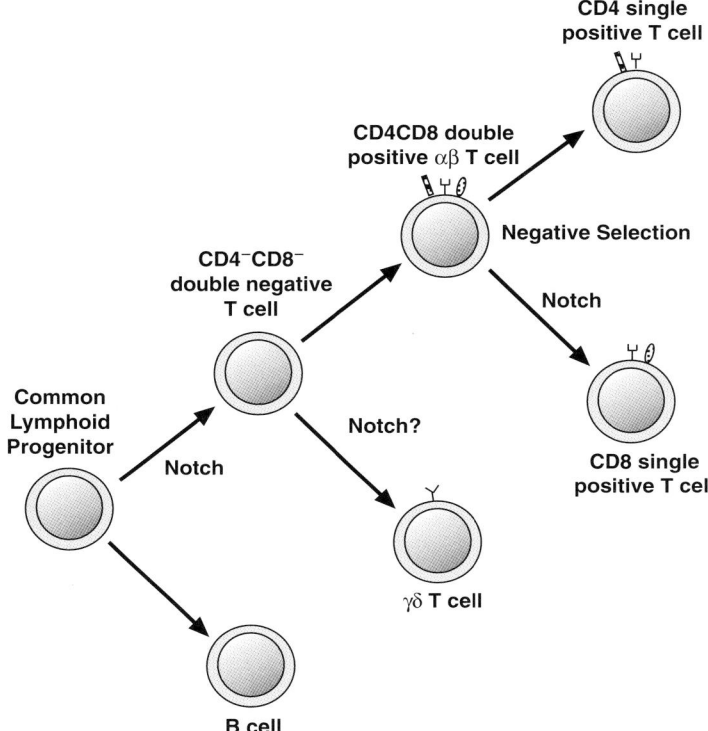

Fig. 1 Notch signaling in T cell development. T cells arise from common lymphoid progenitors that migrate to the thymus under an instructive Notch signal. At that point, they become double-negative cells, because they are doubly negative for the expression of the cell surface markers CD4 and CD8. As these developing thymocytes rearrange their T cell receptors they become either γδ-bearing or αβ-bearing. There are some reports that Notch signaling may affect this decision, although there is not consensus as to whether Notch biases toward αβ or γδ T cells. Cells with an αβ T cell receptor go on to become doubly positive for CD4 (*rectangle*) and CD8 (*oval*). It is at this point that negative and positive selection occurs. There is some preliminary data implicating the involvement of Notch signaling in negative selection (central tolerance). Cells that pass these critical tests become either CD8 single-positive or CD4 single-positive effector cells that enter the peripheral circulation. There is some evidence supporting the involvement of Notch signaling in CD8 vs CD4 lineage commitment

and genetic heterogeneity both contribute. New insight has recently come from spontaneous or induced monogenic mouse models of autoimmune disease. These animal models provide a system where environmental conditions can be precisely regulated and signaling pathways essential in breaching tolerance can be thoroughly characterized in order to translate these findings to human disease. One such model animal system that has helped in our understanding of some of the mechanisms involved in the genesis of autoimmune disease is the *itchy* mouse.

The *Itchy* Mouse

Phenotype of Itchy Mice

On a C57BL/6J background, homozygous a^{18H} mice (also referred to as *itchy* mice or *itch⁻/⁻* mice) are dark agouti in color with black pinna hairs. However, unlike all other alleles of *nonagouti* (*a*), *itchy* mice also develop an autoimmune-like disease characterized histologically by a mixed infiltrate (consisting of lymphocytes, eosinophils, and histiocytes) in nearly every organ system, lymphoproliferation resulting in splenomegaly and lymphadenopathy, and cortical atrophy of the thymus with medullary proliferation (Hustad et al. 1995). Furthermore, these animals produce antinuclear antibodies, and IgG deposits can be detected in the glomeruli as early as 8 weeks of age (Matesic et al. 2006). At about 5 months of age, *itchy* mice develop dermatitis and ulcerations that are especially prevalent on the head and neck region. These mice eventually die between 6 and 9 months of age from asphyxiation, as their lung function becomes compromised from alveolar proteinosis and interstitial inflammation composed of mostly B220⁺ cells. This phenotype can be recapitulated by transplantation of *itchy*-derived bone marrow into a lethally irradiated syngeneic host. However, the mutation is no longer lethal when moved onto a $RagI^{-/-}$ background where mature lymphocytes are lacking (L.E. Matesic, N.G. Copeland, N.A. Jenkins, unpublished observations). These results suggest that the autoimmune-like disease is cell autonomous to a bone marrow-derived cell, most likely a lymphocyte.

The Molecular Basis of the Itchy Mutation

The molecular defect responsible for the *itchy* phenotype is a small inversion on distal mouse chromosome 2. The breakpoints of this inversion affect the expression of two genes, *Agouti* and *Itch*. Specifically, there is a decrease in the amount of *Agouti* message, the consequence of which is a dark agouti coat color, as well as a complete abrogation of the expression of *Itch*, which presumably accounts for the immune dysfunction (Perry et al. 1998). The *Itch* gene has an open reading frame of 2,562 nucleotides, encoding a protein of 854 amino acids with a molecular weight of approximately 113 kDa. Itch is ubiquitously expressed in all adult tissues as well as throughout development. Sequence alignments of the predicted amino acid sequence demonstrates that Itch contains three important motifs: a C2 domain, four WW domains, and a HECT (homologous to E6-AP carboxy terminus) domain. The C2 domain can be found in a multitude of proteins with diverse biological functions. This motif is thought play a role in membrane targeting or subcellular localization, in some cases responding to increases in levels of intracellular Ca^{2+} (Nalefski and Falke 1996). The WW domain is named for the presence of two conserved tryptophan residues that guide the folding of this protein module. WW domains have been implicated in protein–protein interactions, with high binding affinity for PPLP, PPXY, or phospho-serine/threonine motifs (Sudol 1996). HECT domains have been shown to have ubiquitin ligase (E3) activity and, as such, serve important roles in regulating protein stability, function, and subcellular localization in diverse cellular processes such as signal transduction, regulation of transcription, DNA repair, cell cycle progression, antigen presentation, and apoptosis (Hershko and Ciechanover 1998).

Ubiquitination

Ubiquitination is a posttranslational modification that directly conjugates a highly conserved 76-amino acid ubiquitin (Ub) molecule to a lysine residue on a target protein. The sequential action of three enzymes mediates this reversible process. First, Ub is activated in an ATP-dependent manner by an Ub-activating enzyme (E1) to form a thioester bond between the active site cysteine in the E1 and the C-terminal glycine residue of Ub. The activated Ub is then transferred to an Ub-conjugating enzyme (E2) to form a similar thioester linkage. This process comes to fruition when the E3 recruits both the E2–Ub complex and the target protein substrate in order to facilitate the transfer of the Ub from the E2 to the target protein. As such, it is the E3 that confers substrate specificity in ubiquitination. Consequently, it is not surprising that E3s are encoded by several hundred genes in the mammalian genome and often contain protein–protein interaction motifs in addition to the E3 catalytic site (Semple 2003). There are two major classes of mammalian E3s: the HECT and RING (really interesting new gene) families, which differ from one another not only in their sequence but also in their mode of action. RING E3s act as a scaffold for the transfer of Ub to the target protein, while HECT E3s have intrinsic enzymatic activity and the Ub is transferred from the E2 to a conserved cysteine residue in the HECT domain before being attached to the target protein (Liu 2007). Itch is a member of the HECT family of E3s.

In addition to the regulation offered by controlling the timing of ubiquitination as well as its reversibility, there are diverse biological outcomes associated with the ubiquitination signature affixed to a substrate. A target protein can be monoubiquitinated at a single lysine residue or serially monoubiquitinated at several different lysine residues via the lysine 63 residue of Ub. Such modifications usually signal for altered protein trafficking (e.g., internalization of membrane receptors). Alternatively, a substrate protein can be polyubiquitinated with a chain of four or more Ub molecules on one or more lysine residues via the lysine 48 residue, which leads to degradation by the 26S proteasome (Wang et al. 2006).

Itch Function in T Cells

Since the molecular lesion responsible for the *itchy* mutation was cloned, much progress has been made in understanding the physiological role of Itch. Numerous targets that are regulated by Itch have been identified. These are summarized in Table 1. A few of these have particular relevance to T cell function and are discussed here in greater detail.

Table 1 Targets of itch binding and ubiquitination

Target	Action of Itch	Function	Reference
LMP2A	PolyUb	EBV infection	Ikeda et al. 2001
ErbB–4	polyUb	Receptor tyrosine kinase	Omerovic et al. 2007
Trpv4 and Trpc4	MonoUb	Ion channels	Wegierski et al. 2006
NF-E2	Acts as transcriptional co-repressor	Heterodimeric transcription factor	Chen et al. 2001
CXCR4	MonoUb	Chemokine receptor	Marchese et al. 2003
Hrs	MonoUb; CXCR4-dependent	Endocytosis	Marchese et al. 2003
p63	PolyUb	Transcription factor involved in epidermal differentiation	Rossi et al. 2006
p73	PolyUb	DNA damage response	Rossi et al. 2005
RNF11	Not determined	RING E3	Kitching et al. 2003
p68	PolyUb	Subunit of Im	Ingham et al. 2005
Smac2	Proteolysis-independent Ub	TGF-β signaling	Bai et al. 2004
HEF1	PolyUb	TGF-β signaling	Feng et al. 2004
JunB	PolyUb	Th2 differentiation	Fang et al. 2002
c-Jun	PolyUb	T cell activation	Fang et al. 2002
Endophilin-A	MonoUb	Clathrin-mediated endocytosis	Angers et al. 2004
Cbl-c	PolyUb	RING E3	Magnifico et al. 2003
Atrophin–1	Not determined	DRPLA gene	Wood et al. 1998
Occludin	PolyUb	Sertoli tight junctions	Traweger et al. 2002
Notch1	MonoUb and polyUb	Various developmental processes	Qiu et al. 2000
Deltex	K29 polyUb	Regulation of Notch signaling	Chastagner et al. 2006
c-FLIP	PolyUb	NF-κB induced anti-apoptotic protein	Chang et al. 2006
Bcl10	PolyUb	Important for activation of NF-κB	Scharschmidt et al. 2004
PLC-γ1	PolyUb	Induced by Ca^{2+}/calcineurin signaling	Heissmeyer et al. 2004
PKC-θ	PolyUb	Induced by Ca^{2+}/calcineurin signaling	Heissmeyer et al. 2004
Gli1	PolyUb facilitated by Numb	Transcription factor in hedgehog signaling	Di Marcotullio et al. 2006
FAM/USP9X	Reverses Itch auto-polyUb	Ub protease	Mouchantaf et al. 2006

EBV Epstein–Barr virus; MonoUB, monoubiquitination; NF-κB, nuclear factor-κB; PolyUB, polyubiquitination; TGF, transforming growth factor; Th, T helper

Itch in T Cell Differentiation

JunB is a transcription factor that plays an important role in T cell differentiation. Subsequent to antigen exposure, naïve CD4 T cells can differentiate into either T helper (Th)1 or Th2 cells, depending on their cytokine profiles and effector functions (Mosmann and Coffman 1989). JunB is preferentially expressed in Th2 cells and activates the transcription of interleukin (IL)-4 and IL-5 (Li et al. 1999). The increased levels of these cytokines results in an allergic response and antibody class switching to IgG1, IgA, and IgE, as well as the recruitment of eosinophils via IL-5 (Neurath et al. 2002). JunB is polyubiquitinated by Itch, and without proper regulation of this transcription factor, *itchy* mice develop a Th2 bias in T cell differentiation, have increased IgG1 and IgE levels in the serum, and experience eosinophil activation (Fang et al. 2002).

The function of Itch in T cell differentiation is regulated by phosphorylation and interaction with other proteins. The activation of c-Jun NH_2-terminal kinase 1 (JNK1) by MAP/ERK kinase kinase 1 (MEKK1) results in the phosphorylation of Itch on serine or threonine sites (Gao et al. 2004). This induces a structural change in the Itch ligase, so that it adopts a more open and active conformation, which allows for more efficient recruitment and degradation of the JunB substrate (Gallagher et al. 2006). In contrast, Fyn-mediated tyrosine phosphorylation of Itch negatively regulates JunB ubiquitination and turnover (Yang et al. 2006). Finally, Itch has recently been shown to coimmunoprecipitate and colocalize with Nedd4 family interacting protein 1 (Ndfip1) in T cells (Oliver et al. 2006). *Ndfip1*$^{-/-}$ mice have a similar phenotype to *itchy* mice, with severe skin and lung inflammation and a Th2 bias. Furthermore, levels of JunB are increased in *Ndfip1*$^{-/-}$ T cells, suggesting that Ndfip1 is required for efficient ubiquitination of JunB by Itch. Since Ndfip1 is a membrane-bound protein, it may act to recruit Itch to the appropriate subcellular compartment for Itch to exert its effects.

Itch in T Cell Anergy

Itch also plays an important role in T cell anergy, a process that renders a lymphocyte functionally inactive but alive following an encounter with antigen. Itch is upregulated in anergizing conditions and polyubiquitinates phospholipase C (PLC)-γ1 and protein kinase C (PKC)-θ, two key molecules induced by Ca^{2+}/calcineurin signaling; this, in turn, destabilizes the immunological synapse and induces T cell unresponsiveness after T cell receptor engagement in response to restimulation with antigen together with antigen-presenting cells (Heissmeyer et al. 2004). The failure to induce anergy may account for the inability to establish peripheral tolerance and the development of autoimmune disease in *itch*$^{-/-}$ mice. This hypothesis has recently been proved in an in vivo system that measures Th2 tolerance in airway inflammation. In that animal model, the lack of Itch leads to a breach in tolerance of Th2 cells and to the development of allergic responses under experimental conditions that would induce anergy in normal Th2 cells (Venuprasad et al. 2006).

Notch Signaling

Itch has been shown to mono- and polyubiquitinate Notch1 in vitro (Qiu et al. 2000). Notch signaling plays a number of important roles in the immune system, influencing everything from hematopoiesis to T cell lineage commitment to the function of peripheral T cells (reviewed in Radtke et al. 2004). Notch signaling is also known to mediate critical steps of T cell development (Fig. 1). As such, the mechanism by which Itch may regulate Notch signaling in vivo is of particular interest in the genesis of autoimmune disease.

Canonical Notch Signaling

Notch proteins are evolutionarily conserved transmembrane receptors that play important roles in cellular differentiation, proliferation, and apoptosis (Artavanis-Tsakonas et al. 1999; Miele and Osborne 1999). In mammals, there are four Notch receptors (Notch1–4) and five ligands (Jagged1 and 2; Delta1, 3, and 4) which function through direct cell-to-cell contact since both the ligands and the receptors are integral membrane proteins. The Notch receptors exist at the cell surface as a functional heterodimer, resulting from a furin-like processing event in the *trans* Golgi (Blaumueller et al. 1997). Upon ligand binding, ADAM10 or ADAM17 cleaves the Notch receptor extracellularly, releasing the extracellular domain (Brou et al. 2000). This is followed by another cleavage event mediated by γ-secretase (whose catalytic site is thought to be in presenilin subunits), which generates the intracellular fragment of Notch (ICN). The ICN translocates into the nucleus where it becomes a transcriptional coactivator for recombination signal-binding protein for immunoglobulin κJ region (RBP-Jκ), initiating the transcription of HES (hairy and enhancer of split) and HEY (HES-related with YRPW motif) target genes (Lai 2004). ICN is ubiquitinated in the nucleus by FBXW7 (F-box and WD repeat domain containing 7) and rapidly degraded (Gupta-Rossi et al. 2001; Wu et al. 2001). Studies in *Drosophila* have identified two additional E3s, Suppressor of *deltex* [*Su(dx)*] and DNedd4, which regulate the level of endogenous Notch. Specifically, these C2-WW-HECT E3s ubiquitinate full-length (FL), unactivated Notch in the endosome to target it for proteolysis. In the absence of these E3s, more FL Notch is present in the cell and can either be spuriously activated in the endosome by γ-secretase or recycled back to the plasma membrane, thus effectively lowering the threshold for Notch signaling (Sakata et al. 2004; Wilkin et al. 2004).

Noncanonical Notch Signaling

Through the extensive study of Notch signaling in various model organisms, some exceptions to the rule of canonical Notch signaling have been described. Noncanonical Notch signaling can involve the use of alternative ligands, alternative transcriptional coactivators, or nonnuclear mediators. In the vertebrate nervous system, F3/contactin acts as a Notch ligand to initiate a signal that promotes oligodendrocyte maturation and myelination (Hu et al. 2003). There are a number of other noncanonical ligands that can activate Notch signaling (e.g., NB3, NOV,

MAGP1, and MAGP2), but they have not been shown to have activity in the immune system (Osborne and Minter 2007). In *Drosophila*, Notch can signal through some members of the Wingless pathway (Axelrod et al. 1996; Ramain et al. 2001) instead of through Suppressor of Hairless (the ortholog of RBP-Jκ).

With respect to nonnuclear mechanisms of Notch signaling, there is a growing body of evidence that such pathways do exist under physiological conditions. In neuronal growth cones, Notch signaling has been proposed to directly regulate the actin cytoskeleton via a protein complex containing the tyrosine kinase Abl to regulate axon guidance (Giniger 1998). The cytoplasmic protein Deltex has also been shown to initiate Notch signaling in the late endosome of *Drosophila* (Hori et al. 2004). In Jurkat T cells, FL Notch1 coimmunoprecipitates with p56[lck] and with phosphatidylinositol 3-kinase (PI3K). This interaction was observed to activate AKT signaling and mediate an antiapoptotic effect (Sade et al. 2004).

Noncanonical Notch Signaling in Autoimmune Disease

The first connection between Notch signaling and autoimmune disease was the description of the combined *presenilin1* and *2* loss-of-function phenotype. Animals that are heterozygous for a knockout allele of *presenilin1* and homozygous for a knockout allele of *presenilin2* develop seborrheic keratosis and an autoimmune disease similar to that seen in *itchy* mice. Specifically, these animals display IgG deposition in the kidneys, produce antinuclear antibodies, and have splenomegaly as well as dermatitis consisting of a mixed inflammatory infiltrate that is predominantly B220+ (Tournoy et al. 2004). This was originally interpreted as resulting from a reduction in Notch signaling through the canonical pathway, which caused an excess of B lymphocytes and of CD4 T cells, since canonical Notch signaling is required for T cell lineage commitment and perhaps for progressing from a double positive to a single-positive CD8 T cell (Fig. 1). This autoimmune phenotype, however, could instead result from the increased amount of FL Notch1–4 present in the T cells of these mice, which could then signal through a noncanonical pathway. Since that initial report, there have been a number of studies confirming that ligand-activated Notch signaling in T cells can occur without cleavage of Notch. Specifically, Notch-mediated suppression in human T cells (Kostianovsky et al. 2007), cytokine production by primary CD4 T cells and dendritic cells (Stallwood et al. 2006), and activation and proliferation of peripheral helper T cells (Rutz et al. 2005) all occurred in the presence of γ-secretase inhibitors where there was a complete inhibition of the canonical signaling pathway.

Increased Notch signaling was directly linked to autoimmune disease when it was discovered that some *lck–Notch1* transgenic mice, which overexpress the *Notch1* ICN exclusively in developing T cells, develop a systemic and progressive autoimmune disease (Matesic et al. 2006). Furthermore, this disease is similar to that observed in *itch*[−/−] animals, having approximately the same age of onset. *Notch1* transgenic animals with autoimmune disease have splenomegaly and lymphadenopathy. There is a mixed inflammation in most organ systems with severe kidney involvement, including membranoproliferative glomerulonephropathy and interstitial inflammation that is almost exclusively CD3⁺. Additionally, the diseased animals display a progressive deposition of IgG complexes in the glomeruli as well the production of antinuclear antibodies.

The similarity of the *itchy* phenotype to that of the Notch transgenics implies that these proteins may function in the same pathway in the genesis of autoimmune disease. This is supported by the fact that Itch can target Notch1 for ubiquitination in vitro (Qiu et al. 2000) and by phylogenetic analysis suggesting that *Itch* is the mouse ortholog of *Drosophila Su(dx)* (Matesic et al. 2006). In *Drosophila*, a class of gain-of-function *Notch* alleles (Ax^{E2}) is enhanced by a loss-of-function *Su(dx)* mutation (Fostier et al. 1998), suggesting that *Su(dx)* is a negative regulator of *Notch* signaling. To determine whether a similar genetic interaction also occurs in mammals, *itch*⁻/⁻ mice were bred to the *lck–Notch1* transgenic mice.

All *itchy* mice carrying the *Notch1* transgene are considerably smaller than their littermates and die between 8 and 12 weeks of age. Examination of these animals reveals lymphoproliferation and massive amounts of chronic, active inflammation with eosinophils in almost every organ system examined. As with *lck–Notch1 tg⁺* mice, some membranoproliferative glomerulonephropathy is present in the kidneys. Consistent with the autoimmune-like disease aspect of the phenotype, the sera of *itchy* animals carrying the *Notch1* transgene contain antinuclear antibodies, and more IgG deposition can be detected in the glomeruli of 8-week-old *itch*⁻/⁻; *lck–Notch1 tg⁺* mice (i.e., mice that carry the Notch1 transgene and are homozygous for the itchy mutation) when compared to age- and gender-matched wildtype or single mutant animals. Thus, *itch*⁻/⁻; *lck-Notch1 tg⁺* animals develop a similar autoimmune-like disease as *itch*⁻/⁻ or *lck-Notch1 tg⁺* mice but with more severe lesions and a much earlier age of onset. The fact that the mutations in concert yield severe early-onset disease, which was not seen with either mutation alone, supports the hypothesis that these alleles genetically interact. In addition, the combination of these mutations produces novel phenotypes including a perturbation in T cell development, with a reduction in the number of double-positive and an increase in the number of double-negative and single-positive T cells. TUNEL (terminal deoxynucleotidyl transferase biotin dUTP nick end labeling) staining shows reduced apoptosis in the thymi of *itch* animals that carry the *Notch1* transgene (Matesic et al. 2006).

Mechanistically, this reduction in apoptosis can be explained by an increase in noncanonical Notch signaling. Quantitative analysis of transcriptional targets of canonical Notch signaling such as *Hes1* reveals no correlation with the severity of the autoimmune disease. Antibody staining, however, displays increased levels of FL Notch1 in diseased animals, and the scale of the increase correlates with the severity of the autoimmune phenotype. In the *itchy* mice there is increased FL Notch1 due to the lack of ubiquitination and degradation of Notch1 by Itch. This makes more FL Notch1 available for signaling. In contrast, in the transgenic animals there is increased canonical Notch signaling. One of the transcriptional targets of this signaling cascade is *Notch1* itself. This causes an increase in the amount of FL Notch1 at the cell surface, lowering the signaling threshold. Thus, when the effects of these two mutations are combined, the amount of FL Notch1 increases to an even greater degree, effectively lowering the Notch signaling threshold. This is manifest in the earlier age of onset and greater severity of the autoimmune disease (Matesic et al. 2006).

Increased levels of FL Notch1 can be found specifically in the double-positive thymocyte population prior to the onset of overt pathology. There are also corresponding increases in phospho-AKT in double-positive thymocytes but no change in other signaling pathways including mitogen-activated protein kinase (MAPK), p38, and JNK. Since AKT is known to provide a cell survival signal, it was hypothesized that the increased FL Notch1 complexes with p56[lck] and PI3K to activate the phosphorylation of AKT, which delivers a survival signal to double-positive thymocytes (Matesic et al. 2006). Normally 95% of double-positive thymocytes will die in the thymus, due to failure to meet the criteria for positive and negative selection (Strasser 1995). In these double mutants, however, there are decreased amounts of apoptosis correlating with the increase in phospho-AKT. It is tempting to speculate that, in these double mutant animals, the noncanonical Notch signal is allowing autoreactive cells to persist, thus providing a breach in central tolerance. However, this remains to be formally demonstrated. A similar noncanonical signaling mechanism has been noted at the point of β selection to promote the survival and glucose uptake/metabolism of pre-T cells via AKT signaling (Ciofani and Zuniga-Pflucker 2005).

Are There Other Aspects of Noncanonical Notch Signaling Involved in Autoimmune Disease?

Studies of *itchy* mice have brought to light many signaling pathways that are altered in this autoimmune disease state. Perhaps one of the most exciting findings is the link between noncanonical AKT-mediated Notch signaling and autoimmunity. It will be interesting to see if other mediators of noncanonical Notch signaling such as Abl and Deltex also play a role in the genesis of autoimmune disease. Recent reports have shown that c-Abl can phosphorylate c-Jun and protect it from Itch-mediated degradation (Gao et al. 2006). What remains to be demonstrated is whether Notch can regulate c-Abl in T cells in a manner analogous to that observed in growth cones. If this is the case, then there should be increased c-Abl activity in T cells derived from the *Notch1* transgenic animals, which would yield the stabilization of c-Jun protein (Fig. 2).

There are also studies linking Itch to Deltex. Specifically, Itch has been shown to ubiquitinate Deltex1 (Dtx1), a RING E3, through an unusual K29 linkage (Chastagner et al. 2006). Deltex, in turn, can catalyze the ubiquitination and degradation of MEKK1 (Liu and Lai 2005). MEKK1 has been shown to phosphorylate Itch and augment its ability to ubiquitinate JunB via JNK1 (Gao et al. 2004). These observations offer the tantalizing possibility that there may be a connection between the Th2 bias and noncanonical Notch signaling (Fig. 3). However, there are some outstanding questions: (1) Do T cells from Notch1 transgenics have a Th2 bias? If

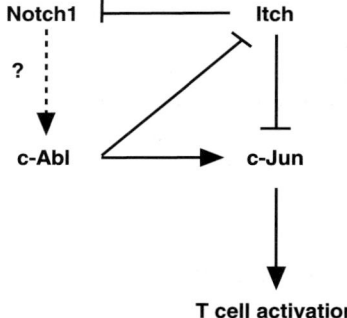

Fig. 2 A hypothetical role for c-Abl-mediated noncanonical Notch signaling in T cell activation. Notch has been shown to signal via a protein complex containing Abl in growth cones. Abl can also phosphorylate c-Jun and protect it from Itch-mediated ubiquitination and degradation during T cell activation. It remains to be determined whether Notch can signal via c-Abl in this cellular context (*dashed line*). (*Arrows* represent activation and *bars* represent inhibitory effects)

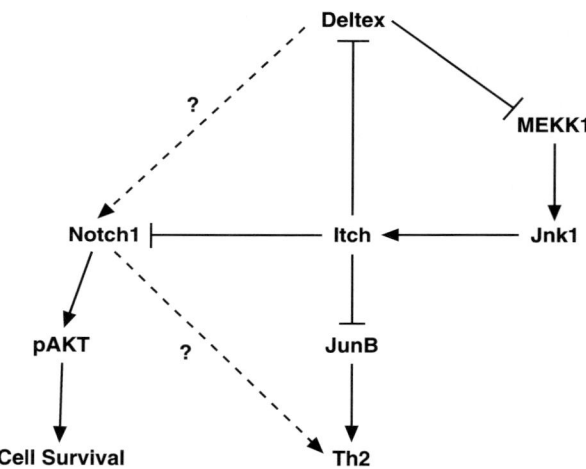

Fig. 3 Deltex could connect noncanonical Notch signaling to T cell differentiation. Deltex is a RING E3 and has been shown to target MEKK1 for ubiquitination and degradation by the 26S proteasome. MEKK1 can activate JNK1, which can phosphorylate Itch and increase its ability to ubiquitinate JunB. Itch can also ubiquitinate Deltex via an unconventional Ub linkage. In this way, Itch and Deltex antagonistically regulate one another. It remains to be determined if the overexpression of Deltex could result in autoimmune disease (*dashed line*). Furthermore, it is not known whether the increased Notch signaling in the Notch1 transgenic leads to a bias in Th2 differentiation (*dashed line*; *arrows* represent activation and *bars* represent inhibitory effects)

so, what is the connection between increased Notch and the Th2 bias, and (2) will overexpression of Dtx1 in developing T cells yield an autoimmune phenotype? The answers will likely be complex since the translation between Deltex function in *Drosophila* and mammals has been confusing at best. Although Deltex has been shown to be a positive regulator of Notch signaling in *Drosophila*, when Deltex1 is overexpressed in hematopoietic stem cells, a phenotype mimicking Notch inactivation is observed, suggesting that *Dtx1* negatively regulates Notch signaling (Izon et al. 2002). Knockout mice lacking the function of just *Dtx1* (Storck et al. 2005) or both *Dtx1 and Dtx2* (Lehar and Bevan 2006) display normal immune development and normal immune responses. T cells from these animals, however, were not assayed for any bias in Th1 vs Th2 differentiation, so the possibility remains that Deltex could have some physiological function in the immune system.

Conclusions

As our understanding of the *itchy* phenotype continues to grow, one of the remaining challenges we face is the integration of all of these signaling pathways in the explanation of the mutant phenotype. That is, why do *itchy* mice develop autoimmune disease? Is it due to a breach in central tolerance, in peripheral tolerance, or both? Mechanistically, how does this happen? As we arrive at answers to these questions, we will gain a greater understanding of the pathogenesis of autoimmune disease. This will allow for the design of better therapeutics that might be able to benefit a large number of people suffering from a number of diseases characterized by the loss of self-tolerance.

Acknowledgements This research was supported by the Intramural Research Program of the NIH, National Cancer Institute, Center for Cancer Research.

References

Angers A, Ramjaun AR, McPherson PS (2004) The HECT domain ligase itch ubiquitinates endophilin and localizes to the trans-Golgi network and endosomal system. J Biol Chem 279:11471–11479

Artavanis-Tsakonas S, Rand MD, Lake RJ (1999) Notch signaling: cell fate control and signal integration in development. Science 284:770–776

Axelrod JD, Matsuno K, Artavanis-Tsakonas S, Perrimon N (1996) Interaction between Wingless and Notch signaling pathways mediated by disheveled. Science 271:1826–1832

Bai Y, Yang C, Hu K, Elly C, Liu YC (2004) Itch E3 ligase-mediated regulation of TGF-beta signaling by modulating smad2 phosphorylation. Mol Cell 15:825–831

Blaumueller CM, Qi H, Zagouras P, Artavanis-Tsakonas S (1997) Intracellular cleavage of Notch leads to a heterodimeric receptor on the plasma membrane. Cell 90:281–291

Brou C, Logeat F, Gupta N, Bessia C, LeBail O, Doedens JR, Cumano A, Roux P, Black RA, Israel A (2000) A novel proteolytic cleavage involved in Notch signaling: the role of the disintegrin-metalloprotease TACE. Mol Cell 5:207–216

Chang L, Kamata H, Solinas G, Luo JL, Maeda S, Venuprasad K, Liu YC, Karin M (2006) The E3 ubiquitin ligase itch couples JNK activation to TNFalpha-induced cell death by inducing c-FLIP(L) turnover. Cell 124:601–613

Chastagner P, Israel A, Brou C (2006) Itch/AIP4 mediates Deltex degradation through the formation of K29-linked polyubiquitin chains. EMBO Rep 7:1147–1153

Chen X, Wen S, Fukuda MN, Gavva NR, Hsu D, Akama TO, Yang-Feng T, Shen CK (2001) Human ITCH is a coregulator of the hematopoietic transcription factor NF-E2. Genomics 73:238–241

Ciofani M, Zuniga-Pflucker JC (2005) Notch promotes survival of pre-T cells at the beta-selection checkpoint by regulating cellular metabolism. Nat Immunol 6:881–888

Di Marcotullio L, Ferretti E, Greco A, De Smaele E, Po A, Sico MA, Alimandi M, Giannini G, Maroder M, Screpanti I, Gulino A (2006) Numb is a suppressor of Hedgehog signalling and targets Gli1 for Itch-dependent ubiquitination. Nat Cell Biol 8:1415–1423

Fang D, Elly C, Gao B, Fang N, Altman Y, Joazeiro C, Hunter T, Copeland N, Jenkins N, Liu YC (2002) Dysregulation of T lymphocyte function in itchy mice: a role for Itch in TH2 differentiation. Nat Immunol 3:281–287

Feng L, Guedes S, Wang T (2004) Atrophin-1-interacting protein 4/human Itch is a ubiquitin E3 ligase for human enhancer of filamentation 1 in transforming growth factor-beta signaling pathways. J Biol Chem 279:29681–29690

Foster M, Evans DA, Artavanis-Tsakonas S, Baron M (1998) Genetic characterization of the Drosophila melanogaster Suppressor of *deltex* gene: a regulator of notch signaling. Genetics 150:1477–1485

Gallagher E, Gao M, Liu YC, Karin M (2006) Activation of the E3 ubiquitin ligase Itch through a phosphorylation-induced conformational change. Proc Natl Acad Sci USA 103:1717–1722

Gao B, Lee SM, Fang D (2006) The tyrosine kinase c-Abl protects c-Jun from ubiquitination-mediated degradation in T cells. J Biol Chem 281:29711–29718

Gao M, Labuda T, Xia Y, Gallagher E, Fang D, Liu YC, Karin M (2004) Jun turnover is controlled through JNK-dependent phosphorylation of the E3 ligase Itch. Science 306:271–275

Giniger E (1998) A role for Abl in Notch signaling. Neuron 20:667–681

Gupta-Rossi N, Le Bail O, Gonen H, Brou C, Logeat F, Six E, Ciechanover A, Israel A (2001) Functional interaction between SEL-10, an F-box protein, and the nuclear form of activated Notch1 receptor. J Biol Chem 276:34371–34378

Heissmeyer V, Macian F, Im SH, Varma R, Feske S, Venuprasad K, Gu H, Liu YC, Dustin ML, Rao A (2004) Calcineurin imposes T cell unresponsiveness through targeted proteolysis of signaling proteins. Nat Immunol 5:255–265

Hershko A, Ciechanover A (1998) The ubiquitin system. Annu Rev Biochem 67:425–479

Hori K, Fostier M, Ito M, Fuwa TJ, Go MJ, Okano H, Baron M, Matsuno K (2004) Drosophila deltex mediates suppressor of Hairless-independent and late-endosomal activation of Notch signaling. Development 131:5527–5537

Hu QD, Ang BT, Karsak M, Hu WP, Cui XY, Duka T, Takeda Y, Chia W, Sankar N, Ng YK, Ling EA, Maciag T, Small D, Trifonova R, Kopan R, Okano H, Nakafuku M, Chiba S, Hirai H, Aster JC, Schachner M, Pallen CJ, Watanabe K, Xiao ZC (2003) F3/contactin acts as a functional ligand for Notch during oligodendrocyte maturation. Cell 115:163–175

Hustad CM, Perry WL, Siracusa LD, Rasberry C, Cobb L, Cattanach BM, Kovatch R, Copeland NG, Jenkins NA (1995) Molecular genetic characterization of six recessive viable alleles of the mouse agouti locus. Genetics 140:255–265

Ikeda M, Ikeda A, Longnecker R (2001) PY motifs of Epstein-Barr virus LMP2A regulate protein stability and phosphorylation of LMP2A-associated proteins. J Virol 75:5711–5718

Ingham RJ, Colwill K, Howard C, Dettwiler S, Lim CS, Yu J, Hersi K, Raaijmakers J, Gish G, Mbamalu G, Taylor L, Yeung B, Vassilovski G, Amin M, Chen F, Matskova L, Winberg G, Ernberg I, Linding R, O'Donnell P, Starostine A, Keller W, Metalnikov P, Stark C, Pawson T (2005) WW domains provide a platform for the assembly of multiprotein networks. Mol Cell Biol 25:7092–7106

Ishikawa A, Kitajima S, Takahashi Y, Kokubo H, Kanno J, Inoue T, Saga Y (2004) Mouse Nkd1, a Wnt antagonist, exhibits oscillatory gene expression in the psm under the control of notch signalling. Mech Dev 121:1443–1453

Izon DJ, Aster JC, He Y, Weng A, Karnell FG, Patriub V, Xu L, Bakkour S, Rodriguez C, Allman D, Pear WS (2002) Deltex1 redirects lymphoid progenitors to the B cell lineage by antagonizing Notch1. Immunity 16:231–243

Jacobson DL, Gange SJ, Rose NR, Graham NM (1997) Epidemiology and estimated population burden of selected autoimmune diseases in the United States. Clin Immunol Immunopathol 84:223–243

Kitching R, Wong MJ, Koehler D, Burger AM, Landberg G, Gish G, Seth A (2003) The RING-H2 protein RNF11 is differentially expressed in breast tumours and interacts with HECT-type E3 ligases. Biochim Biophys Acta 1639:104–112

Kostianovsky AM, Maier LM, Baecher-Allan C, Anderson AC, Anderson DE (2007) Up-regulation of gene related to anergy in lymphocytes is associated with Notch-mediated human T cell suppression. J Immunol 178:6158–6163

Lai EC (2004) Notch signaling: control of cell communication and cell fate. Development 131:965–973

Lehar SM, Bevan MJ (2006) T cells develop normally in the absence of both Deltex1 and Deltex2. Mol Cell Biol 26:7358–7371

Li B, Tournier C, Davis RJ, Flavell RA (1999) Regulation of IL-4 expression by the transcription factor JunB during T helper cell differentiation. EMBO J 18:420–432

Liu WH, Lai MZ (2005) Deltex regulates T-cell activation by targeted degradation of active MEKK1. Mol Cell Biol 25:1367–1378

Liu YC (2007) The E3 ubiquitin ligase Itch in T cell activation, differentiation, and tolerance. Semin Immunol 19:197–205

Magnifico A, Ettenberg S, Yang C, Mariano J, Tiwari S, Fang S, Lipkowitz S, Weissman AM (2003) WW domain HECT E3s target Cbl RING finger E3s for proteasomal degradation. J Biol Chem 278:43169–43177

Marchese A, Raiborg C, Santini F, Keen JH, Stenmark H, Benovic JL (2003) The E3 ubiquitin ligase AIP4 mediates ubiquitination and sorting of the G protein-coupled receptor CXCR4. Dev Cell 5:709–722

Matesic LE, Haines DC, Copeland NG, Jenkins NA (2006) Itch genetically interacts with Notch1 in a mouse autoimmune disease model. Hum Mol Genet 15:3485–3497

Miele L, Osborne B (1999) Arbiter of differentiation and death: Notch signaling meets apoptosis. J Cell Physiol 181:393–409

Mosmann TR, Coffman RL (1989) TH1 and TH2 cells: different patterns of lymphokine secretion lead to different functional properties. Annu Rev Immunol 7:145–173

Mouchantaf R, Azakir BA, McPherson PS, Millard SM, Wood SA, Angers A (2006) The ubiquitin ligase itch is auto-ubiquitylated in vivo and in vitro but is protected from degradation by interacting with the deubiquitylating enzyme FAM/USP9X. J Biol Chem 281:38738–38747

Nalefski EA, Falke JJ (1996) The C2 domain calcium-binding motif: structural and functional diversity. Protein Sci 5:2375–2390

Neurath MF, Finotto S, Glimcher LH (2002) The role of Th1/Th2 polarization in mucosal immunity. Nat Med 8:567–573

Oliver PM, Cao X, Worthen GS, Shi P, Briones N, MacLeod M, White J, Kirby P, Kappler J, Marrack P, Yang B (2006) Ndfip1 protein promotes the function of itch ubiquitin ligase to prevent T cell activation and T helper 2 cell-mediated inflammation. Immunity 25:929–940

Omerovic J, Santangelo L, Puggioni EM, Marrocco J, Dall'armi C, Palumbo C, Belleudi F, Di Marcotullio L, Frati L, Torrisi MR, Cesareni G, Gulino A, Alimandi M (2007) The E3 ligase Aip4/Itch ubiquitinates and targets ErbB-4 for degradation. FASEB J 21:2849–2862

Osborne BA, Minter LM (2007) Notch signalling during peripheral T-cell activation and differentiation. Nat Rev Immunol 7:64–75

Perry WL, Hustad CM, Swing DA, O'Sullivan TN, Jenkins NA, Copeland NG (1998) The itchy locus encodes a novel ubiquitin protein ligase that is disrupted in a18H mice. Nat Genet 18:143–146

Qiu L, Joazeiro C, Fang N, Wang HY, Elly C, Altman Y, Fang D, Hunter T, Liu YC (2000) Recognition and ubiquitination of Notch by Itch, a hect-type E3 ubiquitin ligase. J Biol Chem 275:35734–35737

Radtke F, Wilson A, Mancini SJ, MacDonald HR (2004) Notch regulation of lymphocyte development and function. Nat Immunol 5:247–253

Ramain P, Khechumian K, Seugnet L, Arbogast N, Ackermann C, Heitzler P (2001) Novel Notch alleles reveal a Deltex-dependent pathway repressing neural fate. Curr Biol 11:1729–1738

Rossi M, De Laurenzi V, Munarriz E, Green DR, Liu YC, Vousden KH, Cesareni G, Melino G (2005) The ubiquitin-protein ligase Itch regulates p73 stability. EMBO J 24:836–843

Rossi M, De Simone M, Pollice A, Santoro R, La Mantia G, Guerrini L, Calabro V (2006) Itch/AIP4 associates with and promotes p63 protein degradation. Cell Cycle 5:1816–1822

Rutz S, Mordmuller B, Sakano S, Scheffold A (2005) Notch ligands Delta-like1, Delta-like4 and Jagged1 differentially regulate activation of peripheral T helper cells. Eur J Immunol 35:2443–2451

Sade H, Krishna S, Sarin A (2004) The anti-apoptotic effect of Notch-1 requires p56lck-dependent, Akt/PKB-mediated signaling in T cells. J Biol Chem 279:2937–2944

Sakaguchi S (2004) Naturally arising CD4+ regulatory t cells for immunologic self-tolerance and negative control of immune responses. Annu Rev Immunol 22:531–562

Sakata T, Sakaguchi H, Tsuda L, Higashitani A, Aigaki T, Matsuno K, Hayashi S (2004) Drosophila Nedd4 regulates endocytosis of notch and suppresses its ligand-independent activation. Curr Biol 14:2228–2236

Scharschmidt E, Wegener E, Heissmeyer V, Rao A, Krappmann D (2004) Degradation of Bcl10 induced by T-cell activation negatively regulates NF-kappa B signaling. Mol Cell Biol 24:3860–3873

Schwartz RH (2003) T cell anergy. Annu Rev Immunol 21:305–334

Semple CA (2003) The comparative proteomics of ubiquitination in mouse. Genome Res 13:1389–1394

Stallwood Y, Briend E, Ray KM, Ward GA, Smith BJ, Nye E, Champion BR, McKenzie GJ (2006) Small interfering RNA-mediated knockdown of notch ligands in primary CD4+ T cells and dendritic cells enhances cytokine production. J Immunol 177:885–895

Storck S, Delbos F, Stadler N, Thirion-Delalande C, Bernex F, Verthuy C, Ferrier P, Weill JC, Reynaud CA (2005) Normal immune system development in mice lacking the Deltex-1 RING finger domain. Mol Cell Biol 25:1437–1445

Strasser A (1995) Life and death during lymphocyte development and function: evidence for two distinct killing mechanisms. Curr Opin Immunol 7:228–234

Sudol M (1996) Structure and function of the WW domain. Prog Biophys Mol Biol 65:113–132

Tournoy J, Bossuyt X, Snellinx A, Regent M, Garmyn M, Serneels L, Saftig P, Craessaerts K, De Strooper B, Hartmann D (2004) Partial loss of presenilins causes seborrheic keratosis and autoimmune disease in mice. Hum Mol Genet 13:1321–1331

Traweger A, Fang D, Liu YC, Stelzhammer W, Krizbai IA, Fresser F, Bauer HC, Bauer H (2002) The tight junction-specific protein occludin is a functional target of the E3 ubiquitin-protein ligase itch. J Biol Chem 277:10201–10208

Venuprasad K, Elly C, Gao M, Salek-Ardakani S, Harada Y, Luo JL, Yang C, Croft M, Inoue K, Karin M, Liu YC (2006) Convergence of Itch-induced ubiquitination with MEKK1-JNK signaling in Th2 tolerance and airway inflammation. J Clin Invest 116:1117–1126

Wang M, Cheng D, Peng J, Pickart CM (2006) Molecular determinants of polyubiquitin linkage selection by an HECT ubiquitin ligase. EMBO J 25:1710–1719

Wegierski T, Hill K, Schaefer M, Walz G (2006) The HECT ubiquitin ligase AIP4 regulates the cell surface expression of select TRP channels. EMBO J 25:5659–5669

Wilkin MB, Carbery AM, Fostier M, Aslam H, Mazaleyrat SL, Higgs J, Myat A, Evans DA, Cornell M, Baron M (2004) Regulation of notch endosomal sorting and signaling by Drosophila Nedd4 family proteins. Curr Biol 14:2237–2244

Wood JD, Yuan J, Margolis RL, Colomer V, Duan K, Kushi J, Kaminsky Z, Kleiderlein JJ, Sharp AH, Ross CA (1998) Atrophin-1, the DRPLA gene product, interacts with two families of WW domain-containing proteins. Mol Cell Neurosci 11:149–160

Wu G, Lyapina S, Das I, Li J, Gurney M, Pauley A, Chui I, Deshaies RJ, Kitajewski J (2001) SEL-10 is an inhibitor of notch signaling that targets notch for ubiquitin-mediated protein degradation. Mol Cell Biol 21:7403–7415

Yang C, Zhou W, Jeon MS, Demydenko D, Harada Y, Zhou H, Liu YC (2006) Negative regulation of the E3 ubiquitin ligase itch via Fyn-mediated tyrosine phosphorylation. Mol Cell 21:135–141

Zhang J, Xu X, Liu Y (2004) Activation-induced cell death in T cells and autoimmunity. Cell Mol Immunol 1:186–192

TIM Gene Family and Their Role in Atopic Diseases

D.T. Umetsu(✉), S.E. Umetsu, G.J. Freeman, R.H. DeKruyff

Contents

Abstract The TIM gene family was discovered seven years ago by positional cloning in a mouse model of asthma and allergy. Three of the family members (TIM-1, TIM-3, and TIM-4) are conserved between mouse and man, and have been shown to critically regulate adaptive immunity. In addition, TIM-1 has been shown to play a major role as a human susceptibility gene for asthma, allergy and autoimmunity. Recently, TIM-4 has been identified as a ligand of phosphatidylserine and to control the uptake of apoptotic cells. These studies together suggest that the TIM gene family evolved to regulate immune responses by managing survival and cell death of hematopoetic cells.

D.T. Umetsu
Harvard Medical School, Division of Immunology and Allergy, Children's Hospital,
Karp Laboratories, Boston, Rm 10127, 1 Blackfan Circle, Boston, MA 02115, USA
dale.umetsu@childrens.harvard.edu

B. Beutler (ed.), *Immunology, Phenotype First: How Mutations Have Established*   201
New Principles and Pathways in Immunology. Current Topics in Microbiology
and Immunology 321. © Springer-Verlag Berlin Heidelberg 2008

Introduction

Bronchial asthma is an inflammatory disease of the lungs that has increased dramatically in prevalence over the past two decades in industrialized countries, doubling in prevalence since 1980, so that one in five individuals is now affected. In addition, other atopic diseases, including respiratory allergies (allergic rhinitis) and a skin disease known as atopic dermatitis, have increased greatly in prevalence over the past 20 years. As a result, current healthcare expenditures for the atopic diseases in industrialized countries are enormous. The large increase in prevalence is thought to be due to the dramatic changes in the environment of industrialized countries that have occurred over the past 20 years, but the specific environmental changes that are responsible for driving the increased development of allergic inflammation and asthma are not yet clear. Possible environmental changes that have affected the prevalence of asthma, allergy, and atopy include reductions in the frequency of infections (e.g., measles, mumps, rubella, tuberculosis, hepatitis A virus, and others) (Bach 2002; Matricardi et al. 1997, 2002) due to improved public health measures, increased use of vaccines and antibiotics (Umetsu et al. 2002), smaller family size (Strachan 1989), increased exposure to indoor allergens (Platts-Mills et al. 1996), and changes in diet (Devereux 2006), to name a few.

Allergy and asthma are complex genetic traits caused by environmental factors in genetically susceptibility individuals. It is estimated that a dozen or so susceptibility genes affect the development of asthma. Because each of the atopic diseases occurs in the same families and each has similar pathogenic mechanisms (affecting body surfaces that interact with the environment and involving eosinophilic inflammation), many of the susceptibility genes for asthma, allergic rhinitis, and atopic dermatitis are shared, although disease-specific genes (lung-, skin- or nasal mucosa-specific) may be involved as well. However, the identification of specific asthma, allergic rhinitis, atopic dermatitis, or atopy susceptibility genes has been difficult, because each susceptibility gene exerts only a small effect in the overall disease pathogenesis, and because each susceptibility gene interacts both with other genes on other chromosomes and with the environment in nonadditive ways. Furthermore, each susceptibility gene segregates independently, complicating the identification of these susceptibility genes. Thus, although multiple genome-wide scans have linked numerous chromosomal regions to asthma and allergy, only a few specific susceptibility genes within these chromosomal regions have been identified with any degree of certainty (Cookson and Moffatt 2000).

Several years ago our laboratory set out to identify an atopy susceptibility gene that might regulate the development of asthma and allergy, and which might provide important insight into the regulation of allergic inflammatory responses. Because of the genetic complexity of asthma and allergy, however, we first sought to simplify the problem by reducing the number of interacting atopy susceptibility genes. We therefore developed a unique mouse model of asthma through the use of congenic mice, generated by genetically moving discrete chromosomal segments from one mouse strain, DBA/2 (asthma resistant), into another strain, BALB/c (asthma susceptible), by repeated backcrossing (Ruscetti et al. 1985). In our mouse model, the BALB/c strain produces high levels of interleukin (IL)-4 and develops severe airway hyperreactivity (AHR), a cardinal feature of asthma, on exposure to allergen. In contrast, the DBA/2 mice develop low IL-4 responses and have normal airway reactivity when exposed to the same allergen. The congenic strains we developed had discrete chromosomal segments from the DBA/2 on the BALB/c background, and thus converted a complex genetic trait (asthma and allergy) into a single locus trait, thereby eliminating interference from other atopy susceptibility genes on other chromosomes. These mice were then screened for the development of AHR and IL-4 on exposure to allergen. One congenic strain, called C.D2/Es-3/Hba, stood out in that it exhibited the DBA/2 phenotype of resistance to AHR and produced low levels of IL-4. Moreover, the DBA/2 chromosome segment that the C.D2/Es-3/Hba strain inherited from the DBA/2 chromosome 11 was syntenic to human chromosome 5q23–35, a region that has been repeatedly linked to asthma and allergy in humans (Marsh et al. 1994). Using the congenic C.D2/Es-3/Hba strain along with BALB/c mice and traditional positional cloning techniques (powerful for identification of single gene but not multigenic traits), we identified a novel atopy susceptibility gene locus called *Tapr* (T cell and airway phenotype regulatory). Within the *Tapr* locus, we then positionally cloned the TIM (T cell, Ig domain, and mucin domain) gene family (McIntire et al. 2001).

TIM Gene Family

The TIM family of genes consists of eight members (*Tims 1–8*) on mouse chromosome 11B1.1, and three members (*TIM-1, -3,* and *-4*) on human chromosome 5q33.2 (McIntire et al. 2001). All of the mouse and human TIM genes encode a type 1 membrane protein, consisting of an N-terminal Cys-rich IgV-like domain, a mucin-like domain, a transmembrane domain, and an intracellular tail. The intracellular tails of TIM-1, TIM-2, and TIM-3, but not TIM-4, contain predicted tyrosine phosphorylation motifs, suggesting that these TIMs are involved in transmembrane signaling. Whereas TIM-3 has only three predicted glycosylation sites, human TIM-1 has 60, which are primarily *O*-linked glycosylation motifs located within the mucin-like domain. The N-terminal Cys-rich regions of the TIM homologs have a sequence identity of about 40%, whereas sequence identity between the mouse and human orthologs is around 60% (Santiago et al. 2007a). The structural similarities between all the TIMs suggest that they arose from an ancestral gene by successive gene duplication events.

Human TIM-1 as an Atopy Susceptibility Gene

TIM-1 (HUGO designation HAVCR1) is highly polymorphic in monkeys and humans as it is in mice [with single nucleotide polymorphisms (SNPs) as well as insertion/deletion variants occurring primarily in the mucin-like domain in both mice and humans], suggesting that human TIM-1 might serve as a susceptibility gene on human chromosome 5q23–35, a chromosomal region that has been repeatedly linked with asthma. Association analysis of the insertion/deletion variants of TIM-1 in human subjects with asthma and allergy demonstrated that allelic variation of TIM-1 contributes to the risk of atopy, but that this association depended upon past exposure to the hepatitis A virus (HAV). Specifically, the 157insMTTTVP and 195celT were associated with protection from atopy, but this protection was only observed in individuals who were seropositive to HAV (McIntire et al. 2003). The relationship to HAV is important, particularly since TIM-1 was previously discovered as the cellular receptor for HAV (HAVcr-1) in African green monkeys (Kaplan et al. 1996) and in humans (Feigelstock et al. 1998). Moreover, previous epidemiological studies in several distinct populations indicated that the prevalence of allergy and asthma was significantly lower in HAV seropositive individuals compared to that in HAV seronegative individuals (Matricardi et al. 1997, 2002).

The association analyses of TIM-1 and atopy, among the first to demonstrate a link between environmental factors (HAV infection) with an important susceptibility gene (TIM-1), provides a molecular mechanism for the hygiene hypothesis. The hygiene hypothesis attempts to explain the dramatic increase in the prevalence of atopic diseases that has occurred over the past 20 years, and states that infections, which have decreased substantially in industrialized countries over the past two decades, stimulate the immune system in such a way as to protect against asthma and allergy. The specific infectious agents that might be responsible for protection against allergy in the hygiene hypothesis are unclear, although infection with HAV has been associated with a reduced risk for developing atopy (Matricardi et al. 1997, 2002). Initially, the protection against atopy associated with HAV infection was assumed to be due to poor hygiene, because infection with HAV was thought to be a marker of poor hygiene, as the virus is transmitted through fecal–oral routes. However, the discovery of TIM-1 as an atopy susceptibility gene and of TIM-1 as the receptor for HAV suggests HAV has direct and long-lasting effects on T cells and on the immune system. As such, childhood infection with HAV, which occurred in nearly all children two decades ago, protects children from the development of asthma and allergy. In the past, childhood infection with HAV was for the most part mild and clinically inapparent, but recognized by the presence of antibodies to HAV, which approached 100% prevalence in Western countries prior to 1970 (Bach 2002). In contrast, the prevalence of infection with HAV today is less than 5% in young children in the United States, and this great reduction in the prevalence of infection may contribute to the increase in the prevalence of atopic diseases. Of note, currently in the United States, infection with HAV occurs primarily during food-borne epidemics or in daycare settings (Haaheim et al. 2002). Since protection against the development of atopy is also associated with early entrance into daycare (Ball et al. 2000), it is possible that in daycare settings HAV may be the important microbe that protects against atopy, although other infectious agents may also contribute to protection.

The association between polymorphic variants of TIM-1 and protection against atopic diseases has been reproduced in a number of studies, including one in African-American asthmatics (Gao et al. 2005), and others in children with atopic dermatitis in Arizona (Graves et al. 2005) and in Australia (Page et al. 2006), in Koreans with asthma and atopic dermatitis (Chae et al. 2003), but not in Japanese children with asthma (Noguchi et al. 2003). The lack of association of TIM-1 in Japanese children with asthma may be due to a reduced incidence of HAV infection in Japan, which is now close to zero in young Japanese children. However, the precise immunological mechanisms by which HAV infection alters TIM-1 and the immune system to protect against atopy are not yet clear. The immunology of TIM-1 is only beginning to be understood (see below), and the results so far indicate that TIM-1 potently regulates immune responses through novel mechanisms.

The powerful effects of TIM-1 on the immune system and in atopy may reflect the high degree of polymorphisms that occur in TIM-1, primarily in exon 4. In exon 4 of TIM-1, nonsynonymous nucleotide substitutions occur much more frequently than synonymous substitutions, similar to patterns observed in major histocompatibility complex loci (McIntire et al. 2001; Nakajima et al. 2005). Together with the fact that the sequence variability in TIM-1 occurs in humans, chimps, and gorillas, these results suggest that the gene sequence variability of TIM-1 is driven by evolutionary natural selection, presumably due to pressures from infection with HAV. Further investigation of the differential functions of the TIM-1 polymorphic variants will provide important insight into immune regulation and potentially into the understanding of host defense against HAV.

Human TIM-1 in Autoimmune Disease

TIM-1 has been associated not only with atopic diseases, but also with several autoimmune diseases, suggesting that TIM-1 regulates the immune system more globally. For example, rheumatoid arthritis was associated with polymorphisms in exon 4 (5509_5511delCAA) of TIM-1 (Chae et al. 2004a), while in patients with rheumatoid arthritis, C-reactive protein or rheumatoid factor levels were associated with polymorphisms in the promoter region of TIM-1 (Chae et al. 2005). How TIM-1 regulates autoimmune disease is not known, nor is it known whether HAV infection is associated with protection from autoimmunity. However, TIM-1 mRNA is expressed in the cerebrospinal fluid mononuclear cells of patients with multiple sclerosis (MS), primarily in patients in remission rather than in patients in relapse, suggesting that TIM-1 regulates the development of MS, possibly as a beneficial element, perhaps associated with tolerance (Khademi et al. 2004).

Role of TIM-3 as a Susceptibility Gene

Both human and mouse TIM-3 are polymorphic with several SNPs present in the coding regions of the IgV regions. These polymorphisms have not been associated with atopic disease (Page et al. 2006), although a promoter polymorphism may be associated with allergic rhinitis (Chae et al. 2004b). SNPs in the coding regions of the IgV regions of TIM-3, however, have been associated with rheumatoid arthritis (Chae et al. 2004b). The immunological mechanisms by which TIM-3 functions to regulate Th1 biased immune responses and autoimmunity will be discussed below.

TIMs as Costimulatory Molecules on T Cells

TIM-1 is a type 1 cell surface molecule expressed on CD4$^+$ but not on CD8$^+$ T cells, and initial studies indicated that TIM-1 is preferentially expressed on CD4$^+$ Th2 cells (McIntire et al. 2001). In contrast, TIM-3 is preferentially expressed on Th1 cells (Monney et al. 2002). Naïve CD4$^+$ T cells do not express either TIM-1 or TIM-3, but upon activation with specific antigen and dendritic cells or with anti-CD3 and CD28 monoclonal antibody (mAb), CD4$^+$ T cells express TIM-1. On further differentiation, TIM-1 expression is maintained on Th2 cells, but not on Th1 cells (Umetsu et al. 2005), although TIM-3 expression increases on differentiating Th1 cells (Monney et al. 2002).

Cross-linking of TIM-1 on T cells with an agonist mAb provides a very potent costimulatory signal to CD4$^+$ T cells that increases T cell proliferation and cytokine production [IL-4, interferon (IFN)-γ, and IL-10] (Umetsu et al. 2005). The costimulatory effect is seen only in the presence of T cell receptor (TCR) signaling, and could not be observed with monomeric Fab fragments of the anti-TIM-1 mAb. In vivo administration of the agonist anti-TIM-1 mAb along with antigen also greatly increased antigen-specific T cell proliferation and cytokine production, indicating that the agonistic anti-TIM-1 mAb provided a potent adjuvant effect. The adjuvant effect of anti-TIM-1 mAb potently blocked the development of respiratory tolerance (Umetsu et al. 2005), consistent with the idea that TIM-1 costimulation potently activates T cells. Normally, respiratory exposure to antigen induces T cell unresponsiveness, and is associated with the development of antigen-specific regulatory T cells expressing FoxP3 (Akbari et al. 2002; Stock et al. 2004), but treatment with an agonist anti-TIM-1 mAb prevented this tolerance induction. It is possible that distinct regions of TIM-1 interact with different receptors or molecules, and mAbs recognizing these distinct regions may have different effects on the immune response, or that the affinity of an antibody for TIM-1 on different cell types may affect the type of response that is induced. Thus, for example, anti-TIM-1 mAbs recognizing exon 4 of the mucin/stalk domain greatly exacerbated airway inflammation and Th2 cytokine production, but another mAb blocked inflammation in a mouse model of asthma (Sizing et al. 2007). However, the precise events that regulate the various outcomes of TIM-1 signaling by distinct mAbs are not yet known.

The molecular signal transduction mechanisms by which TIM-1 costimulates T cell activation are also not fully known. It is known, however, that overexpression of TIM-1 in T cells results in an increase in production of IL-4 but not IFN-γ (de Souza et al. 2005). Furthermore, transfection of D10 cells with TIM-1 results in increased transcription from the IL-4 promoter and activation of NFAT/AP1 elements (de Souza et al. 2005), suggesting that TIM-1 preferentially enhances Th2 cytokine production, which is consistent with the preferential expression of TIM-1 on Th2 cells (McIntire et al. 2001). Activation of T cells appears to result in the phosphorylation of a conserved tyrosine in the cytoplasmic tail (Y276) of TIM-1 (de Souza et al. 2005). In studies of TIM-1 utilizing overexpression of TIM-1 on Jurkat T cells, which normally do not express TIM-1 proteins, investigators have found that TIM-1 colocalizes on the T cell surface with CD3 (Binne et al. 2007). TIM-1 coimmunoprecipitates with the TCR complex upon TCR cross-linking and T cell activation, and TCR signaling increases upon TIM-1 cross-linking. Furthermore, TIM-1 cross-linking caused rapid tyrosine phosphorylation of TIM-1, as well as phosphorylation of Zap70 and ITK.

TIM-1 Ligands

Several approaches have been taken to determine the natural ligands of TIM-1, and these approaches have identified TIM-1 itself, TIM-4, and IgAλ as molecules that can bind to TIM-1. The structure of TIM-1 includes a glycosylated mucin domain, which imparts a degree of promiscuity to the TIM-1 molecule. This may explain the identification of multiple ligands, and has made it difficult to determine which if any of the already identified ligands is the primary ligand of TIM-1. Staining with TIM-1-Ig fusion proteins (consisting of the TIM-1 IgV domain with or without the mucin domain coupled to the Fc portion of IgG) as well as with a TIM-1 tetramer demonstrated that TIM-1 binds to CD11c⁺ splenocytes and more weakly to B220⁺ B cells and CD11b⁺ splenocytes (Meyers et al. 2005; Wilker et al. 2007). This binding was dependent on divalent cations for high-affinity binding as the addition of EGTA significantly reduced binding (Wilker et al. 2007). TIM-1-Ig and TIM-1 tetramer bound to CHO cells transfected with TIM-4 (Meyers et al. 2005), and this interaction could be specifically inhibited by anti-TIM-1 mAb, indicating that TIM-4 was a ligand of TIM-1. In addition, TIM-1-Ig and TIM-1 tetramers bound to cells expressing TIM-1, and this binding was dependent on the presence of the glycosylated mucin stalk, although the mucin stalk alone was insufficient for TIM binding, indicating that homotypic TIM-1-TIM-1 binding also occurred.

Administration of TIM-4-Ig in vivo along with antigen induced high levels of splenocyte proliferation and cytokine production. The interpretation was that TIM-4-Ig bound to TIM-1 on T cells resulting in T cell activation (Meyers et al. 2005). TIM-4 is expressed on CD11b⁺ and CD11c⁺ cells, including macrophages and dendritic cells (DCs), particularly on lymphoid CD8α⁺ DCs or on splenic stromal cells, but not on T cells (Shakhov et al. 2004). Administration of a TIM-1-Ig fusion protein, however, produced similar results, which was initially difficult to understand. Nevertheless, it is likely that TIM-1 may bind to itself, which is suggested by clumping of TIM-1 transfectants (Umetsu et al. 2005) and by the crystal structure of TIM-1, which was solved in 2007 (Santiago et al. 2007a).

IgAλ was also recently described as a putative ligand of human TIM-1 (Tami et al. 2007). This ligand was identified using an expression cloning strategy based on binding of a human TIM-1-Fc fusion protein to cells transfected with a human lymph node cDNA library. The interaction of TIM-1 with IgAλ was blocked by mAbs against IgA, Igλ, and human TIM-1. Since IgA did not inhibit HAV infection of African green monkey kidney cells, it is likely that the IgA and virus binding sites on TIM-1 are distinct. The precise physiological implications of this finding are not yet clear, though it is possible that the IgA-TIM-1 interaction has a synergistic effect in host defense against HAV.

TIM-1 Crystal Structure

Crystal structure analysis of TIM-1 confirmed the homotypic TIM-1–TIM-1 interactions, which are conserved in mice and humans, suggesting that this interaction is an important immunoregulatory mechanism. The TIM family members share a common structural organization with other Ig superfamily members. The IgV domain of TIM-1 has two antiparallel β-sheets, bridged by the first and last of six Cys residues in the IgV domain, similar to the structure of Ig superfamily members. The remaining four Cys residues link two loops, forming a cleft in the IgV domain. One loop connects two β-strands (the FG loop) and another loop connects two other β-strands (the CC′ loop). The six conserved Cys residues in all of the TIM molecules appear to provide a distinctive structural feature of TIM IgV domains. The major differences between the IgV domains of TIM-1 and TIM-2, which display high sequence identity (66%), occur mainly in this cleft region, suggesting that the cleft provides important functionality to the TIMs. Importantly, the HAV appears to bind to human TIM-1 at this cleft region, with Ser37 in the CC′ loop possibly the critical virus-binding residue (Santiago et al. 2007a).

The TIM-1 IgV domains crystallized in asymmetric pairs, such that each TIM-1 domain was related by a rotation angle of about 180°, with their C-terminal ends extending in opposite directions. This suggested that two TIM-1 molecules on two different cells might interact through two Thr17 residues at TIM-1 molecular surfaces opposite the clefts. This idea is supported by the observation that TIM-1 transfected cells tend to aggregate in clumps (Umetsu et al. 2005), and that TIM-1 molecules on transfected cells cluster at intercellular junctions (Santiago et al. 2007a). In addition, soluble TIM-1-Ig fusion proteins bind to cells transfected with TIM-1 (Umetsu et al. 2005) and to plastic surfaces coated with TIM-1–Ig. The homophilic binding in BIAcore assays was about 0.6 μM, and required contributions from the mucin domains and divalent cations (Santiago et al. 2007a). It is therefore possible that the homophilic binding of TIM-1 at intercellular junctions could facilitate phosphorylation of TIM-1, resulting in T cell activation. Since TIM-1 is also overexpressed after ischemic kidney injury (Han et al. 2002), and in renal carcinoma (Vila et al. 2004), the homophilic interactions of TIM-1 could also mediate cell adhesion interactions for renal cell regeneration and tumor development. Importantly, most of the TIM-1 molecules in transfected cells accumulated in intracellular vesicles, but trafficked to the cell surface after treatment with ionomycin or PMA (Santiago et al. 2007a). This may explain the observation of the presence of TIM-1 mRNA in lymphocytes that express minimal levels of TIM-1 cell surface protein (Mesri et al. 2006).

TIM-4, a Receptor for Phosphatidylserine

Although TIM-4 can bind to TIM-1, TIM-4 appears to have a critical role in other settings, notably in facilitating the uptake of apoptotic cells by macrophages and dendritic cells. Macrophages in the peritoneum and subsets of macrophages and DCs in the spleen express TIM-4, which has been shown recently by two independent groups to be an important and specific receptor for phosphatidylserine, a membrane phospholipid expressed by apoptotic cells (Kobayashi et al. 2007; Miyanishi et al. 2007). The specificity of the binding was confirmed by crystallographic studies of TIM-4 with phosphatidylserine binding in the cleft of the IgV domain (Santiago et al. 2007b). Moreover, cells expressing TIM-4 avidly phagocytized apoptotic cells (expressing PS), and this process was specifically blocked by anti-TIM-4 mAb (Kobayashi et al 2007). These studies suggest that TIM-4, by controlling the uptake of apoptotic cells, may regulate the development of tolerance and autoimmunity.

TIM-2, an Inhibitory Costimulatory Molecule

Murine TIM-2, which has no counterpart in humans, has sequence similarities to TIM-1, although their crystal structures indicate that the two molecules are quite distinct (see below). TIM-2 is expressed by B cells and by epithelial cells in bile ducts and renal tubules (Chen et al. 2005), as well as by activated Th2 cells (detected by mRNA analysis) (Chakravarti et al. 2005). A number of reports have suggested several distinct ligands for TIM-2. These ligands include Sema4A, which is expressed on activated macrophages, B cells, and DCs (Kumanogoh et al. 2002), and H-ferritin, which could act as an immune regulator by inhibiting T cell proliferation or impairing B cell maturation (Chen et al. 2005). Sema4A plays an important role in T cell activation, and Sema4A-deficient mice exhibit defective Th1 responses (Kumanogoh et al. 2005). In addition, blockade of TIM-2 signaling by administration of a TIM-2–Ig fusion protein results in enhanced Th2 responses (IL-4 and IL-10) and inhibition of IFN-γ production (Chakravarti et al. 2005). Furthermore, administration of the TIM-2–Ig fusion protein during the induction phase inhibits the severity of experimental autoimmune encephalomyelitis. TIM-2-deficient mice develop increased Th2 responses (Rennert et al. 2006), suggesting that TIM-2 activation provides an inhibitory signal to T cells which would normally produce Th2 cytokines. Thus, T cells from TIM-2-deficient mice immunized with antigen proliferate more vigorously and produce increased quantities of Th2 as well as Th1 cytokines, and develop increased airway inflammation in an asthma model. On the other hand, overexpression of TIM-2 in human T cell lines (Jurkat cells) results in a reduction in NFAT and AP-1 transcriptional activity (Knickelbein et al. 2006). Together, these studies indicate that TIM-2, which is preferentially expressed on Th2 cells, signals to inhibit the development of Th2 responses.

The crystal structure of TIM-2 has also been solved and indicates that TIM-2 IgV molecules readily form homodimers. The IgV domain of TIM-2, like that of TIM-1, has six Cys residues, which stabilizes two β-sheets and a cleft formed by the FG loop and the CC′ loop (Santiago et al. 2007a). In contrast to the homodimers of TIM-1, the angle between the two TIM-2 IgV domains was 60°, suggesting that dimerization of molecules occurs in a *cis* manner on the same cell surface, rather than between TIM-2 molecules on two different cells, as appears to occur with TIM-1 IgV molecules. IgV dimerization creates an extended glycan-free surface at the top, which allows accessibility to ligands. It is possible that the ligands of TIM-2 may differ depending on whether monomeric versus dimeric TIM-2 is available.

TIM-3, Another Inhibitory Costimulatory Molecule

Mouse TIM-3 (HUGO designation HAVCR-2) was independently identified using an expression cloning strategy of Th1 cells, and is expressed by Th1 cells after two to three rounds of polarizing stimulation in vitro (Monney et al. 2002; Sanchez-Fueyo et al. 2003). Mouse TIM-3 encodes a 281-amino acid protein, while human TIM-3 encodes a 302-amino acid protein that shares 63% homology with mouse TIM-3 (McIntire et al. 2001; Monney et al. 2002). TIM-3 is preferentially expressed on Th1 cells and CD8[+] T cells, as well as macrophages, DCs, and natural killer (NK) cells (Khademi et al. 2004). TIM-3 appears to provide a negative signal to T cells, and thus, blockade of TIM-3 signaling with a blocking anti-TIM-3 mAb in mice developing experimental autoimmune encephalopathy greatly worsens disease, increases IFN-γ production, and is associated with an increase in the activation status of macrophages (Monney et al. 2002). Similarly, administration of a TIM-3–Ig fusion protein, which blocks TIM-3 activation signals, resulted in greatly increased Th1 cell development with increased IFN-γ and IL-2 production, and blockade of peripheral tolerance (Sabatos et al. 2003). Furthermore, blockade of TIM-3 signaling accelerated diabetes in NOD mice, and prevented acquisition of transplantation tolerance induced by costimulation blockade (Sanchez-Fueyo et al. 2003). The proinflammatory effects of TIM-3 blockade were mediated in part by dampening of the antigen-specific immunosuppressive function of CD4[+] CD25[+] regulatory T cell populations. On the other hand, enhancing TIM-3 signaling appears to cause rapid Th1 cell death, inhibits Th1-mediated allo-immune responses, and enhances transplantation tolerance. Thus, TIM-3 signaling downregulates Th1-dependent immune responses, and facilitates the development of tolerance.

Th1 cell clones generated from the cerebrospinal fluid of patients with MS produced increased amounts of IFN-γ but expressed lower levels of TIM-3 and T-bet, suggesting that the failure to upregulate expression of TIM-3 might represent an intrinsic defect that contributes to the pathogenesis of MS (Koguchi et al. 2006). In addition, blockade of TIM-3 signaling during coxsackievirus infection resulted in increased myocarditis and reduced regulatory T cell activity (Frisancho-Kiss et al. 2006). Furthermore, in a model of asthma induced by the pulmonary transfer of ovalbumin (OVA)-specific Th2 cells, TIM-3 blockade significantly enhanced IFN-γ production, decreased eosinophils and Th2 cells in the lung, and greatly reduced AHR, presumably because Th1 responses can inhibit allergen-induced AHR (Kearley et al. 2007). However, since Th1 responses can also play a proinflammatory role in asthma, the precise role of TIM-3 or of TIM-3 blockade in the regulation or treatment of asthma is unclear.

TIM-3 Ligands

Using TIM-3-Ig and an expression cloning strategy, galectin-9 was identified as a ligand of TIM-3 (Zhu et al. 2005). Galectins are mammalian protein lectins recognizing conserved carbohydrates (Liu and Rabinovich 2005). Galectin-9 has been known to induce T cell apoptosis, and it appears that binding to TIM-3 mediates this process, although galectin-9 inhibits apoptosis in eosinophils, presumably through a non-TIM-3-mediated pathway (Hsu et al. 2006). Galectin-9 is expressed on endothelial cells, fibroblasts, and astrocytes, and it attaches to TIM-3 on T cells resulting in rapid Th1 but not Th2 cell clumping and cell death. This suggests that induction of galectin-9 by IFN-γ helps to resolve Th1 inflammatory responses.

Analysis of the crystal structure of the IgV domain of TIM-3 demonstrates that TIM-3 has a structure very similar to TIM-1 and TIM-2, in having six Cys residues in the IgV domain, resulting in a cleft formed by two β-strands, the FG loop and the CC′ loop, which are stabilized by two of the disulfide bonds (Cao et al. 2007). This cleft is critical for the binding of TIM-3 to a ligand(s) other than galectin-9, as binding of TIM-3 to cell lines [and the presumed ligand(s)] was abolished by site-directed mutagenesis of residues located in proximity to the cleft. These results suggest that there may be at least two independent TIM-3 ligands: galectin-9, which does not bind to the cleft region, and another ligand(s) that binds to the cleft region. As with TIM-1 and TIM-2, ligands may bind specifically to the conserved FG-CC′ cleft of TIM-3 or the cleft may contribute to local structural or dynamic changes associated with the recognition of ligand epitopes on the target molecules. The TIM-3 ligands may include specific carbohydrate moieties, as suggested by a recent report indicating that TIM ligands might be promiscuous (Wilker et al. 2007). Finally, polymorphisms in the sequence of mouse TIM-3 all occur in the IgV domain, and may affect ligand binding. Since these polymorphisms occur distal to the FG-CC′ cleft of TIM-3, the polymorphisms are unlikely to directly affect ligand recognition associated with the FG-CC′ cleft, but they might affect the binding to galectin-9, or could modulate the interactions between the IgV and mucin domains, thus altering the overall presentation of the ligand-binding surfaces.

Summary and Conclusions

The TIM gene family, which includes eight murine and three human members, was identified using a genetic approach and a unique congenic mouse model of allergic asthma. This model converted a complex genetic trait (allergic asthma) into a monogenic problem, allowing the positional cloning of the TIM gene family in 2001, and using AHR and Th2 cytokine production as readouts. This approach proceeded without knowledge or assumptions of the previously unknown TIM genes, which turn out to code for distinctive proteins with previously unsuspected structures and function. TIM-1 in particular, but TIM-3 as well, are polymorphic and both are associated with development of atopy and autoimmunity, and play important roles in regulating T cell function. Importantly, TIM-1 is the receptor for the hepatitis A virus, infection with which had previously been shown to protect against the development of allergy and asthma. Since improved hygiene and public health measures over the past two decades have considerably reduced the prevalence of HAV infection, TIM-1 provides a molecular explanation for the hygiene hypothesis.

The mechanisms by which the TIM molecules function in the immune system are now the focus of a large number of investigations. TIM-1 and TIM-2 are preferentially expressed on Th2 cells, while TIM-3 is preferentially expressed on Th1 cells, consistent with the idea that the TIMs play important roles in the immunoregulation and biology of T cells. TIM-1 costimulatory signaling causes enhanced T cell activation, whereas TIM-2 and TIM-3 costimulation generates inhibitory signals in T cells. The precise mechanisms by which TIM-1 affects the development of atopy or how HAV affects T cell signaling, however, are still unknown. The answers to these questions will generate important new information about the TIM molecules and their ligands in immune regulation. Although several TIM ligands have been identified already, knowledge of the crystal structure of mouse TIM-1, TIM-2, and TIM-3 has helped us to understand the specific function of known ligands, and explain how different ligands might each bind to the TIMs. We believe that future studies of the TIMs will lead to a much improved understanding of the regulation of atopy and autoimmunity, and lead to novel and effective immunotherapies for these diseases.

Acknowledgements Supported by grants AI054456 and HL062348 from the National Institutes of Health.

References

Akbari O, Freeman GJ, Meyer EH, Greenfield EA, Chang TT, Sharpe AH, Berry G, DeKruyff RH, Umetsu DT (2002) Antigen-specific regulatory T cells develop via the ICOS-ICOS-ligand pathway and inhibit allergen-induced airway hyperreactivity. Nat Med 8:1024–1032

Bach J (2002) The effect of infections on susceptibility to autoimmune and allergic diseases. N Engl J Med 347:911–920

Ball TM, Castro-Rodriguez JA, Griffith KA, Holberg CJ, Martinez FD, Wright AL (2000) Siblings, day-care attendance, and the risk of asthma and wheezing during childhood. N Engl J Med 343:538–543

Binne LL, Scott ML, Rennert PD (2007) Human TIM-1 associates with the TCR complex and up-regulates T cell activation signals. J Immunol 178:4342–4350

Cao E, Zang X, Ramagopal UA, Mukhopadhaya A, Fedorov A, Fedorov E, Zencheck WD, Lary JW, Cole JL, Deng H, Xiao H, Dilorenzo TP, Allison JP, Nathenson SG, Almo SC (2007) T cell immunoglobulin mucin-3 crystal structure reveals a galectin-9-independent ligand-binding surface. Immunity 26:311–321

Chae S, Song J, Lee Y, Kim J, Chung H (2003) The association of the exon 4 variations of Tim-1 gene with allergic diseases in a Korean population. Biochem Biophys Res Commun 12:346–350

Chae SC, Song JH, Shim SC, Yoon KS, Chung HT (2004a) The exon 4 variations of Tim-1 gene are associated with rheumatoid arthritis in a Korean population. Biochem Biophys Res Commun 315:971–975

Chae SC, Park YR, Lee YC, Lee JH, Chung HT (2004b) The association of TIM-3 gene polymorphism with atopic disease in Korean population. Hum Immunol 65:1427–1431

Chae SC, Park YR, Song JH, Shim SC, Yoon KS, Chung HT (2005) The polymorphisms of Tim-1 promoter region are associated with rheumatoid arthritis in a Korean population. Immunogenetics 56:696–701

Chakravarti S, Sabatos CA, Xiao S, Illes Z, Cha EK, Sobel RA, Zheng XX, Strom TB, Kuchroo VK (2005) Tim-2 regulates T helper type 2 responses and autoimmunity. J Exp Med 202:437–444

Chen TT, Li L, Chung DH, Allen CD, Torti SV, Torti FM, Cyster JG, Chen CY, Brodsky FM, Niemi EC, Nakamura MC, Seaman WE, Daws MR (2005) TIM-2 is expressed on B cells and in liver and kidney and is a receptor for H-ferritin endocytosis. J Exp Med 202:955–965

Cookson WO, Moffatt MF (2000) Genetics of asthma and allergic disease. Hum Mol Genet 9:2359–2364

de Souza AJ, Oriss TB, O'Malley KJ, Ray A, Kane LP (2005) T cell Ig and mucin 1 (TIM-1) is expressed on in vivo-activated T cells and provides a costimulatory signal for T cell activation. Proc Natl Acad Sci U S A 102:17113–17118

Devereux G (2006) The increase in the prevalence of asthma and allergy: food for thought. Nat Rev Immunol 6:869–874

Feigelstock D, Thompson P, Mattoo P, Zhang Y, Kaplan GG (1998) The human homolog of HAVcr-1 codes for a hepatitis A virus cellular receptor. J Virol 72:6621–6628

Frisancho-Kiss S, Nyland JF, Davis SE, Barrett MA, Gatewood SJ, Njoku DB, Cihakova D, Silbergeld EK, Rose NR, Fairweather D (2006) Cutting edge: T cell Ig mucin-3 reduces inflammatory heart disease by increasing CTLA-4 during innate immunity. J Immunol 176:6411–6415

Gao PS, Mathias RA, Plunkett B, Togias A, Barnes KC, Beaty TH, Huang SK (2005) Genetic variants of the T-cell immunoglobulin mucin 1 but not the T-cell immunoglobulin mucin 3 gene are associated with asthma in an African American population. J Allergy Clin Immunol 115:982–988

Graves PE, Siroux V, Guerra S, Klimecki WT, Martinez FD (2005) Association of atopy and eczema with polymorphisms in T-cell immunoglobulin domain and mucin domain-IL-2-inducible T-cell kinase gene cluster in chromosome 5 q 33. J Allergy Clin Immunol 116:650–656

Haaheim L, Pattison J, Whitley R (2002) A practical guide to clinical virology. John Wiley and Sons, Chichester

Han WK, Bailly V, Abichandani R, Thadhani R, Bonventre JV (2002) Kidney Injury Molecule-1 (KIM-1): a novel biomarker for human renal proximal tubule injury. Kidney Int 62:237–244

Hsu DK, Yang RY, Liu FT (2006) Galectins in apoptosis. Methods Enzymol 417:256–273

Kaplan G, Totsuka A, Thompson P, Akatsuka T, Moritsugu Y, Feinstone SM (1996) Identification of a surface glycoprotein on African green monkey kidney cells as a receptor for hepatitis A virus. EMBO J 15:4282–4296

Kearley J, McMillan SJ, Lloyd CM (2007) Th2-driven, allergen-induced airway inflammation is reduced after treatment with anti-Tim-3 antibody in vivo. J Exp Med 204:1289–1294

Khademi M, Illes Z, Gielen AW, Marta M, Takazawa N, Baecher-Allan C, Brundin L, Hannerz J, Martin C, Harris RA, Hafler DA, Kuchroo VK, Olsson T, Piehl F, Wallstrom E (2004) T Cell Ig- and mucin-domain-containing molecule-3 (TIM-3) and TIM-1 molecules are differentially expressed on human Th1 and Th2 cells and in cerebrospinal fluid-derived mononuclear cells in multiple sclerosis. J Immunol 172:7169–7176

Knickelbein JE, de Souza AJ, Tosti R, Narayan P, Kane LP (2006) Cutting edge: inhibition of T cell activation by TIM-2. J Immunol 177:4966–4970

Kobayashi N, Karisola P, Pena-Cruz V, Dorfman DM, Jinushi M, Umetsu SE, Butte MJ, Nagumo H, Chernova I, Zhu B, et al (2007) TIM-1 and TIM-4 glycoproteins bind phosphatidylserine and mediate uptake of apoptotic cells. Immunity 27:927–940

Koguchi K, Anderson DE, Yang L, O'Connor KC, Kuchroo VK, Hafler DA (2006) Dysregulated T cell expression of TIM3 in multiple sclerosis. J Exp Med 203:1413–1418

Kumanogoh A, Marukawa S, Suzuki K, Takegahara N, Watanabe C, Ch'ng E, Ishida I, Fujimura H, Sakoda S, Yoshida K, Kikutani H (2002) Class IV semaphorin Sema4A enhances T-cell activation and interacts with Tim-2. Nature 419:629–633

Kumanogoh A, Shikina T, Suzuki K, Uematsu S, Yukawa K, Kashiwamura S, Tsutsui H, Yamamoto M, Takamatsu H, Ko-Mitamura EP, Takegahara N, Marukawa S, Ishida I, Morishita H, Prasad DV, Tamura M, Mizui M, Toyofuku T, Akira S, Takeda K, Okabe M, Kikutani H (2005) Nonredundant roles of Sema4A in the immune system: defective T cell priming and Th1/Th2 regulation in Sema4A-deficient mice. Immunity 22:305–316

Liu FT, Rabinovich GA (2005) Galectins as modulators of tumour progression. Nat Rev Cancer 5:29–41

Marsh DG, Neely JD, Breazeale DR, Ghosh B, Freidhoff LR, Ehrlich-Kautzky E, Schou C, Krishnaswamy G, Beaty TH (1994) Linkage analysis of IL4 and other chromosome 5q31.1 markers and total serum immunoglobulin E concentrations. Science 264:1152–1156

Matricardi PM, Rosmini F, Ferrigno L, Nisini R, Rapicetta M, Chionne P, Stroffolini T, Pasquini P, D'Amelio R (1997) Cross sectional retrospective study of prevalence of atopy among Italian military students with antibodies against hepatitis A virus. BMJ 314:999–1003

Matricardi PM, Rosmini F, Panetta V, Ferrigno L, Bonini S (2002) Hay fever and asthma in relation to markers of infection in the United States. J Allergy Clin Immunol 110:381–387

McIntire J, Umetsu S, Macaubas C, Hoyte E, Cinnioglu C, Cavalli-Sforza L, Barsh G, Hallmayer J, Underhill P, Risch N, Freeman G, DeKruyff R, Umetsu D (2003) Immunology: hepatitis A virus link to atopic disease. Nature 425:576

McIntire JJ, Umetsu SE, Akbari O, Potter M, Kuchroo VK, Barsh GS, Freeman GJ, Umetsu DT, DeKruyff RH (2001) Identification of Tapr (an airway hyperreactivity regulatory locus) and the linked Tim gene family. Nat Immunol 2:1109–1116

Mesri M, Smithson G, Ghatpande A, Chapoval A, Shenoy S, Boldog F, Hackett C, Pena CE, Burgess C, Bendele A, Shimkets RA, Starling GC (2006) Inhibition of in vitro and in vivo T cell responses by recombinant human Tim-1 extracellular domain proteins. Int Immunol 18:473–484

Meyers J, Chakravarti S, Schlesinger D, Illes D, Waldner H, Umetsu S, Kenny J, Zheng X, Umetsu D, DeKruyff R, Strom T, Kuchroo V (2005) Tim-4 is the ligand for Tim-1, and the Tim-1-Tim-4 interaction regulates T cell expansion. Nature Immunol

Miyanishi M, Tada K, Koike M, Uchiyama Y, Kitamura T, Nagata S (2007) Identification of Tim4 as a phosphatidylserine receptor. Nature 450:435–439

Monney L, Sabatos CA, Gaglia JL, Ryu A, Waldner H, Chernova T, Manning S, Greenfield EA, Coyle AJ, Sobel RA, Freeman GJ, Kuchroo VK (2002) Th1-specific cell surface protein Tim-3 regulates macrophage activation and severity of an autoimmune disease. Nature 415:536–541

Nakajima T, Wooding S, Satta Y, Jinnai N, Goto S, Hayasaka I, Saitou N, Guan-Jun J, Tokunaga K, Jorde LB, Emi M, Inoue I (2005) Evidence for natural selection in the HAVCR1 gene: high degree of amino-acid variability in the mucin domain of human HAVCR1 protein. Genes Immun 6:398–406

Noguchi E, Nakayama J, Kamioka M, Ichikawa K, Shibasaki M, Arinami T (2003) Insertion/deletion coding polymorphisms in hHAVcr-1 are not associated with atopic asthma in the Japanese population. Genes Immun 4:170–173

Page NS, Jones G, Stewart GJ (2006) Genetic association studies between the T cell immunoglobulin mucin (TIM) gene locus and childhood atopic dermatitis. Int Arch Allergy Immunol 141:331–336

Platts-Mills TA, Woodfolk JA, Chapman MD, Heymann PW (1996) Changing concepts of allergic disease: the attempt to keep up with real changes in lifestyles. J Allergy Clin Immunol 98: S297–306

Rennert PD, Ichimura T, Sizing ID, Bailly V, Li Z, Rennard R, McCoon P, Pablo L, Miklasz S, Tarilonte L, Bonventre JV (2006) T cell, Ig domain, mucin domain-2 gene-deficient mice reveal a novel mechanism for the regulation of Th2 immune responses and airway inflammation. J Immunol 177:4311–4321

Ruscetti S, Matthai R, Potter M (1985) Susceptibility of BALB/c mice carrying various DBA/2 genes to development of Friend murine leukemia virus-induced erythroleukemia. J Exp Med 162:1579–1587

Sabatos CA, Chakravarti S, Cha E, Schubart A, Sanchez-Fueyo A, Zheng XX, Coyle AJ, Strom TB, Freeman GJ, Kuchroo VK (2003) Interaction of Tim-3 and Tim-3 ligand regulates T helper type 1 responses and induction of peripheral tolerance. Nat Immunol 4:1102–1110

Sanchez-Fueyo A, Tian J, Picarella D, Domenig C, Zheng X, Sabatos C, Manlongat N, Bender O, Kamradt T, Kuchroo V, Gutierrez-Ramos J, Coyle A, Strom T (2003) Tim-3 inhibits T helper type 1-mediated auto- and alloimmune responses and promotes immunological tolerance. Nat Immunol 4:1093–1101

Santiago C, Ballesteros A, Tami C, Martinez-Munoz L, Kaplan GG, Casasnovas JM (2007a) Structures of T cell immunoglobulin mucin receptors 1 and 2 reveal mechanisms for regulation of immune responses by the TIM receptor family. Immunity 26:299–310

Santiago C, Ballesteros A, Martinez-Munoz L, Mellado M, Kaplan GG, Freeman GJ, Casasnovas JM (2007b) Structures of T cell immunoglobulin mucin protein 4 show a metal-ion-dependent ligand binding site where Phosphatidylserine binds. Immunity 27:941–951

Shakhov AN, Rybtsov S, Tumanov AV, Shulenin S, Dean M, Kuprash DV, Nedospasov SA (2004) SMUCKLER/TIM4 is a distinct member of TIM family expressed by stromal cells of secondary lymphoid tissues and associated with lymphotoxin signaling. Eur J Immunol 34:494–503

Sizing ID, Bailly V, McCoon P, Chang W, Rao S, Pablo L, Rennard R, Walsh M, Li Z, Zafari M, Dobles M, Tarilonte L, Miklasz S, Majeau G, Godbout K, Scott ML, Rennert PD (2007) Epitope-dependent effect of anti-murine TIM-1 monoclonal antibodies on T cell activity and lung immune responses. J Immunol 178:2249–2261

Stock P, Akbari O, Berry G, Freeman G, DeKruyff R, Umetsu DT (2004) Induction of TH1-like regulatory cells that express Foxp3 and protect against airway hyperreactivity. Nat Immunol 5:1149–1156

Strachan DP (1989) Hay fever, hygiene, and household size. BMJ 299:1259–1260

Tami C, Silberstein E, Manangeeswaran M, Freeman GJ, Umetsu SE, DeKruyff RH, Umetsu DT, Kaplan GG (2007) Immunoglobulin A (IgA) is a natural ligand of hepatitis A virus cellular receptor 1 (HAVCR1), and the association of IgA with HAVCR1 enhances virus-receptor interactions. J Virol 81:3437–3446

Umetsu D, McIntire J, Macaubas C, Akbari O, DeKruyff R (2002) Asthma: an epidemic of dysregulated immunity. Nat Immunol 3:715–720

Umetsu S, Lee W, McIntire J, Downey L, Sanjanwala B, Akbari O, Berry G, Nagumo H, Freeman G, Umetsu D, DeKruyff R (2005) TIM-1 induces T cell activation and inhibits the development of peripheral tolerance. Nat Immunol 6:447–454

Vila MR, Kaplan GG, Feigelstock D, Nadal M, Morote J, Porta R, Bellmunt J, Meseguer A (2004) Hepatitis A virus receptor blocks cell differentiation and is overexpressed in clear cell renal cell carcinoma. Kidney Int 65:1761–1773

Wilker PR, Sedy JR, Grigura V, Murphy TL, Murphy KM (2007) Evidence for carbohydrate recognition and homotypic and heterotypic binding by the TIM family. Int Immunol 19:763–773

Zhu C, Anderson AC, Schubart A, Xiong H, Imitola J, Khoury SJ, Zheng XX, Strom TB, Kuchroo VK (2005) The Tim-3 ligand galectin-9 negatively regulates T helper type 1 immunity. Nat Immunol 6:1245–1252

Index

Current Topics in Microbiology and Immunology

Volumes published since 2002

Vol. 295: **Sullivan, David J.; Krishna Sanjeew (Eds.):** Malaria: Drugs, Disease and Post-genomic Biology. 2005. 40 figs., XI, 446 pp. ISBN 3-540-25363-7

Vol. 296: **Oldstone, Michael B. A. (Ed.):** Molecular Mimicry: Infection Induced Autoimmune Disease. 2005. 28 figs., VIII, 167 pp. ISBN 3-540-25597-4

Vol. 297: **Langhorne, Jean (Ed.):** Immunology and Immunopathogenesis of Malaria. 2005. 8 figs., XII, 236 pp. ISBN 3-540-25718-7

Vol. 298: **Vivier, Eric; Colonna, Marco (Eds.):** Immunobiology of Natural Killer Cell Receptors. 2005. 27 figs., VIII, 286 pp. ISBN 3-540-26083-8

Vol. 299: **Domingo, Esteban (Ed.):** Quasispecies: Concept and Implications. 2006. 44 figs., XII, 401 pp. ISBN 3-540-26395-0

Vol. 300: **Wiertz, Emmanuel J.H.J.; Kikkert, Marjolein (Eds.):** Dislocation and Degradation of Proteins from the Endoplasmic Reticulum. 2006. 19 figs., VIII, 168 pp. ISBN 3-540-28006-5

Vol. 301: **Doerfler, Walter; Böhm, Petra (Eds.):** DNA Methylation: Basic Mechanisms. 2006. 24 figs., VIII, 324 pp. ISBN 3-540-29114-8

Vol. 302: **Robert N. Eisenman (Ed.):** The Myc/Max/Mad Transcription Factor Network. 2006. 28 figs., XII, 278 pp. ISBN 3-540-23968-5

Vol. 303: **Thomas E. Lane (Ed.):** Chemokines and Viral Infection. 2006. 14 figs. XII, 154 pp. ISBN 3-540-29207-1

Vol. 304: **Stanley A. Plotkin (Ed.):** Mass Vaccination: Global Aspects – Progress and Obstacles. 2006. 40 figs. X, 270 pp. ISBN 3-540-29382-5

Vol. 305: **Radbruch, Andreas; Lipsky, Peter E. (Eds.):** Current Concepts in Autoimmunity. 2006. 29 figs. IIX, 276 pp. ISBN 3-540-29713-8

Vol. 306: **William M. Shafer (Ed.):** Antimicrobial Peptides and Human Disease. 2006. 12 figs. XII, 262 pp. ISBN 3-540-29915-7

Vol. 307: **John L. Casey (Ed.):** Hepatitis Delta Virus. 2006. 22 figs. XII, 228 pp. ISBN 3-540-29801-0

Vol. 308: **Honjo, Tasuku; Melchers, Fritz (Eds.):** Gut-Associated Lymphoid Tissues. 2006. 24 figs. XII, 204 pp. ISBN 3-540-30656-0

Vol. 309: **Polly Roy (Ed.):** Reoviruses: Entry, Assembly and Morphogenesis. 2006. 43 figs. XX, 261 pp. ISBN 3-540-30772-9

Vol. 310: **Doerfler, Walter; Böhm, Petra (Eds.):** DNA Methylation: Development, Genetic Disease and Cancer. 2006. 25 figs. X, 284 pp. ISBN 3-540-31180-7

Vol. 311: **Pulendran, Bali; Ahmed, Rafi (Eds.):** From Innate Immunity to Immunological Memory. 2006. 13 figs. X, 177 pp. ISBN 3-540-32635-9

Vol. 312: **Boshoff, Chris; Weiss, Robin A. (Eds.):** Kaposi Sarcoma Herpesvirus: New Perspectives. 2006. 29 figs. XVI, 330 pp. ISBN 3-540-34343-1

Vol. 313: **Pandolfi, Pier P.; Vogt, Peter K. (Eds.):** Acute Promyelocytic Leukemia. 2007. 16 figs. VIII, 273 pp. ISBN 3-540-34592-2

Vol. 314: **Moody, Branch D. (Ed.):** T Cell Activation by CD1 and Lipid Antigens, 2007, 25 figs. VIII, 348 pp. ISBN 978-3-540-69510-3

Vol. 315: **Childs, James, E.; Mackenzie, John S.; Richt, Jürgen A. (Eds.):** Wildlife and Emerging Zoonotic Diseases: The Biology, Circumstances and Consequences of Cross-Species Transmission. 2007. 49 figs. VII, 524 pp. ISBN 978-3-540-70961-9

Vol. 316: **Pitha, Paula M. (Ed.):** Interferon: The 50th Anniversary. 2007. VII, 391 pp. ISBN 978-3-540-71328-9

Vol. 317: **Dessain, Scott K. (Ed.):** Human Antibody Therapeutics for Viral Disease. 2007. XI, 202 pp. ISBN 978-3-540-72144-4

Vol. 318: **Rodriguez, Moses (Ed.):** Advances in Multiple Sclerosis and Experimental Demyelinating Diseases. 2008. XIV, 376 pp. ISBN 978-3-540-73679-9

Vol. 319: **Manser, Tim (Ed.):** Specialization and Complementation of Humoral Immune Responses to Infection. 2008. XII, 174 pp. ISBN 978-3-540-73899-2

Vol. 320: **Paddison, Patrick J.; Vogt, Peter K. (Eds.):** RNA Interference. 2008. VIII, 273 pp. ISBN 978-3-540-75156-4

Vol. 321: **Beutler, Bruce (Ed.):** Immunology, Phenotype First: How Mutations Have Established New Principles and Pathways in Immunology. 2008. XIV, 221 pp. ISBN 978-3-540-75202-8

Printing: Krips bv, Meppel, The Netherlands
Binding: Stürtz, Würzburg, Germany